DIFFERENTIAL DIAGNOSIS OF INTRAOCULAR TUMORS

A stereoscopic presentation

DIFFERENTIAL DIAGNOSIS OF INTRAOCULAR TUMORS

A stereoscopic presentation

J. DONALD M. GASS, M.D.

Associate Professor of Ophthalmology,
Bascom Palmer Eye Institute,
University of Miami School of Medicine,
Miami, Florida

RC280
E9
G37
1974

With 794 illustrations and 112 stereoscopic views in full color
on 16 View-Master® reels keyed to labeled drawings and figures,
and a View-Master® compact viewer

THE C. V. MOSBY COMPANY

Saint Louis   1974

303329

Copyright © 1974 by The C. V. Mosby Company

All rights reserved. No part of this book may be reproduced in any manner without written permission of the publisher.

Printed in the United States of America

Distributed in Great Britain by Henry Kimpton, London

Library of Congress Cataloging in Publication Data

Gass, John Donald M   1928-
   Differential diagnosis of intraocular tumors.

   1. Eye—Tumors. 2. Diagnosis, Differential.
I. Title. [DNLM: 1. Diagnosis, Differential—Atlases.
2. Eye neoplasms—Diagnosis—Atlases. WW17 G251d]
RC280.E9G37   616.9'92'84   74-8614
ISBN 0-8016-1750-2

GW/U/B   9 8 7 6 5 4 3 2 1

To:

Dr. A. Edward Maumenee

Dr. Frank B. Walsh

Dr. Lorenz E. Zimmerman
   and

Dr. Edward W. D. Norton

PREFACE

A great variety of neoplastic, hamartomatous, and other tumefactions may occur in the eye. Primary malignant intraocular tumors occur infrequently; so many ophthalmologists have seen relatively few of them during their residency training and early years of practice. The fate of any eye, and indeed of the patient, depends on the physician's ability to differentiate malignant tumors originating in the eye from all the other intraocular tumors. Although special diagnostic procedures such as ultrasonography, radioactive uptake studies, and fluorescein angiography may be of some value, no diagnostic examination provides as much valuable information as does direct binocular visualization of the tumor through the indirect ophthalmoscope and slit lamp. Utilizing these tools, the clinician is able to make detailed observations concerning the gross anatomy of most intraocular tumors. These observations, coupled with a thorough knowledge of ocular pathology, enable him to make an accurate diagnosis in most cases. Despite the importance of the appearance of tumors in making a correct diagnosis, most of the available literature to date has had to rely on drawings or paintings of the fundus and black and white photographs to supplement verbal descriptions of intraocular tumors.

The purpose of this atlas is to utilize color fundus stereophotographs, black and white fluorescein angiographs, and photomicrographs to correlate the in vivo and histopathologic features of intraocular tumors and to acquaint the physician with the characteristic appearance of the various neoplastic and developmental intraocular tumors as well as lesions that may simulate them.

All but a few of the tumors depicted in this book were observed in patients examined at the Bascom Palmer Eye Institute during the past ten years. I have included variations of intraocular tumors that are frequently encountered as well as some of the rarer tumors. The histopathologic condition of the tumors illustrated is included when available. When not available, the histopathologic findings in other tumors believed to be similar to the tumor illustrated have been used. I recognize that there will be disagreement concerning the diagnosis of those patients in whom the eye was unavailable for histopathologic examination. I hope that many of these eyes will be obtained in the future as part of the Special Eye Bank Program at the Bascom Palmer Eye Institute. A number of important intraocular tumors have not been observed and were necessarily omitted from the atlas. Other tumors were omitted because of the limitations of fundus photography, particularly in regard to lesions in the peripheral fundus.

Chapter 1 is concerned with the value and techniques of fundus stereophotographs and fluorescein stereoangiography in the diagnosis and management of intraocular tumors. The principles of interpretation of fluorescein angiography are discussed. The remaining chapters in the first half of the atlas are concerned primarily with malignant melanomas of the choroid and ciliary body and neoplastic, hamartomatous, and other tumors that may be misdiagnosed as malignant melanomas. The chapters in the second half of the atlas deal primarily with retinal vascular and glial hamartomas that may simulate either retinoblastoma or uveal melanomas. The final chapter concerns a variety of neoplastic and nonneoplastic tumors of the iris.

Statistics gathered at the Armed Forces Institute of Pathology over the past twelve years indicate that in eyes with clear media one in five enucleated with the clinical diagnosis of malignant melanoma proved to have other lesions.[1,2] A batting average of only 80% accuracy deserves our attention. I hope that this atlas will be of aid in improving that average.

I wish to thank Dr. Edward W. D. Norton, Chairman of the Department of Ophthalmology, the members of the full-time and resident staff, and the many other physicians whose patients are illustrated in this book. I am particularly indebted to Mr. Johnny Justice, Jr., Mrs. Dixie Sparks Gilbert, Mr. Kenneth Peterson, Mr. Earl Choromokos, Mrs. Jessica Eichrodt, Mr. R. Dean Clark, Mrs. Nancy Hechlinski, Mr. William Milam, Mr. Ilan Hadar, Mr. Arthur Smialowski, and Mr. Ajendra Macker for their skill in fundus photography, and Mr. Joseph Goren and Miss Barbara French for preparation of the illustrations. Finally, I wish to thank Mrs. Margaret Bertolami, Mrs. Andrea Roberts, Mrs. Reva Hurtes, Dr. Kay Ellen Frank, Dr. Dwain Fuller, and Dr. Rolando Chanis, Jr., for their help in preparing and editing the manuscript.

J. DONALD M. GASS

1. Ferry, A. P.: Lesions mistaken for malignant melanomas of the posterior uvea: A clinicopathologic analysis of 100 cases with ophthalmoscopically visible lesions, Arch. Ophthal. **72:**463-469, 1964.
2. Shields, J. A., and Zimmerman, L. E.: Lesions simulating malignant melanomas of the posterior uvea, Arch. Ophthal. **89:**466-471, 1973.

CONTENTS

Fundus stereophotography and fluorescein angiography in patients with intraocular tumors

During the last decade the techniques of fundus stereophotography and fluorescein angiography have provided much new and practical information concerning diseases of the inner eye. These techniques are of particular value in the diagnosis, treatment, and follow-up care of patients with intraocular tumors. In the near future fundus stereophotography and fluorescein angiography will be part of the diagnostic armamentarium of every ophthalmologist.

VALUE OF FUNDUS PHOTOGRAPHY AND ANGIOGRAPHY

Increased accuracy in diagnosis. Fundus stereophotographs permit deliberate study of the tumor in question for details that are often overlooked during the course of patient examination. The stereopsis provided in photographs usually exceeds that observed by direct visualization, and the anatomy of the lesion and its relationship to overlying and surrounding structures is more easily appreciated. Fluorescein stereoangiography provides additional anatomic information not apparent either by direct examination or by fundus stereophotography. Most importantly, it provides information concerning some of the physiologic alterations within the tumor and surrounding structures.

Consultation. Photographs provide an easy means to obtain rapid consultation by mail.

Follow-up. Photographs provide an invaluable part of a patient's permanent record, particularly in regard to the detection of future anatomic and physiologic changes occurring naturally in the tumor or in following therapy. Photographic supplementation of handwritten diagrams and notes is of particular importance when the patient is under the care of two or more physicians. Copies of photographs of suspicious or unusual lesions may be given to the patient for his own personal record.

Clinicopathologic correlation. The availability of photographs for comparison of detailed funduscopic and angiographic findings with histopathologic findings is invaluable in the improvement of one's diagnostic skills.

Education. Serial photographic studies illustrating the natural course and posttherapeutic course of intraocular tumors are extremely useful for instructing others in accurate tumor diagnosis and proper patient management.

EQUIPMENT AND TECHNIQUE OF FLUORESCEIN ANGIOGRAPHY

Equipment. A variety of fundus cameras are available (Zeiss, West German; Zeiss, East German; Topcon; Nikon; Kowa; and Olympus). The photographs in this atlas were made primarily with various models of the Zeiss West German fundus camera. A few were made with the Topcon camera. The illumination diaphragm of the camera contains two different filters: (1) a no. 58 Wratten green filter for black and white fundus photographs, and (2) a B-4 Baird-Atomic blue exciter filter for black and white or color angiograms. Two Zeiss-Contax camera backs are used. One contains Kodachrome II film for color stereophotographs; the other contains Kodak Tri-X film for black and white angiography. In this latter camera back either a B-5 Baird Atomic yellow interference filter or a no. 12 Wratten yellow filter is taped within the bayonet fitting just in front of the focal plane shutter. High-speed Ektachrome film may be used in lieu of the Kodak Tri-X film for color angiography. A flash recycling speed exceeding one per second is

2

unnecessary for adequate angiography of intraocular tumors. For infrared-color fundus photographs Ektachrome infrared film and a no. 15 Wratten yellow filter are used.

Technique. (Zeiss, West German fundus camera). The patient's pupils are widely dilated with several instillations of 10 percent phenylephrine and 1 percent cyclopentolate drops prior to photography. Tonometry, in particular the applanation type, should be avoided prior to the photographic study. The eyepiece must be adjusted to the photographer's eye. Plain and stereoscopic color photographs of the lesion are made. Stereophotographs are made simply by taking rapidly paired photographs through two different portions of the widely dilated pupil by shifting the camera laterally with the joy stick. The Allen stereoseparator may also be used to obtain stereophotographs. Color photographs are made with the camera back loaded with Kodachrome II film at a shutter speed of 50. The strobe power control on the Zeiss transformer is set at II and the viewing lamp at II. The corrective lens switch is set at $-16/+17$ ($-7/+22$ on the Zeiss fundus flash II) for all photographs except those of aphakic patients when it should be changed to $+16/+33$ ($+20/+40$ on the Zeiss fundus flash II). The camera back containing Tri-X film and the yellow B-5 Baird Atomic or no. 12 Wratten yellow filter replaces the previous camera back. The shutter speed is set on 50, the synchronization at FX, the strobe setting at 1, and the view lamp at 4, and the illuminating diaphragm is rotated to the no. 58 Wratten green filter to make black and white photographs of the lesion.

The illumination diaphragm is changed to the B-4 Baird Atomic blue filter. The strobe is set at III or IV depending upon the media and the viewing lamp is set at 4. After the patient and the photographer are seated comfortably at the camera, the physician injects either 10 milliliters of 5 percent or 5 milliliters of 10 percent, sodium fluorescein rapidly into the antecubital vein through a 21-gauge needle. Lesser amounts of fluorescein are used in children. Approximately 5 to 10 seconds after initial injection of the dye, serial stereophotographs are recorded at rates as high as one frame per second during the first 2 minutes. Stereophotographs are recorded intermittently thereafter, usually at 5, 15, 30, and 60 minute intervals after dye injection. The Baird Atomic filters have recently been replaced by Spectrotech SE4 excitation and Spectrotech SB5 barrier filters.

Film processing. Kodak Kodachrome II and High-speed Ektachrome film are processed in the standard way described by the Kodak Company. The Kodak Tri-X is developed in Kodak D-11 stock solution for 7 minutes at 72° Fahrenheit. A contact sheet of the Tri-X negative is made on an 8 x 10 inch Dupont Cronar A film for the patient's record. Cronar S is used if higher contrast is desired. Rapid automatic processing units such as the Pako Pakorol are available for development of the black and white film at a cost of under $5,000.

Stereoscopic viewing. Stereoscopic viewing of the fluorescein negatives and paired color photographs is possible with +8.00 sphere spectacles or, if preferred, the pictures can be placed in permanent stereomounts.

Safety precautions. Intravenous injection of sodium fluorescein has been widely used in humans for approximately 10 years and is a safe procedure. Nevertheless, a rare individual may have an unfavorable reaction to the injection, and the clinician must be prepared to manage such a patient. Inquiry into previous unfavorable reactions to fluorescein or other types of injections should be made. Nausea and less often vomiting may occur in 5 to 10 percent of patients receiving very rapid injections of fluorescein. In the majority of instances, this reaction is attributable to a reflex vasovagal effect. The incidence of this complication can be reduced by using slow injections of fluorescein in those patients in whom the early phases of angiography are not critical for diagnosis. The use of a smaller volume of more concentrated fluorescein, when it becomes commercially available, will also reduce this complication. Syncope may rarely occur. Urticaria is a rare occurrence and usually requires no specific therapy. Wheezing, respiratory collapse, or anaphylactic shock have been reported in only a few patients. Adrenaline and cortisone for injection and emergency respiratory apparatus should be readily available for such emergencies. Routine skin testing or administration of test doses is not done unless there is some reason to suspect a possible reaction to the injection. If the patient has had a previous reaction to fluorescein, the injection should not be repeated.

GENERAL PRINCIPLES OF INTERPRETATION OF FLUORESCEIN ANGIOGRAPHY

Fluorescein angiography provides a means of detecting alterations of (1) blood flow to the eye, (2) blood flow within the eye, (3) retinovascular permeability, and (4) the normal pattern of overall intraocular fluorescence. Before consideration is given to those alterations caused by intraocular tumors, a brief review of important anatomic and physiologic features of the ocular fundus and their relationship to the angiographic appearance of the normal fundus, is presented.

Anatomy and physiology of the choroid and retina. The neurosensory retina is a transparent, multilayered tissue composed of neuronal cells, supporting neuroepithelial cells (Mueller cells), and blood vessels derived from the central retinal artery. The retinal blood vessels are lined by endothelium with electron-microscopically tight cellular junctions. This peculiar endothelial structure, not present outside of the central nervous system, probably plays an important role in maintaining the extracellular spaces of the retina free from serous transudate. The pigment epithelium (RPE) is a monocellular layer of neuroepithelial cells tightly bound to each other by means of a system of terminal bars that preclude the passage of fluid or particulate matter between the cells. Their apical processes are loosely interdigitated with retinal receptor elements. This interdigitation serves more as a means of transporting substances between the RPE and retina than as a means of firm attachment. The RPE is in turn tightly adherent to the collagen portion of Bruch's membrane by means of the RPE basement membrane or basal lamina. The collagen and elastic tissue comprising Bruch's membrane is a condensation of the stroma of the choroid and as such it probably plays no role in controlling the passage of metabolites or fluid between the choroidal vessels and retina. The endothelial cells lining the inner wall of the choriocapillaris are separated by numerous large pores. Thus, unlike retinal endothelial cells, they provide no barrier to the passage of fluid or particulate matter from the choriocapillaris into Bruch's membrane. It is probable, therefore, that the RPE, like the retinovascular endothelium, contains an intracellular pumping mechanism that plays a major role in maintaining the subretinal space and extracellular spaces of the retina in a relative state of deturgescence while at the same time permitting the free flow of electrolytes, nutrients, and waste products between the retina and the choroidal vessels. Thus, permeability alterations of the RPE and not the choriocapillaris are primarily responsible for exudative retinal detachment. The RPE cells contain pigment granules that in the Caucasian impart an orange color to the fundus. The concentration of pigment in the

RPE varies according to the pigmentary characteristics of the individual, and the concentration is always sufficiently great in the macular region to obscure details of the choroidal structure from view. The xanthochromic pigment concentrated in the outer retinal layers in the macular area may also play some role in obscuring the choroidal details from view.

Normal angiogram. Fluorescein dye injected into the antecubital vein enters the choroidal and optic nerve head vessels by way of the short ciliary arteries, usually one second or less ahead of that entering the retinal circulation by way of the central retinal artery. The dye is confined to the intravascular spaces in the normal retina and central nervous system. The choroidal and other tissue capillaries outside the central nervous system, however, are quite permeable to fluorescein. The dye rapidly escapes from the choriocapillaris and stains the collagen and elastic portion of Bruch's membrane, the stroma of the choroid, and the sclera. For the purposes of interpretation the entire choroid may be considered as one large vascular space lined on its inner surface by the RPE, which, like the retinal capillary endothelium, is impermeable to fluorescein. Fluorescein permeates the choroidal tissue and when viewed through the pigment epithelial filter produces the mottled background choroidal fluorescence, which is usually visible everywhere throughout the fundus except the central macular area during the early phases of angiography. In the macular area the yellow intraretinal pigment and the heavily pigmented pigment epithelium completely obscure the background choroidal fluorescence. In the early stages of angiography the details of the retinal circulation are clearly outlined on a background of mottled choroidal fluorescence. The retinal and choroidal fluorescence progressively decreases during excretion of dye by the kidneys and liver. One hour after injection the choroidal and retinal fluorescence has disappeared or is barely visible.

Angiographic abnormalities produced by intraocular tumors. Since a major function of the retinovascular endothelium and the RPE is to maintain the extracellular space of the retina and the subretinal space in a state of relative deturgescence, damage to either of these tissues by a tumor may be accompanied by escape of serous exudation from the retinal vessels into the intercellular spaces of the retina and from the choroidal compartment into the subretinal space. Fluorescein dye will likewise diffuse from the retinal vessels and the choroidal compartment into the extravascular exudate.

From the angiographic point of view a tumor may be described as being hypofluorescent, hyperfluorescent, or invisible (causing no alteration in the normal angiogram), or as showing a combination of these three elements. It may appear hyperfluorescent because of (1) the unusual accumulation of extravascular dye within, around, or on its surface; (2) depigmentation or atrophy of the overlying pigment epithelium causing greater visibility of the underlying choroidal fluorescence; or (3) the presence of an unusual number of blood vessels within or near the inner surface of the tumor. In the first instance the zone of hyperfluorescence usually increases in size, changes in pattern, and is visible 1 hour after injection. In the last two instances the fluorescence reaches the maximum very early in the study, usually remains constant in pattern, fades rapidly, and is barely visible after 1 hour. Some choroidal tumors show a combination of these three types of fluorescence.

A tumor may appear hypofluorescent by obscuring either or both the normal choroidal and retinal fluorescence from view. A fluorescent lesion may appear relatively hypofluorescent when it is surrounded by an area of intense fluorescence. In the broad sense of the word, a tumor is any mass lesion regardless of its makeup. It may be solid, or nonsolid. A nonsolid tumor may be composed of a focal collection of transudate, exudate, blood, or a combination of these elements (Figs. 1-1 and 1-2). A localized rhegmatogenous detachment is an example of what might be broadly categorized as a transudative mass. Here vitreal fluid migrates passively through a retinal hole into the subretinal space. Angiography typically shows no evidence of retinal vascular or RPE permeability alterations and not staining of the subretinal fluid in rhegmatogenous retinal detachment (Fig. 1-1, A). In the case of long-standing retinal detachments, whether it be of a primary or secondary type, the area of detachment may appear hyperfluorescent during the early stages of angiography because pigment epithelial flattening and depigmentation permit greater visibility of the underlying choroidal fluorescence (Fig. 1-1, B). Leakage of dye from the retinal capillaries may occur in some long-standing retinal detachments. An intraretinal cyst or retinoschisis is another example of a transudative tumefaction. The

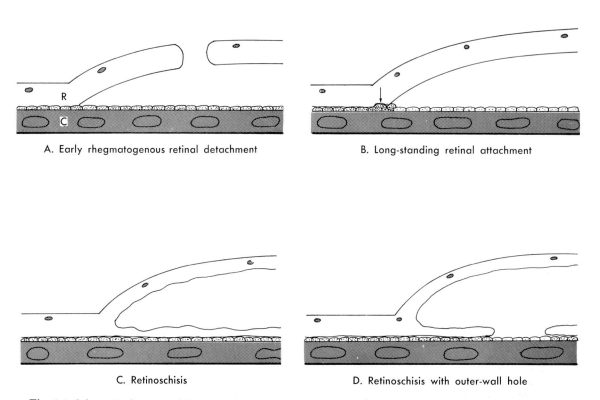

A. Early rhegmatogenous retinal detachment

B. Long-standing retinal attachment

C. Retinoschisis

D. Retinoschisis with outer-wall hole

Fig. 1-1. Schematic diagrams of fluorescein angiographic findings in transudative tumors of the ocular fundus. *Gray areas,* Fluorescein; *R,* retina; *C,* choroid. **A,** When of recent onset, the area of rhegmatogenous retinal detachment appears normal angiographically; if the subretinal fluid is cloudy, it may partially obscure the background choroidal fluorescence. **B,** A retinal detachment of long standing, whether it be rhegmatogenous or secondary, will appear hyperfluorescent during the early phases of angiography because of the increased visibility of the choroidal fluorescence through the flattened and depigmented retinal pigment epithelium. A relatively hypofluorescent demarcation line from hyperplasia of the pigment epithelium *(arrow)* may or may not be present. Perivascular leakage of dye (not shown) from the retinal capillaries occurs in some patients. **C,** An area of retinoschisis appears normal angiographically or may show decreased choroidal fluorescence if the intraretinal transudate is cloudy. **D,** Holes in the outer layer of retinoschisis appear hyperfluorescent because of flattening and depigmentation of the RPE within the area of the hole (see Fig. 7-18).

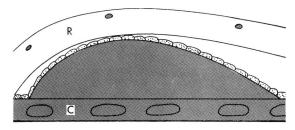

A. Serous pigment epithelial
detachment

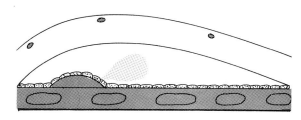

B. Serous retinal detachment secondary
to pigment epithelial detachment

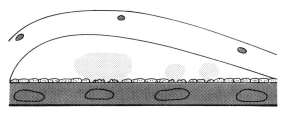

C. Serous retinal detachment secondary
to pigment epithelial defects

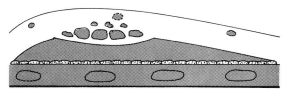

D. Serous retinal detachment secondary
to retinal vascular disease

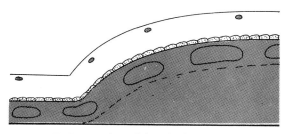

E. Serous choroidal and ciliary body
detachment

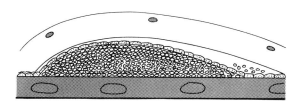

F. Hemorrhagic detachment of the
retina and pigment epithelium

Fig. 1-2. Schematic diagrams of fluorescein angiographic findings in exudative tumors of the ocular fundus. *Gray areas*, Fluorescein; *R*, retina; *C*, choroid. **A,** Serous detachments of the pigment epithelium appear hyperfluorescent during the early and late phases of fluorescein angiography because of the rapid diffusion of dye from the choroid across the full breadth of Bruch's membrane into the subpigment epithelial exudate. The dye often is unable to diffuse through the detached RPE into the subretinal exudate in concentrations adequate for visualization. **B,** Localized serous retinal detachment may be secondary to diffusing of exudate through a localized serous detachment of the RPE. The circumscribed area of RPE detachment appears hyperfluorescent during the early and late phases of angiography. In some patients during the later phases of angiography fluorescein diffuses rapidly through a break in the detached RPE into the subretinal exudate. **C,** A localized serous retinal detachment may be secondary to either an anatomic or functional defect in the RPE. Fluorescein diffuses through the area of damaged RPE into the subretinal exudate. **D,** In a serous retinal detachment secondary to retinal vascular disease fluorescein diffuses out of the retinal vessels into the intraretinal and subretinal exudate. **E,** A serous detachment of the choroid and ciliary body does not appear hyperfluorescent despite the presence of fluorescein-stained exudate in the suprachoroidal space. The incident blue light is unable to penetrate significantly the overlying pigment epithelium and choroidal tissue. **F,** Blood lying beneath the pigment epithelium and retina completely obscures the background choroidal fluorescence from view.

fluid filling the cyst does not stain with fluorescein and is apparently unrelated to abnormal retinal capillary permeability (Fig. 1-1, C). If retinoschisis is associated with a hole in its outer layer or with a long-standing retinal detachment, areas of early hyperfluorescence corresponding to the depigmented pigment epithelium may be apparent in the early course of angiography (Fig. 1-1, D).

Examples of localized exudative tumefactions include serous detachment of the pigment epithelium (Fig. 1-2, A), serous retinal detachment secondary to an underlying serous pigment epithelial detachment (Fig. 1-2, B), and serous retinal detachment secondary to one or more defects in the pigment epithelium (Fig. 1-2, C). In the case of serous pigment epithelial detachment, fluorescein diffuses out of the choroidal vessels across the full width of Bruch's membrane into the subpigment epithelial exudate to produce a discrete area of fluorescein staining that remains constant in size throughout the course of angiography. The dye may (Fig. 1-2, B) or may not (Fig. 1-2, A) be capable of diffusing through the pigment epithelium into the subretinal exudate in concentrations adequate for visualization. In the presence of one or more anatomic or functional defects in the detached pigment epithelium, fluorescein diffuses into the subretinal exudate (Fig. 1-2, C). Localized exudative retinal detachment less frequently occurs secondary to retinovascular disease. In such cases the retina is always thickened by the presence of cystoid retinal edema and exudation. Fluorescein diffuses out of the retinal vessels into the intraretinal and subretinal exudation and produces an intense multiloculated pattern of intraretinal dye overlying a background of less fluorescent subretinal exudate (Fig. 1-2, D). Serous detachment of the choroid and ciliary body is another example of an exudative tumor. Although the exudate is derived from uveal blood vessels and stains heavily with fluorescein, the incident blue light is usually unable to penetrate both the overlying pigment epithelium and the choroidal melanocytes. These lesions, therefore, do not usually appear hyperfluorescent (Fig. 1-2, E). A nonsolid tumor composed primarily of blood or blood pigment in the subretinal or subpigment epithelial space appears as a nonfluorescent subretinal mass throughout the course of angiography (Fig. 1-2, F).

Solid tumors are composed of one or more of the following elements: (1) viable cells, (2) blood vessels, and (3) stroma and, in addition, may contain varying amounts of exudate, including nonviable cells and cellular debris. Most blood vessels within tumors, whether the mass is neoplastic, hamartomatous, choriostomatous, proliferative, or inflammatory in nature, are permeable to fluorescein dye. Although the question is unsettled, the evidence to date suggests that the cell membrane of viable cells, whether neoplastic, hamartomatous, choriostomatous, proliferative, or inflammatory, is a barrier preventing entrance of dye into the cell cytoplasm. Thus, solid viable cellular tumors do not stain with fluorescein. Injured cells, nonviable cells, extracellular matrices (particularly collagen), and exudate within or around cellular tumors do stain with fluorescein.

To be visible angiographically, fluorescein dye must be present in a sufficient amount and must be accessible to the exciting blue light entering the pupil. The fluorescence produced by any tumor, therefore, is largely a function of the number of blood vessels near its anterior surface as well as the extravascular spaces available there for the accumulation of dye. Large lakes of fluorescein-stained exudate located deep within a cellular tumor will not be visible angiographically because the exciting light will not reach the pool of fluorescein. Small solid tumors confined to the outer layers of the choroid will usually not alter the normal background choroidal fluorescence (Fig. 1-3, A). Solid

8

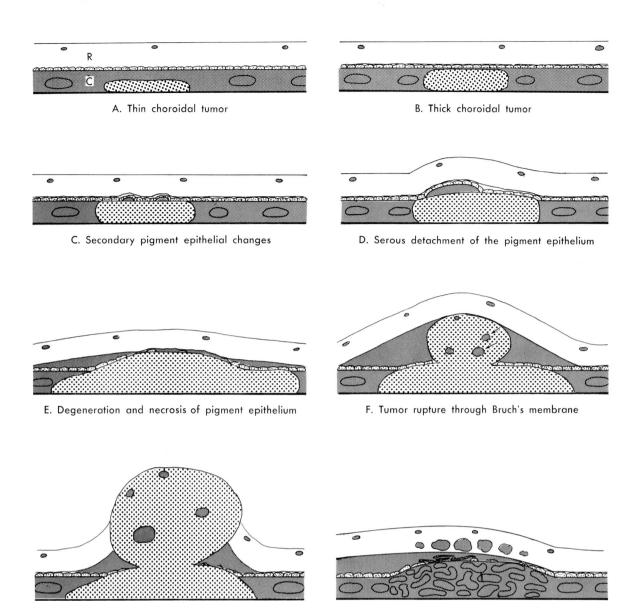

A. Thin choroidal tumor

B. Thick choroidal tumor

C. Secondary pigment epithelial changes

D. Serous detachment of the pigment epithelium

E. Degeneration and necrosis of pigment epithelium

F. Tumor rupture through Bruch's membrane

G. Tumor extension into vitreous

H. Choroidal hemangioma

Fig. 1-3. Schematic diagram of fluorescein angiographic findings in solid cellular choroidal tumors. *Gray areas,* Fluorescein; *dotted areas,* solid cellular tumor; *R,* retina; *C,* choroid. **A,** A tumor confined to the outer choroid may not alter the normal choroidal fluorescence and therefore may not be visible angiographically. **B,** A tumor occupying the full thickness or inner part of the choroid obscures the normal choroidal fluorescence, and, therefore, appears hypofluorescent during the early phases of angiography. **C,** A tumor causing secondary thinning and loss of pigment from the overlying RPE or drusen formation will show irregular areas of early hyperfluorescence corresponding to the RPE changes. Some of the drusen will stain during the course of angiography. **D,** Serous RPE detachment overlying a tumor will show a discrete area of fluorescein staining corresponding to the size of the RPE detachment. **E,** A choroidal tumor causing damage to the overlying RPE and serous retinal detachment will show a pattern of irregular fluorescence early and staining of the subretinal exudate later. **F,** A mushroom-shaped extension of tumor through Bruch's membrane will appear relatively hypofluorescent in contrast to the surrounding fluorescein-stained subretinal exudate. The fluorescein in large vessels near the surface of the tumor may be visible. Fluorescein present in large vessels or lakes within the depth of the tumor (*arrows*), however, will not be visible because the dye is inaccessible to the incident blue light. **G,** That portion of a choroidal tumor extending through the retina into the vitreous appears hypofluorescent because fluorescein diffuses from the retinal surface into the vitreous in relatively low concentrations compared to the high concentration of dye trapped in the surrounding subretinal exudate. **H,** A cavernous hemangioma of the choroid associated with serous retinal detachment and cystic degeneration of the overlying retina shows a prominent vascular pattern angiographically as the dye initially enters the tumor. The dye diffuses from the surface of the tumor and in some cases from the overlying retinal vessels and stains the subretinal and intraretinal exudate as depicted in the diagram. The dye within the cystoid spaces produces a multiloculated pattern of intense fluorescence overlying a background of less intense fluorescence during the late stages of angiography.

9

tumors occupying the full thickness of the choroid but unassociated with changes in the overlying pigment epithelium will appear hypofluorescent by virtue of obscuring the normal choroidal fluorescence from view (Fig. 1-3, *B*). When choroidal tumors cause thinning and depigmentation of the overlying pigment epithelium, irregular hyper-fluorescence may be apparent during the early phases of angiography (Fig. 1-3, *C*). In the case of drusen formation the dye may diffuse from the surface of the tumor through Bruch's membrane and stain the material beneath the elevated pigment epithelium (Fig. 1-3, *C*). In the case of a secondary exudative detachment of the overlying pigment epithelium, the exudate stains heavily (Fig. 1-3, *D*). The tumor may cause multiple small areas of elevation or destruction of the pigment epithelium and subretinal exudation (Fig. 1-3, *E*). These multiple foci of pigment epithelial changes appear angiographically as multiple areas, often pinpoint in size and of intense fluorescence, and the subretinal exudate stains during the late phases of the study. Choroidal tumors that extend through Bruch's membrane into the subretinal space (Fig. 1-3, *F*), or through the retina (Fig. 1-3, *G*), may appear relatively hypofluorescent in contrast to the hyperfluorescence of the subretinal exudate that usually surrounds the base of the tumor. In addition to causing changes in the permeability of the pigment epithelium, tumors may also cause increased retinal vascular permeability and cystoid retinal edema and degeneration (Fig. 1-3, *H*). The exudate within these cystoid spaces stains with fluorescein and produces a typical multi-loculated pattern of intense fluorescence during the late stages of angiography. Cystoid retinal changes may occur secondary to a variety of tumors. They occur most often in association with choroidal hemangiomas. Unlike other solid choroidal tumors, cavernous hemangiomas are composed primarily of large vascular spaces. For this reason they often cause prominent choroidal hyperfluorescence prior to fluorescein entering the retinal circulation.

The presence of pigment, including melanin, hemosiderin, and hemoglobin, as well as optically opaque exudate or tissue within or overlying a tumor, will reduce its degree of fluorescence by denying blue light access to the tumor.

It is apparent that although fluorescein angiography cannot provide the clinician with a definite diagnosis, it can give him valuable information concerning some of the general anatomic and physiologic alterations caused by the tumor in question. This information, when added to his clinical observations, can be important in arriving at a correct diagnosis.

TECHNIQUE OF FLUORESCEIN FUNDUSCOPY

The intraocular events that take place after fluorescein injection may be observed directly by the physician either through the ophthalmoscope or the slit-lamp equipped with an appropriate blue filter. Although this technique has the advantage of requiring few and inexpensive modifications of equipment usually available in the average ophthalmologist's office, it has several major disadvantages when compared with angiographic techniques: (1) The physician must be partly dark adapted; (2) the early events take place rapidly and there is little time for careful study and comparison of the sequential events; (3) the distinction between hyperfluorescence caused by alterations in the pigment epithelium and that caused by escape of fluorescein dye from the choroid and retinal vessels as well as determination of the exact level and location of the fluorescence is more difficult under direct observation; (4) there is no permanent record for comparison of future studies; (5) the technique of fluorescein funduscopy is time consuming for the physician; and (6) the technique requires much practice before the clinician obtains proficiency and competence in his observations and interpretations.

SUGGESTED READINGS

Amalric, P., and Bonin, P.: L'Angiographie fluorescéinique, Bull. Soc. Ophtalmol. Fr. (Numéro spécial):219-318, 1969.

Flindall, R. J., and Gass, J. D. M.: A histopathologic fluorescein angiographic correlative study of malignant melanomas of the choroid, Can. J. Ophthalmol. 6:258-267, 1971.

Gass, J. D. M.: Stereoscopic atlas of macular diseases, St. Louis, 1970, The C. V. Mosby Co., pp. 1-12.

Gass, J. D. M.: Fluorescein angiography: An aid in the differential diagnosis of intraocular tumors, Int. Ophthalmol. Clin. 12(1):85-120, Spring 1972.

Gass, J. D. M., Sever, R. J., Sparks, D., and Goren, J.: A combined technique of fluorescein funduscopy and angiography of the eye, Arch. Ophthalmol. 78:455-461, 1967.

Haining, W. M., and Lancaster, R. C.: Advanced technique for fluorescein angiography, Arch. Ophthalmol. 79:10-15, 1968.

Justice, J., Jr., and Sever, R. J.: Technique of fluorescein fundus photography. In Smith, J. L. (editor): Neuro-ophthalmology. Second Symposium of the University of Miami and the Bascom Palmer Eye Institute, St. Louis, 1965, The C. V. Mosby Co., pp. 82-83.

Norton, E. W. D., Smith, J. L., Curtin, V. T., and Justice, J., Jr.: Fluorescein fundus photography: An aid in the differential diagnosis of posterior ocular lesions, Trans. Am. Acad. Ophthalmol. Otolaryngol. 68:755-765, 1964.

Novotny, H. R., and Alvis, D. L.: A method of photographing fluorescence in circulating blood in the human retina, Circulation 24:82-86, 1961.

Rosen, E. S.: Fluorescence photography of the eye, London, 1969, Appleton-Century-Crofts, pp. 2-5.

Shikano, S., and Shimizu, K.: Atlas of fluorescence fundus angiography, Tokyo, 1968, Igaku Shoin, Ltd., pp. 2-24.

Synder, W. B., Allen, L., and Frazier, O.: Fluorescence angiography of ocular tumors, Trans. Am. Acad. Ophthalmol. Otolaryngol. 71:820-832, 1967.

Suckling, R. D., and Donaldson, K. A.: Detection of melanin in choroidal tumors; use of Ektachrome infrared aero film, Arch. Ophthalmol. 83:700-703, 1970.

Wessing, A. (von Noorden, G. K., translator): Fluorescein angiography of the retina, St. Louis, 1969, The C. V. Mosby Co., pp. 9-30.

CHAPTER TWO

Uveal melanocytic hamartomas

The terms "nevus" and "benign melanoma" are used synonymously to refer to benign melanocytic tumors of the choroid, ciliary body, and iris. Since these tumors are probably present at birth and have a growth potential that rarely is greater than that of normal uveal tissue in which they arise, they properly may be considered hamartomas. Their rate of growth is probably maximum in the prepubertal years. In adulthood their growth rate is extremely slow. Actual growth has rarely been demonstrated, and when it occurs, it should alert the clinician to the possibility of malignant change. During early life most choroidal nevi are hypopigmented and therefore are infrequently observed. They probably achieve their maximum pigmentation by early adulthood.

Although the clinical as well as the pathologic distinction between benign and malignant melanocytic tumors is usually clear-cut, clinical and histopathologic classification of some tumors is difficult or impossible. When the question arises as to whether an intraocular lesion is a benign lesion or an early malignant melanoma, the question should be resolved by careful and frequent serial observations of the lesion rather than resorting to enucleation, x-ray irradiation, or other radical treatment. The use of other ancillary means of investigation of the lesion, such as fluorescein angiography and radioactive phosphorus— ptake studies, is worthwhile, but one must remember that there is no test available to d' ce that can with certainty tell the clinician the malignant potential of a particular tumor.

CHOROIDAL NEVI OR BENIGN MELANOMAS

Choroidal nevi typically are flat or slightly elevated slate-gray tumors that are oval or round and that have well-defined but not sharp margins. They may be located anywhere throughout the fundus. Some clinical studies have suggested an incidence of choroidal nevi to be between 1 and 5 percent in otherwise normal eyes. More recent studies of autopsied eyes have suggested an incidence of at least 10 to 20 percent. Some reports have stated that choroidal nevi are predominantly located in the posterior pole, whereas others have stated that they are randomly distributed. In my experience choroidal nevi occur in approximately 20 percent of adult Caucasians. Most choroidal nevi range in size from one to two disc diameters. They may vary in size, color, and elevation just as do cutaneous nevi. They may be sufficiently large and elevated to cause suspicion of being malignant melanomas. In congenital ocular melanocytosis the entire choroid may be thickened by an increased number of benign melanocytes. In some cases this is associated with a dermal nevus of the lids (nevus of Ota). A similar diffuse nevus of the uveal tract may occasionally occur, usually unilaterally, in patients with neurofibromatosis.

Although typically slate-gray or blue-black in color, the choroidal nevus may vary considerably in color, depending on thickness, melanin content, pigment characteristics of the patient, and the changes in the overlying pigment epithelium. The nevus may be completely pigmented (Fig. 2-1), partly pigmented (Figs. 2-2, *A*, 2-3, *C* and *D*, and 2-4), or nonpigmented (Fig. 2-3, *C*). Nevi composed of a central pigmented portion and a peripheral nonpigmented portion (Fig. 2-4) as well as the reverse (Figs. 2-2, *A*, and 2-17, *E*) may occur.

Retinal and pigment epithelial changes caused by choroidal nevi

DRUSEN. Drusen, which are focal deposits of yellow or white material beneath the pigment epithelium, occur frequently overlying choroidal nevi (Figs. 2-1, 2-2, 2-4, and 2-5). Drusen may vary in size from pinpoint lesions visible only with the contact lens or with fluorescein angiography (Fig. 2-2, *A*) to large lesions that may be considered exudative detachments of the pigment epithelium (Fig. 2-5). In some eyes the subpigment epithelial material is deposited in a nondiscrete or granular fashion overlying choroidal nevi (Fig. 2-1, *E*). Drusen deposition appears to be more common in the larger and more elevated choroidal nevi. The relative thickness of the tumor and its presence within the inner choroidal layers are probably more important than its diameter in regard to its adverse metabolic effects on the overlying choriocapillaris, Bruch's membrane, and pigment epithelium. Although unproved, the degree of drusen deposition is probably also related directly to the age of the patient (Fig. 2-5, *E* and *F*).

SEROUS DETACHMENT OF THE RETINAL PIGMENT EPITHELIUM (RPE) AND RETINA. Drusen deposition is a clinical manifestation of loss of adherence of the basement membrane of the RPE to the collagen portion of Bruch's membrane. Drusen overlying choroidal nevi may enlarge concentrically, often at a slow rate, and may become confluent to form large areas of exudative detachment of the RPE (Fig. 2-5, *A*). The RPE overlying the surface of the drusen may become thin, degenerated, and incompetent as far as preventing the passage of serous fluid from the choriocapillaris into the subretinal space (Figs. 2-6 to 2-11). The area of serous retinal detachment is often limited and may resolve spontaneously. Recurrent and long-standing localized serous retinal detachment secondary to nevi accounts for localized, often apron-shaped, areas of sharply circumscribed thinning of the pigment epithelium extending away from the margin of the nevus (Figs. 2-7 to 2-10, 2-12, and 2-15). Usually only when the serous retinal detachment occurs overlying a nevus near the macula is the patient symptomatic and does the clinician have the opportunity to see the retinal detachment accompanying the nevus (Figs. 2-6 and 2-9). Because of the reparative processes inherent in the pigment epithelium, reattachment of the retina usually occurs spontaneously. If the detachment persists, photocoagulation of the area of leakage after identification with fluorescein angiography is useful in speeding resolution (Figs. 2-6 and 2-9).

CHOROIDAL NEOVASCULARIZATION AND HEMORRHAGIC DETACHMENT OF THE RPE AND RETINA. In addition to drusen deposition and degenerative changes in the RPE, an underlying choroidal nevus may cause degeneration and breaks in the continuity of Bruch's membrane similar to those seen in senile macular degeneration. This may be accompanied by proliferation of neovascular tufts or seafan-like membranes from the choriocapillaris into the subpigment epithelial space (Figs. 2-11 to 2-15). In some patients these small vessel tufts may be visible biomicroscopically as a pinkish or reddish discoloration of a drusen (Fig. 2-11). In others, where the membrane is more fully developed, some of the capillary details of the seafan may be visible (Figs. 2-13 and 2-14). Often, however, details of the neovascular membrane are obscured by a circular or oval, dirty-gray patch of exudate overlying the choroidal nevus (Figs. 2-13 and 2-15). Fluorescein angiography is invaluable in detecting the presence of these choroidal neovascular membranes (Figs. 2-11 to 2-15). When located in the macular area where the choroidal blood supply is maximum, these choroidal neovascular membranes may bleed and produce localized or disciform hemorrhagic detachments of the pigment epithelium and retina (Figs. 2-13 and 2-14). In the early stages hematomas may appear black or may be mistaken for rapid growth of a melanocytic tumor.

OTHER CHANGES IN THE PIGMENT EPITHELIUM AND RETINA. Focal areas of loss of pigment from the pigment epithelium and clumping of pigment, either in the form of dark pigment patches or orange pigment patches, occur overlying choroidal nevi (Figs. 2-7 to 2-9). These latter orange pigment patches or clumps are of particular interest not only because they occur infrequently over choroidal nevi, but also because they are commonly observed overlying choroidal melanomas as well as other choroidal lesions (see page 61). These orange patches are typically irregular in outline and are of variable size (Figs. 2-7 to 2-9). Their color is that of the normal pigment epithelium. The pigment appears to lie at the level of the retinal pigment epithelium. In some cases, it may be finely granular and may extend into the outer retinal layers. These patches of orange pigment appear hypofluorescent during their early stages of angiography (Fig. 2-9, *B*). We do not know whether the presence of this orange pigment has any prognostic significance in regard to neoplastic change in the nevus. There is no evidence to date that drusen have any prognostic significance in this regard.

As discussed above, sharply circumscribed areas of depigmentation of the pigment epithelium may occur adjacent to choroidal nevi secondary to recurrent or long-standing serous retinal detachment. An unusual pigmentary change that may occur within such areas is the migration of pigment-laden cells, presumably pigment epithelial cells, into the inner retinal layers to form bone spicules similar to that in retinitis pigmentosa (Fig. 2-15). The cause of this pigment migration is unknown. There is some evidence to suggest that this pigment migration is possible only in cases where degeneration of the rods and cones leaves naked outer limiting or fenestrated retinal membrane adjacent to the pigment epithelial cells. Such might be the case after spontaneous reattachment of a long-standing retinal detachment.

An infrequent retinal finding overlying large choroidal nevi is ophthalmoscopic and angiographic evidence of cystoid retinal degeneration and edema (Fig. 2-10).

Fluorescein angiography. Choroidal nevi appear hypofluorescent throughout the course of angiography when they occupy either the inner portion or the entire thickness of the choroid and when they are unassociated with alterations in the overlying RPE. If sharply circumscribed and densely pigmented, a pigmented nevus produces a hypofluorescent or dark patch that corresponds roughly in size with that of the tumor (Fig. 2-1). Hypopigmented nevi or nevi that do not involve the inner layers of the choroid will appear less hypofluorescent (Fig. 2-2) and in some cases will not alter the normal background choroidal fluorescence. Most drusen overlying choroidal nevi will fluoresce during the first minute of the angiogram and in many instances will show evidence of progressive staining of the drusen during the course of the study (Figs. 2-1, 2-2, and 2-4). Fluorescein angiography is quite helpful in detecting any abnormalities involving change in the degree of pigmentation (Figs. 2-7 and 2-10) or permeability (Figs. 2-6 to 2-9) of the RPE overlying nevi. It is also of value in detecting the presence of choroidal neovascularization (Figs. 2-11 to 2-15). Fine details of these capillary membranes may be partly or completely obscured because of the relative opacity of the exudate enveloping the membrane. Neovascular membranes usually stain intensely during the course of angiography (Figs. 2-11 to 2-15).

Visual field changes. Relative scotomas corresponding with choroidal nevi have been reported in as high as 85 percent of patients when sophisticated techniques of static perimetry are used. With conventional field techniques, however, these scotomas are difficult to demonstrate in many patients. Scotomas are most likely to occur in those patients with elevated choroidal nevi and particularly when they are associated with visible alterations in the retinal pigment epithelium. The scotoma may involve an area larger than the choroidal nevus when there is evidence of detachment or prior detachment of the surrounding retina.

Malignant change in a nevus. There is some histopathologic evidence that many choroidal and ciliary body melanomas arise from choroidal nevi. Rarely, however, has this been documented clinically (Fig. 2-16).

Histopathology. Choroidal nevi are composed of localized aggregations of melanocytes that may occupy part or the full thickness of the choroid except for the choriocapillaris (Fig. 2-17). In many nevi the choroid is thickened to a varying degree by densely packed melanocytes. Most choroidal nevi examined histopathologically have ranged in size from 1 to 3 millimeters. Localized nevi as large as 11 millimeters have been reported. In some instances portions of the choriocapillaris may be completely obliterated by the nevus (Figs. 2-17, C, and 2-18). In such instances drusen and degenerative changes in Bruch's membrane, pigment epithelium, and neuroreceptor cells of the retina are often present (Fig. 2-18). Cytologically the cells comprising choroidal nevi are similar to those that occur normally in the choroid. Plump polyhedral cells with a small, round, centrally placed, basophilic nucleus without nucleoli are the commonest cell type noted in choroidal nevi (Fig. 2-17, D). The abundant cytoplasm is usually so packed with melanin granules that depigmentation is required to see nuclear details. Except for some tendency for the cells to be elongated, they are indistinguishable from the cells that comprise melanocytomas of the optic nerve head and those that diffusely thicken the choroid in congenital ocular melanocytosis. Small spindle-shaped cells with slender, intensely basophilic nuclei and often with relatively little pigment are another cell type frequently seen in choroidal nevi (Fig. 2-18). They are typically present in the most external portion of these nevi. Plump, fusiform, and dendritic cells and rarely balloon cells with abundant foamy cytoplasm are cell types that occur less frequently in nevi (Fig. 2-17, F). Some tumors that are composed of an admixture of typical nevoid cells and small spindle cells are in the histopathologic gray zone separating typical nevi from spindle-A melanomas. Some of the larger tumors depicted in this chapter as choroidal nevi would probably fall into this category histopathologically.

CILIARY BODY NEVI

Nevi confined to the ciliary body are rarely detected clinically but have been described in approximately 3 percent of patients whose eyes were studied at autopsy. Clinically they usually appear as relatively flat or slightly elevated pigmented lesions involving the pars plana and often the peripheral choroid. Even when they are large, one should observe relatively flat lesions for evidence of growth or the development of secondary retinal detachment or cataract before making a clinical diagnosis of malignant melanoma (Fig. 2-18, F). Ciliary body nevi are histopathologically similar to choroidal nevi except that the cells appear more plump and are less densely packed in the former.

IRIS NEVI

See Chapter 15.

MELANOCYTOMAS OF THE OPTIC NERVE HEAD

These melanocytic hamartomas or nevi are first cousins of uveal tract nevi in that they are derived from similar melanocytes found normally in the region of the lamina cribrosa in darkly pigmented individuals. These deeply pigmented, black, or occasionally dark brown tumors of the optic nerve head occur almost exclusively in Negroes, Orientals, and deeply pigmented Caucasians. They reportedly occur more frequently in females. They vary in size and often arise eccentrically in the optic nerve head, particularly in the lower temporal sector. In 19 patients with this lesion seen at the Bascom Palmer Eye Institute, about one half occurred in Caucasians and there was no predilection in regard to sex or site of involvement in the optic nerve head. The tumor may be confined within the depth of the optic nerve head (Fig. 2-19, C); it may extend into the neighboring choroid (Fig. 2-19, A); and it may extend onto the anterior surface of the optic nerve head (Figs. 2-20, A and D) as well as along the nerve fiber layer of the retina (Figs. 2-19, B, and 2-20, A). When extending into the nerve fiber layer, the tumor has a feathery appearance (Fig. 2-19, B). In some patients the tumor may be quite elevated and involve the entire optic nerve head (Fig. 2-20, A and D). Visual acuity is typically unimpaired. Enlargement of the blind spot is usually present. Less frequently large field defects and slow progression of field loss and visual loss may occur particularly in patients with large melanocytomas (Figs. 2-20, A and D). Progression of field loss usually occurs in the absence of visible changes in the tumor. Small melanocytomas appear hypofluorescent angiographically (Fig. 2-19), and there is minimal evidence of dye leakage. More capillaries are visible in the large tumors, and extravascular leakage of dye may occur (Fig. 2-20).

Although the clinical appearance of melanocytomas may suggest an invasive malignant neoplasm, their cytologic features and clinical course are those of a benign hamartoma (Fig. 2-19, G). Bleaching is required for cytologic study of these heavily pigmented tumors. They are composed of a uniform population of plump polyhedral cells with small basophilic nuclei. These cells are identical with those occurring in congenital ocular melanocytosis and those that comprise the bulk of most choroidal nevi.

These tumors must be differentiated from juxtapapillary choroidal melanomas invading the optic disc (Fig. 3-18) and from retinal pigment epithelial hamartomas (Figs. 8-6 and 8-7). The former are always associated with significant and usually rapidly progressive visual field loss. The presence of field loss or slowly progressive loss of visual acuity, however, does not exclude the possibility of a melanocytoma. A pigmented tumor largely confined to the optic nerve head is unlikely to be a malignant melanoma, since to date there is no well-documented case of a malignant melanoma arising within the optic nerve head. Nevertheless, since the melanocytes comprising a melanocytoma are identical to those that occur commonly in choroidal nevi, it is conceivable that one of these tumors might undergo malignant change.

Fig. 2-1. Angiographic findings in pigmented choroidal nevi.

A, A small, highly-pigmented choroidal nevus (*arrow*) adjacent to the optic disc.

B, Angiogram showing discrete obscuration of the background choroidal fluorescence.

C, Choroidal nevus with overlying discrete drusen (*arrows*).

D, Approximately 10-minute angiogram showing obscuration of choroidal fluorescence by the tumor and fluorescein staining of some of the overlying drusen, as well as staining of several subretinal areas where no drusen are evident (*arrow*).

E, Elevated choroidal nevus with overlying nondiscrete deposition of drusen material. (From Gass.[1])

F, Angiogram reveals irregular hyperfluorescence in the region of the drusen.

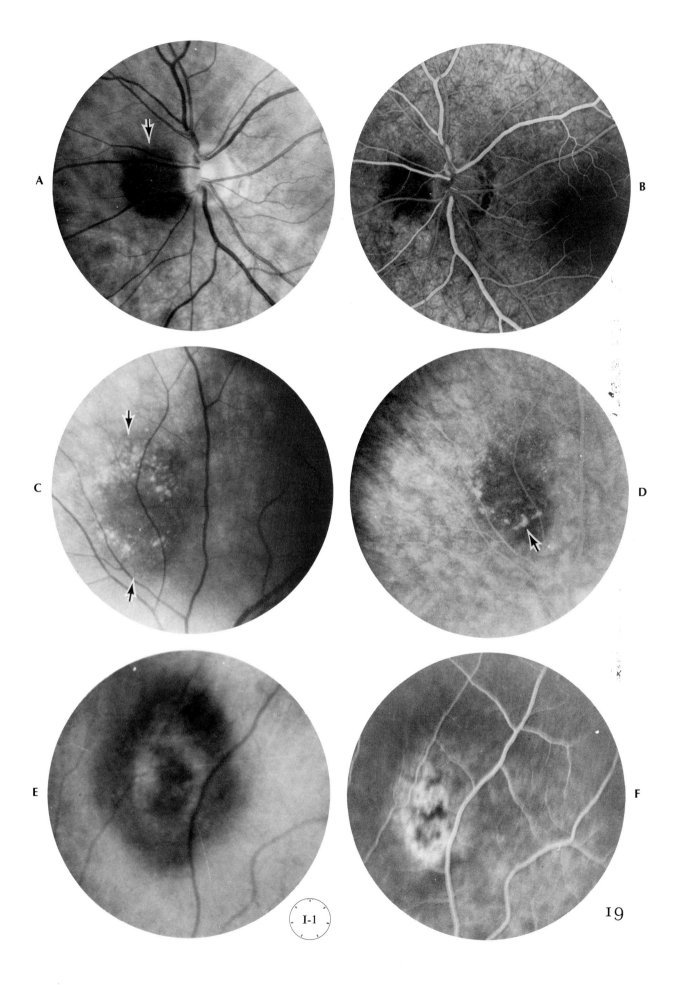

Fig. 2-2. Hypopigmented choroidal nevus with overlying drusen.

A, An elevated, hypopigmented nevus similar to that in Fig. 2-17, **E**. It is nonpigmented centrally and slightly pigmented peripherally. The small drusen on its surface are barely visible.

B, Angiography demonstrating obscuration of the choroidal fluorescence in the peripheral area of pigmentation; punctate staining of the small drusen; and faint diffuse hyper-fluorescence indicative of loss of pigment from the pigment epithelium overlying the center of the tumor. This latter fluorescence disappeared during the later stages of angiography.

C, Nonpigmented choroidal nevus with many drusen, which are present in lesser numbers beyond the confines of the tumor.

D, Angiography showing changes similar to **B**.

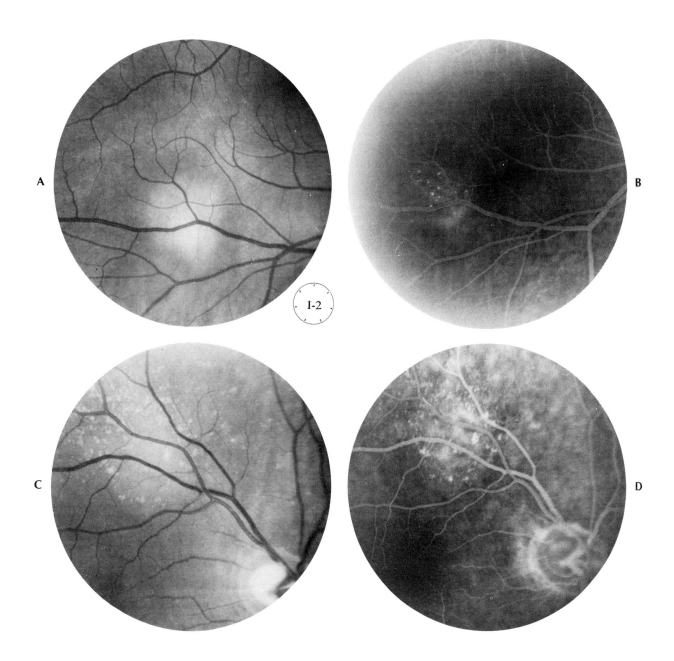

A

B

I-2

C

D

21

Fig. 2-3. Multiple choroidal nevi in a patient with von Recklinghausen's neurofibromatosis.

A, A 12-year-old girl was seen because of right upper lid ptosis, which was first noted at age 3 years. Note the S-shaped deformity of the right upper lid. She had pulsating enophthalmos and radiographic evidence of defects in the orbital wall on the right side.

B, Numerous café-au-lait spots were present.

C and **D,** Partly pigmented choroidal nevi and patches of hypopigmentation of the pigment epithelium and choroid were present in both eyes posteriorly *(arrows)*. The fundus immediately surrounding some of the nevi was hypopigmented.

E and **F,** Angiography revealed patchy areas of hyperfluorescence in the areas of hypopigmentation of the choroid and pigment epithelium. Some of the pigmented nevi were invisible angiographically *(black and white arrow)*. Others partly obscured choroidal fluorescence early *(black arrows)* but were enveloped by choroidal fluorescence later. The angiographic findings indicate that the nevi probably did not involve the full thickness of the choroid. The patient was examined 3 years later and there was no change in the appearance of the fundi.

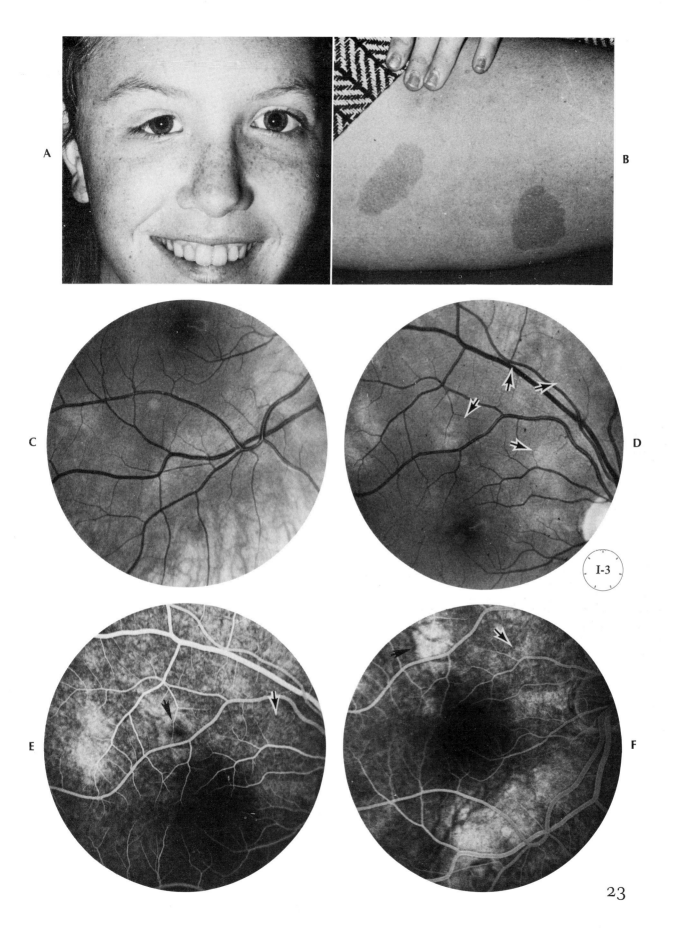

23

Fig. 2-4. Pigmented choroidal nevi surrounded by hypopigmented halo.

A, A slightly elevated pigmented choroidal nevus surrounded by an irregular nonpigmented zone.

B, Fluorescein angiography showing faint hyperfluorescence corresponding to the hypopigmented halo surrounding the nevus.

C, Another nevus similar to that shown in **A**.

D, An elevated pigmented nevus with a broad hypopigmented peripheral zone. Note the many small drusen on its surface.

E and **F,** Fluorescein angiography showing staining of some of the drusen. Three years later this lesion had not changed.

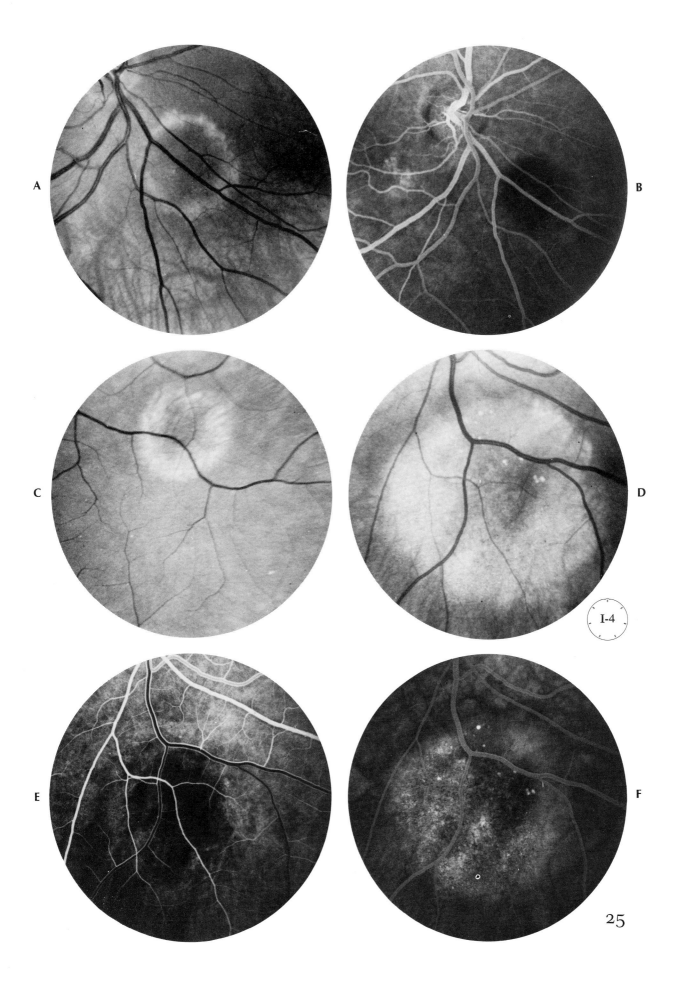

Fig. 2-5. Exudative detachment of the pigment epithelium overlying a choroidal nevus.

A, This large elevated pigmented choroidal nevus (*arrows*) was found on routine eye examination of a 73-year-old woman. Note the multiple drusen and two areas of confluent drusen or exudative detachment of the pigment epithelium overlying the tumor.

B and **C,** Angiography revealed progressive staining of some of the drusen and the subpigment epithelial exudate. There was no change 2½ years later.

D to **F,** Progressive deposition of drusen and possible enlargement of a choidal nevus.

D, This flat pigmented choroidal nevus (*arrows*) was found on a routine eye examination in a 20-year-old white woman. Note the drusen on its surface.

E, Nine years later many new drusen were present and most of the old drusen had faded. There was some evidence of enlargement of the flat nevus in an inferior direction (*arrows*).

F, Infrared fundus photograph of the nevus taken the same day as in **E** outlines its borders more accurately. Of interest is that this patient's mother has widespread metastases from a choroidal melanoma.

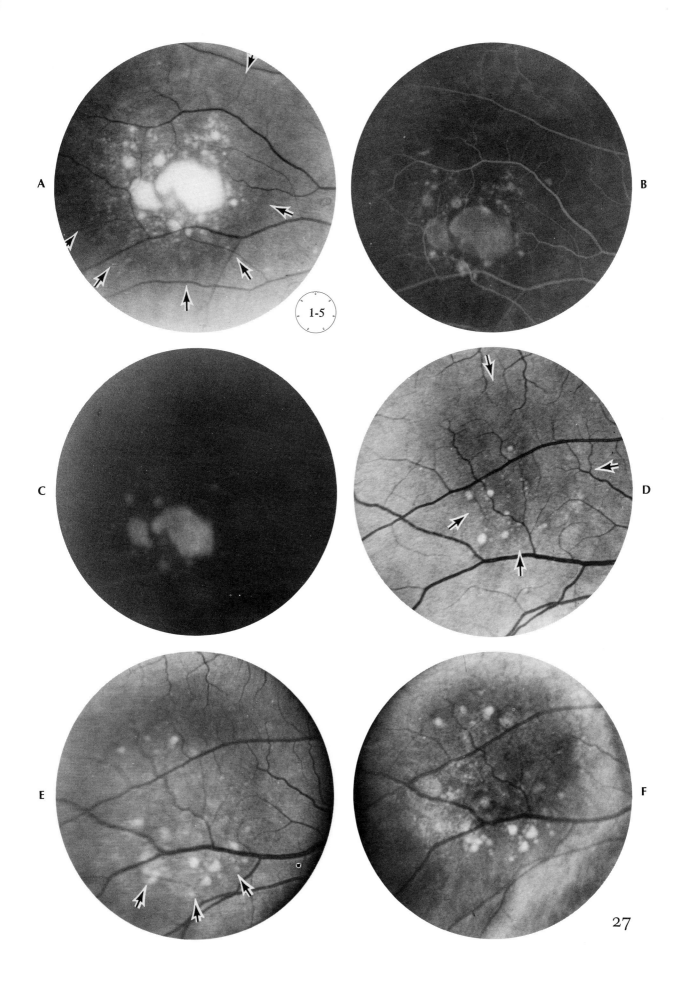

1-5

27

Fig. 2-6. Serous detachment of the macula secondary to a choroidal nevus. A 27-year-old white woman was seen on June 28, 1973, with a 2-week history of blurred vision in the right eye. Visual acuity in the right eye was 20/25 and she demonstrated metamorphosis on the Amsler grid.

A, She had a two-disc-diameter-size, slightly elevated pigmented choroidal nevus. There was a dumb-bell–shaped overlying serous detachment of the retina that extended into the foveal area (*arrows*).

B, Early angiograms revealed evidence of multiple punctate areas of fluorescence indicative of small drusen (*arrow*).

C, Angiography demonstrated a focal leak of fluorescein dye into the subretinal space (*arrow*).

D, Angiogram showing staining of the subretinal exudate.

E, Six applications of 50-micron-size argon laser burns (*arrow*) were made. By July 13, 1972, the serous detachment had resolved and her visual acuity was 20/15. In November 1973, follow-up examination revealed no subretinal fluid and no change in the size of the choroidal nevus.

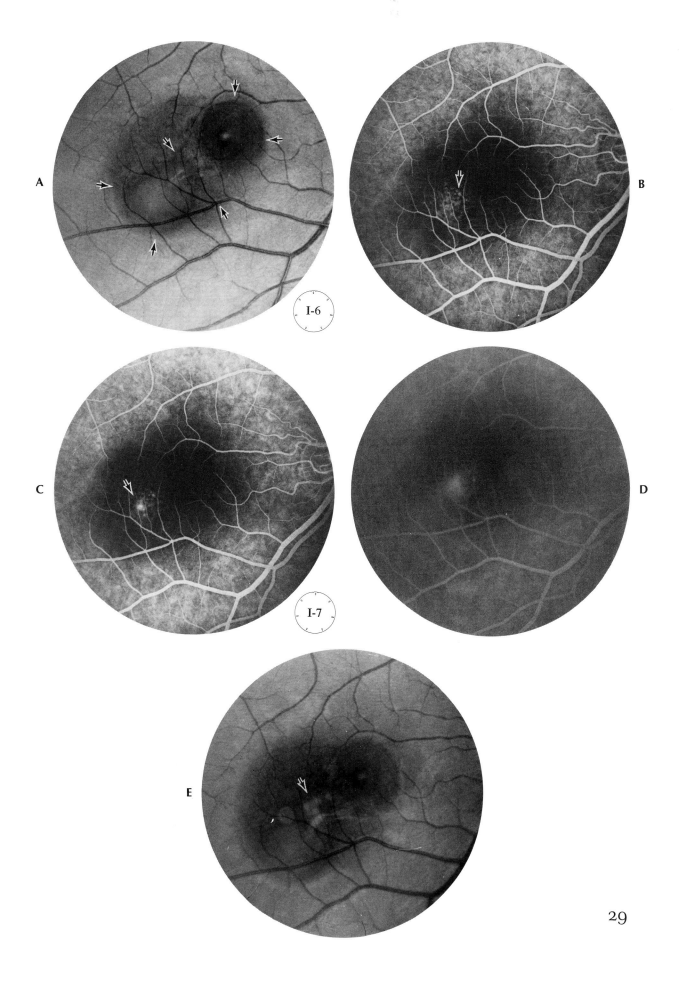

A

B

I-6

C

D

I-7

E

29

Fig. 2-7. Choroidal nevus showing evidence of previous long-standing serous detachment. A 66-year-old white woman was referred to the Bascom Palmer Eye Institute in March 1970, because of an elevated pigmented choroidal tumor in the right eye. Her visual acuity was 20/20.

A, A three-disc-diameter-size pigmented tumor of the choroid was present inferonasal to the right macula. Prominent drusen were present on the surface of the lesion in the region of the major vessels *(black and white arrow).* There was some granular orange pigment scattered on the surface of the lesion. An apron-shaped area of hypopigmentation of the pigment epithelium *(black arrows)* extended inferiorly from the tumor.

B and **C,** Angiography revealed mottled hyperfluorescence over the surface of the lesion as well as in the apron-shaped area inferiorly. The small hypofluorescent area *(arrows)* on the surface of the tumor gradually stained during the course of angiography.

D, Late angiogram revealed that most of the areas of hyperfluorescence disappeared except for the small area of persistent staining *(arrows)* centrally. The apron-shaped area of hypopigmentation inferior to the tumor is indicative of previous prolonged serous retinal detachment that extended downward from the tumor. The focal area of staining on the tumor was probably the site of origin of the subretinal fluid. The uncertainty of the nature of the tumor and the absence of detachment extending outside of the tumor at the time of initial examination were factors considered in not recommending photocoagulation to the site of dye leakage on the tumor surface. The patient has been followed for 3 years with no change in the size of the lesion and no evidence of recurrence of the retinal detachment inferior to the tumor.

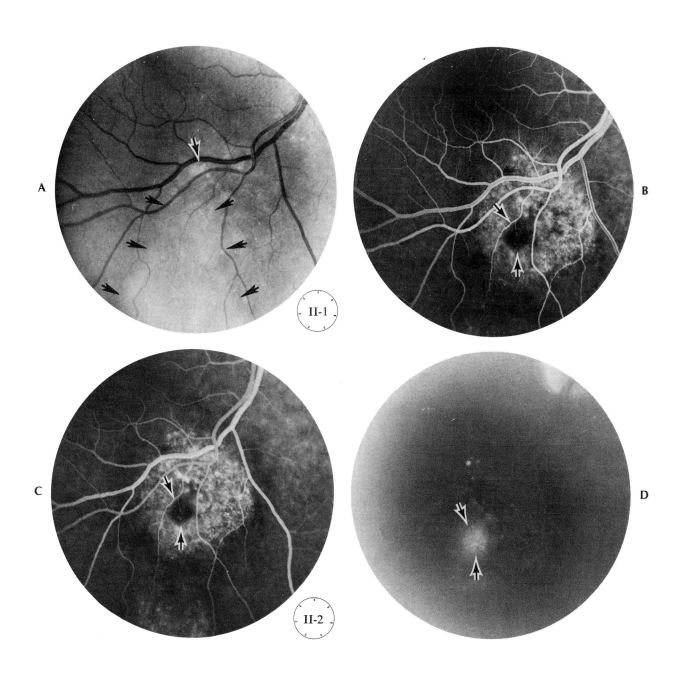

Fig. 2-8. Serous detachment of the retina secondary to a choroidal nevus. A 63-year-old Cuban woman developed blurred vision in January 1965. She was diagnosed as having optic neuritis and evidence of uveitis in both eyes. She was first seen at the Bascom Palmer Eye Institute in May 1965. At that time her visual acuity in the right eye was 20/40 and in the left eye was 20/200. The right fundus was normal. Examination of the left fundus showed a very pale optic disc.

A and **B,** Just superonasal to the optic disc there was a three-disc-diameter-size, elevated pigmented tumor of the choroid *(black arrows)*. There were a number of overlying drusen and patches of yellow-orange pigment. Extending temporally and inferiorly from the edge of the pigmented tumor, there was a localized area of serous detachment *(black and white arrows)*. The subretinal exudate appeared cloudy.

C and **D,** Fluorescein angiography revealed evidence of a pigmentary disturbance overlying the choroidal tumor and in addition showed a prominent focal area of leakage of dye *(arrow)*. The clinical impression at that time was probably an early malignant melanoma of the choroid. The patient was followed at frequent intervals for an 8-year period. The localized retinal detachment resolved spontaneously soon after her initial examination.

E and **F,** She was last examined in July 1973, and at that time there was no change in the appearance of the choroidal lesion. Repeat fluorescein angiogram at this time revealed early hyperfluorescence secondary to pigment epithelial changes but no evidence of a focal leak.

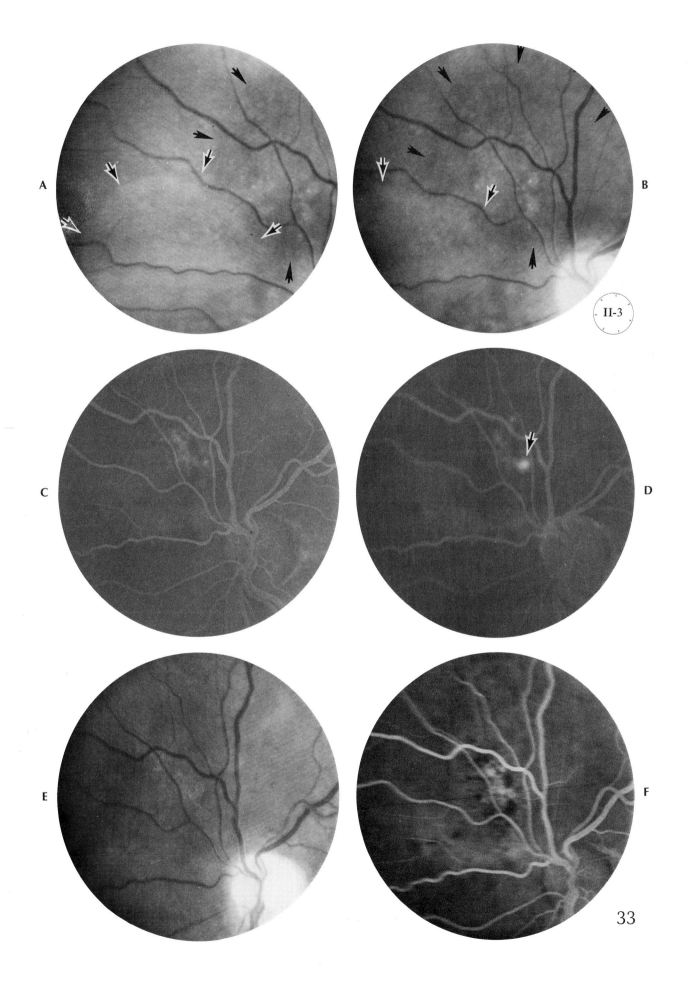

II-3

33

Fig. 2-9. Serous detachment of the macula secondary to a choroidal nevus. A 63-year-old white man was seen on April 28, 1969, and a 2-month history of metamorphopsia and decreased vision in the left eye. Visual acuity in the right eye was 20/20 and in the left eye was 20/50. He had a dense scotoma superior to fixation and a relative scotoma centrally.

A, A one-and-one-half-disc-diameter-size elevated pigmented lesion of the choroid was located on the superotemporal edge of the left macula. Note the small drusen and the irregular patches of orange pigment *(black and white arrows)* overlying the tumor. The detachment of the retina extended nasally from the lesion and involves the macular area *(black arrows).*

B, Early angiogram revealed hyperfluorescence in an area extending nasally from the tumor where the retinal pigment epithelium was depigmented secondary to a long-standing serous detachment. There were several small areas of dye leakage from the choriocapillaris *(arrow).* Note that the orange pigment patches appear hypofluorescent.

C and **D,** The hyperfluorescence attributable to loss of pigment from the pigment epithelium faded from view. *Arrow,* Primary area of staining where serous exudate probably gained entrance into the subretinal space.

E, The patient was observed until May 13, 1969, at which time persistence of the serous macular detachment prompted xenon photocoagulation to the surface of the lesion. The amount of photocoagulation is exessive. It should have been placed only in those areas where leakage was apparent as indicated above.

F, By May 26, 1969, vision in the left eye had recovered to 20/20 and the serous detachment was no longer present. The patient was last seen in November 1972, and there was no evidence of growth of the choroidal lesion.

(**A, B,** and **E** from Gass.[2a])

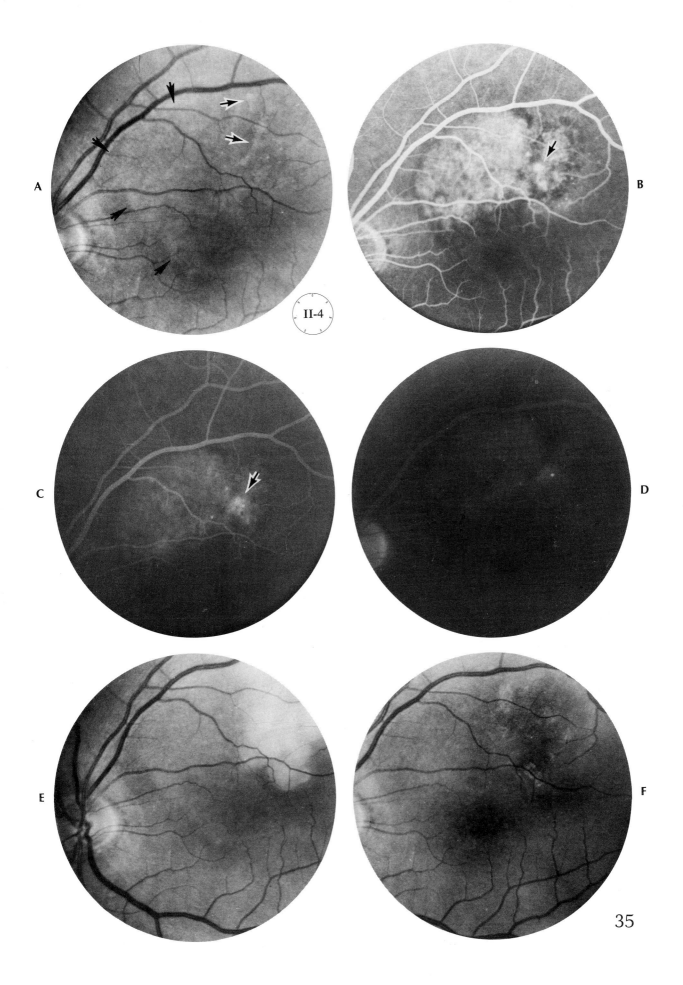

II-4

35

Fig. 2-10. Large pigmented choroidal nevus associated with cystic degeneration of the overlying retina. A 68-year-old man was first seen in May 1965, with the diagnosis of malignant melanoma of the choroid discovered on a routine eye examination. His visual acuity was 20/20 in each eye.

A, A large four-by-six-disc-diameter elevated pigmented tumor of the choroid (*arrows*) was present in the superotemporal portion of the left macula. It extended into the central macular area. A number of fine drusen were present on the surface of the tumor. There was no serous retinal detachment. Note the areas of hypopigmentation of the pigment epithelium extending nasally and inferotemporally from the pigmented tumor.

B and **C,** Early stages of angiography revealed hyperfluorescence attributable to loss of pigment from the pigment epithelium overlying as well as peripheral to the tumor. Two circular areas of hypofluorescence (*arrows*) corresponded to focal areas of cystic changes in the retina.

D, During the course of the study fluorescein gradually leaked into the two hypofluorescent areas shown in **B** and **C,** and into cystic spaces in the overlying retina. Note the multiloculated pattern of staining characteristic of cystoid changes in the outer retinal layers. The broad area of early hyperfluorescence overlying and beyond the margins of the tumor faded from view. This suggests that the patient may have had recurrent or long-standing serous detachment of the retina in this area in the past. The patient has been followed at yearly intervals and was last seen on June 7, 1972. At that time the fundus lesion, visual acuity, and fluorescein angiography were unchanged.

(From Gass.[3])

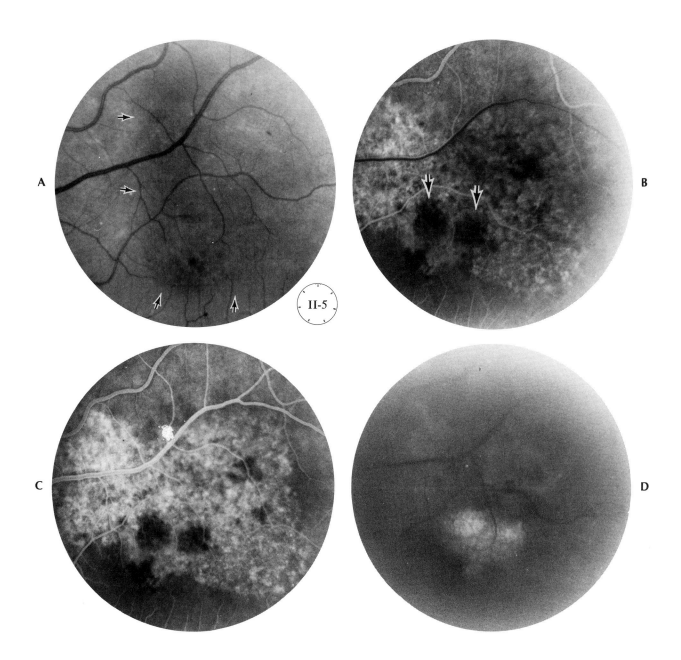

Fig. 2-11. Subpigment epithelial choroidal neovascularization and serous detachment of the macula secondary to a choroidal nevus. A 67-year-old woman developed blurred vision secondary to serous detachment of the right macula.

A, A slightly elevated choroidal nevus was present just superior to the macula of the right eye. The nevus was covered with multiple drusen and a serous detachment of the retina extended downward into the central macular area. There was reddish discoloration of several of the drusen (*arrows*), one of which was surrounded by subretinal blood. Several small subretinal hemorrhages were present. The reddish discoloration appeared to be caused by ingrowth of new capillaries from the choroid beneath the pigment epithelium (see Fig. 2-18).

B to **D,** Angiography revealed evidence of neovascular tufts (*arrows*) beneath the pigment epithelium.

E, Twenty-four months later the size of the nevus was unchanged. A new choroidal neovascular membrane had grown beneath the foveal area (*arrow*). Note the subretinal blood at the margins of the membrane.

F, Angiography confirmed the subfoveal neovascular membrane (*arrow*). Note that there was no evidence of progression of the other neovascular membranes noted in **A.**

(**A** to **D** from Gass.[2b])

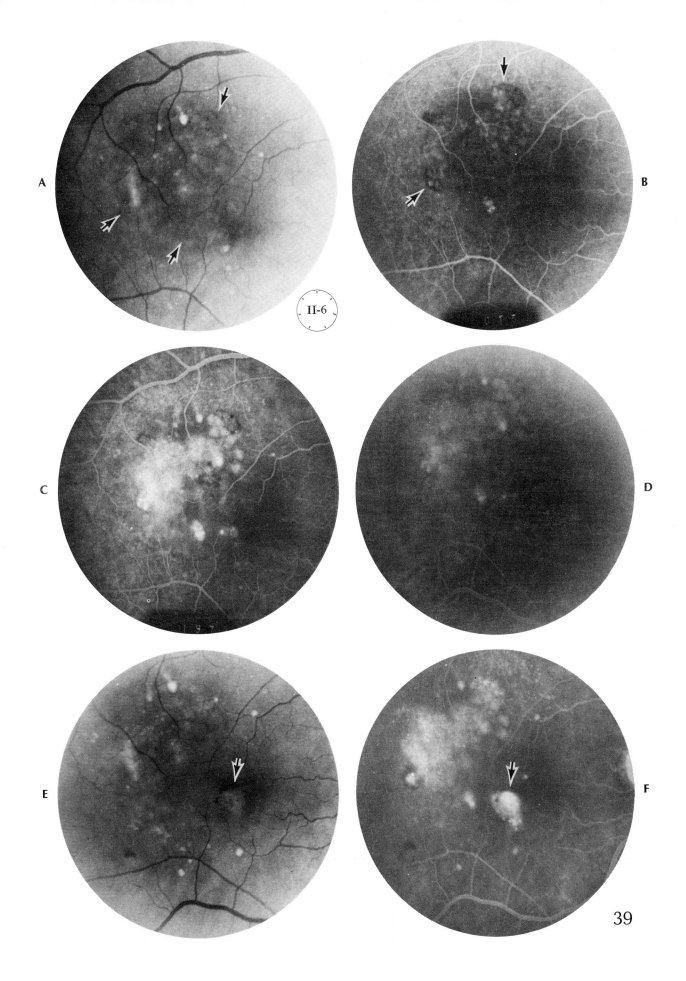

Fig. 2-12. Subretinal blood secondary to choroidal neovascularization overlying a peripheral choroidal nevus. A 56-year-old man reported for routine eye examination. His visual acuity was normal.

A, A two-by-four-disc-diameter-size, flat, pigmented tumor (*black arrows*) of the choroid was present in the periphery of the right eye. It was covered with multiple drusen. In one area there was a small nodular tuft of new vessels (*black and white arrow*) protruding from the choroid beneath the pigment epithelium and retina. A small amount of serous exudate and subretinal blood surrounded this lesion. A circumscribed area of hypopigmentation of the pigment epithelium surrounded part of the tumor. The patient was suspected of having a small malignant melanoma of the choroid.

B to D, Angiography outlined the neovascular tuft (*large arrow*) and revealed extensive staining of the tissues overlying the surface of the lesion. The zone of faint hyperfluorescence extending nasally from the tumor (*small arrows* in **D**) was probably due to hypopigmentation of the pigment epithelium secondary to a previous serous detachment. Because the lesion was relatively flat the patient was followed.

E, Five years later the neovascular tufts and subretinal blood were no longer evident. The choroidal lesion had not changed in size. There was now evidence of a thin subretinal fibrous membrane.

F, Fluorescein angiography showed evidence of some staining of this subretinal fibrous membrane (*arrows*) as well as hyperfluorescence secondary to the pigment epithelial changes.

(**A to D** from Gass.[1])

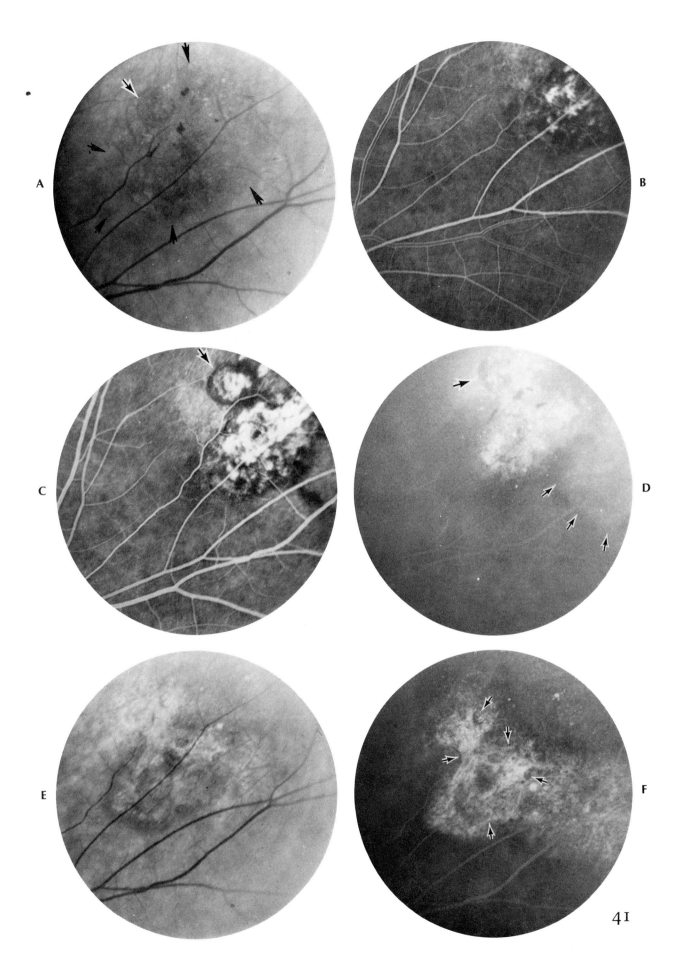

41

Fig. 2-13. Choroidal neovascularization and macular detachment secondary to choroidal nevi. A 73-year-old man was seen in September 1970 for routine eye examination, and a choroidal nevus was noted in the paramacular area of the right eye. Visual acuity at that time was 20/25. In August 1971, he developed blurred vision and metamorphopsia in the right eye.

A, The relatively flat pigmented choroidal nevus involving the temporal half of the macula appeared unchanged in size. A round gray patch of exudate containing new vessels (*arrow*), however, was now present on the surface of the nevus and there was a serous detachment of the retina.

B to **D,** Angiography revealed rapid staining of the neovascular membrane (*arrow*) and staining of the subretinal fluid.

E and **F,** A 61-year-old man had been followed by his local ophthalmologist since age 39 years when a small choroidal nevus was first detected in his left macula. His visual acuity was 20/20 until age 61 years, when he developed blurred vision in that eye. His physician found a serous macular detachment overlying the choroidal nevus, which had not changed in size. Over a period of months the patient developed a progressively enlarging neovascular membrane on the surface of the nevus.

E, A gray choroidal neovascular membrane largely obscured the presence of the underlying choroidal nevus. Note the subretinal blood at the margins of the neovascular membrane.

F, Angiography outlined the details of the choroidal neovascular membrane (*arrows*).

(**A** from Gass[3]; **F,** courtesy Dr. F. J. Heyner, Southfield, Mich.)

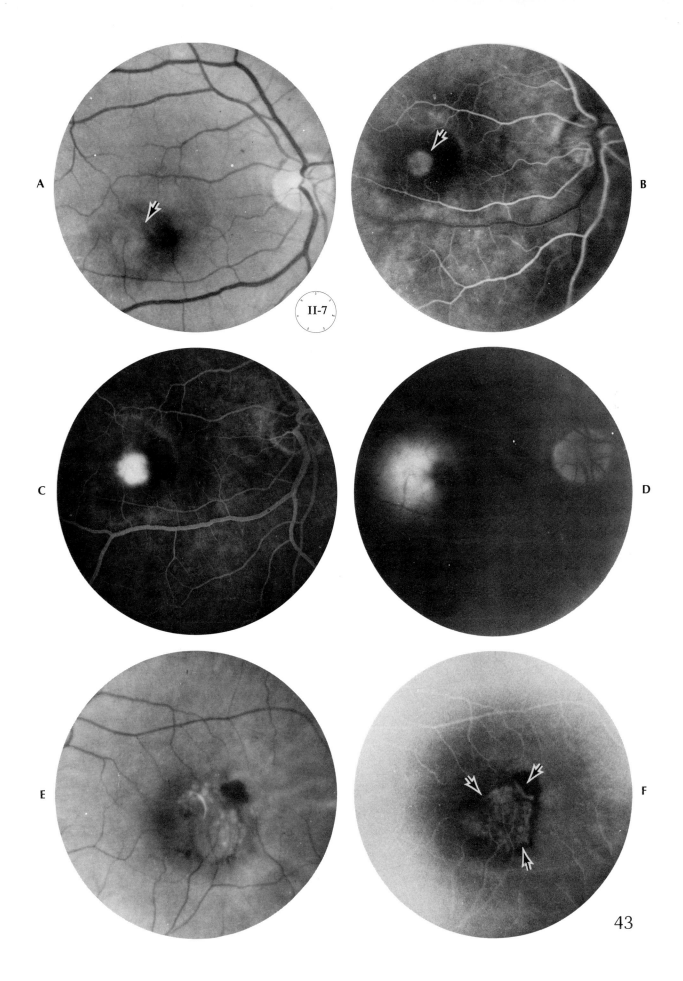

Fig. 2-14. Hemorrhagic detachment of the macula caused by a pigmented choroidal tumor presumed to be a nevus. A 54-year-old white woman was seen on January 12, 1973, with a 6-week history of blurred vision in the right eye. Visual acuity in the right eye was 20/200. Visual acuity and funduscopic examination of the left eye was normal.

A and **B,** A two-and-one-half-disc-diameter-size, slightly elevated, pigmented, choroidal lesion was present just superior to the right macula (*black arrows*). Over the lower edge of this lesion there was an area of circinate retinopathy that surrounded an area of neovascular ingrowth beneath the pigment epithelium and retina. The dilated sheathed new vessels were barely visible (*black and white arrows*). A hemorrhagic detachment of the pigment epithelium and retina extended from the edge of this neovascular membrane into the central macular area. Note the red color of the blood in the subretinal space that surrounds and largely obscures the underlying mound of the hemorrhagic detachment of the pigment epithelium (*gray area, black and white arrows*).

C, Angiography demonstrated new vessels (*arrows*) beneath the retina and pigment epithelium.

D, Angiogram showing evidence of staining in the region of the neovascular membrane as well as in several localized areas over the superior portion of the tumor. Since the hemorrhagic detachment of the pigment epithelium appeared to extend beneath the fovea, photocoagulation of the neovascular membrane was not recommended.

E, The same patient in October 1973. Visual acuity was now 20/400. The choroidal tumor had not changed in size. The subpigment epithelial and subretinal blood had partly resolved and organized.

F, Angiography revealed no evidence of change in the size of the nevus. This patient will be followed at frequent intervals. It is anticipated, however, that this is probably a choroidal nevus and that no growth will be demonstrated.

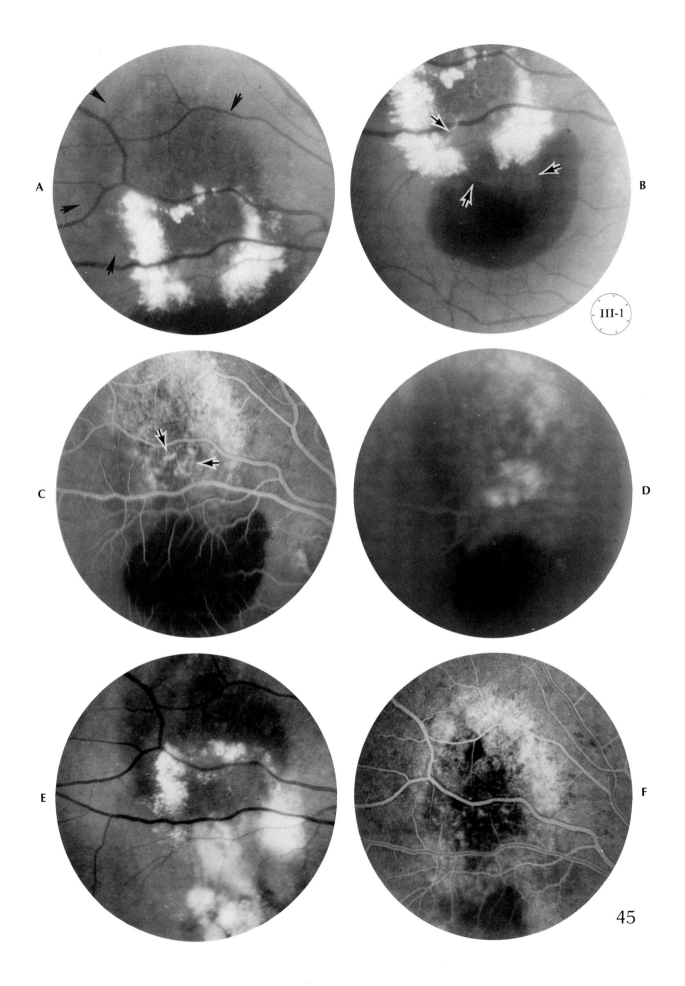

45

Fig. 2-15. Pigmented choroidal tumor presumed to be a choroidal nevus associated with a choroidal neovascular membrane, evidence of previous serous detachment of the retina, and prominent migration of retinal pigment epithelium into the overlying retina. A 54-year-old white woman was seen for a routine eye examination.

A and **B,** In the superotemporal quadrant of the left eye, she had a four-disc-diameter-size elevated pigmented choroidal mass *(black arrows)*. There was a circle of gray subretinal tissue lying on the dome of this mass *(black and white arrows)*. There was an apronlike area of hypopigmentation of the pigment epithelium that extended inferiorly from the edge of this mass. There was heavy intraretinal migration of the retinal pigment epithelium in a bone spicule fashion overlying the tumor as well as the area of depigmentation inferior to the tumor.

C, The apronlike area of hypopigmentation of the pigment epithelium and pigment migration was located inferiorly to the choroidal tumor.

D and **E,** Early phases of fluorescein angiography showed evidence of a choroidal neovascular membrane lying within the gray plaque of tissue noted in **A** and **B** *(arrows)*. Note also the hyperfluorescence secondary to loss of pigment from the pigment epithelium overlying the tumor and in the area inferior to the tumor.

F, Late angiogram showed evidence of fluorescein staining in the region of the choroidal neovascular membrane *(arrows)* as well as staining of the sclera, which can be seen through the depigmented pigment epithelium.

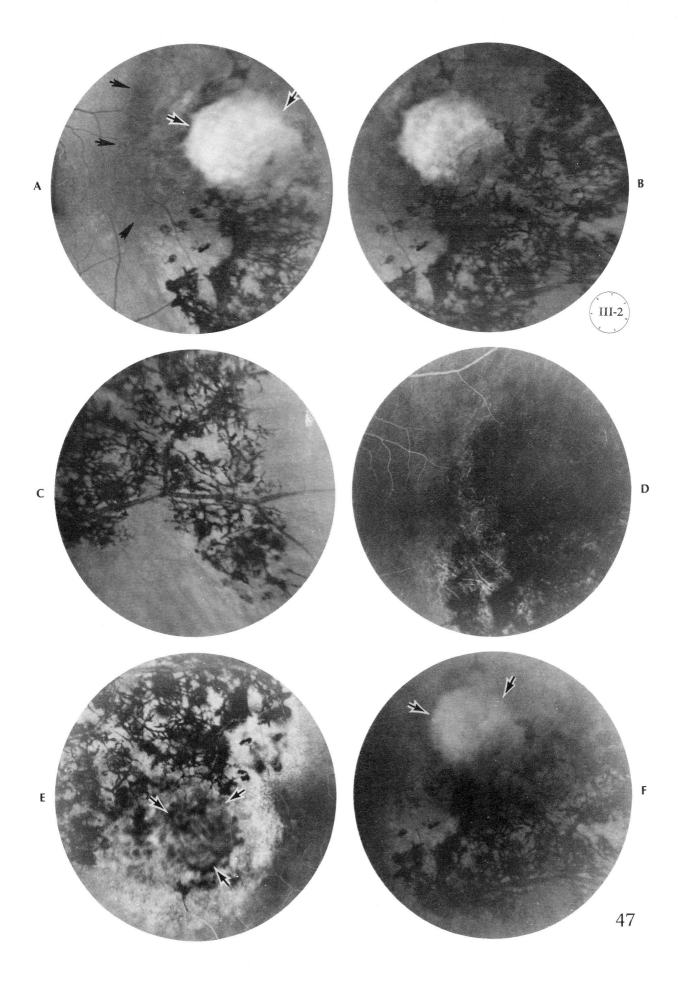

III-2

47

Fig. 2-16. Malignant melanoma of the choroid arising in a choroidal nevus. A 35-year-old man was seen by his local physician for a routine eye examination in 1951.

A, A one-disc-diameter-size pigmented choroidal lesion was present just inferonasal to the left optic disc *(arrows)*. There were a number of drusen present on its surface. The patient was followed at regular intervals by the same physician until 1956. No change in the lesion occurred during that time. He was subsequently followed by another physician at yearly intervals and showed no evidence of change until his examination in 1964.

B, At that time he had a five-by-six-disc-diameter-size, highly elevated melanoma of the choroid in precisely the same area where the nevus had been noted. There was an area of serous detachment of the retina inferiorly.

C and **D,** Angiography revealed leakage of dye from the surface of the tumor into the subretinal fluid.

E, The eye was enucleated and a spindle B melanoma was found.

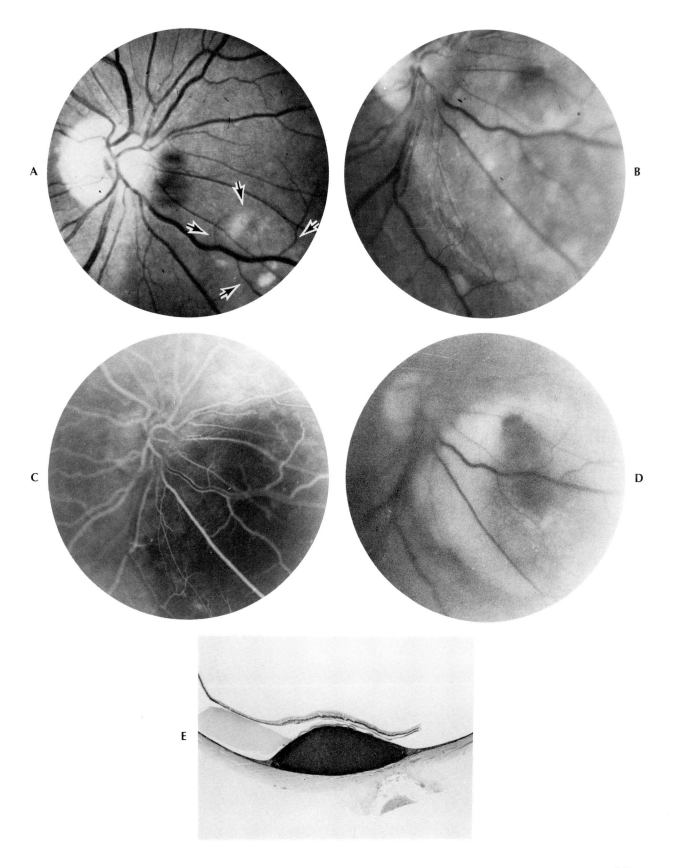

Fig. 2-17. Histopathology of a choroidal nevus.

A, A typical choroidal nevus was followed clinically from 1954 to 1962 without showing any change in size. The three dark areas to the right of the nevus are photographic artifacts.

B, Histopathologic condition of the lesion depicted in **A,** showing slight thickening of the choroid by heavily pigmented benign melanocytes. Note absence of involvement of the choriocapillaris, pigment epithelium, and retina.

C, Choroidal nevus noted on gross examination of an autopsy eye. In some areas the choriocapillaris is compressed and replaced by the tumor *(arrow)*.

D, Bleached section of the same lesion shown in **C.** Note the large fusiform cells with abundant cytoplasm and small nuclei.

E, Hypopigmented choroidal nevus *(arrows)*. Note faint pigmentation of the peripheral portion of this otherwise nonpigmented lesion, which was discovered in an eye at autopsy.

F, Histopathologic condition of lesion depicted in **E.** The section was taken at the midperiphery of the lesion and shows irregular orientation of small spindle and dendritic nevus cells, most of which are nonpigmented. Note sparing of the choriocapillaris. The overlying retina and pigment epithelium were artifactitiously detached but otherwise were normal.

A and **B** from Nauman et al.[4]; respective AFIP Neg. Nos. for **A** and **B,** 65-2263-1 and 65-3147.

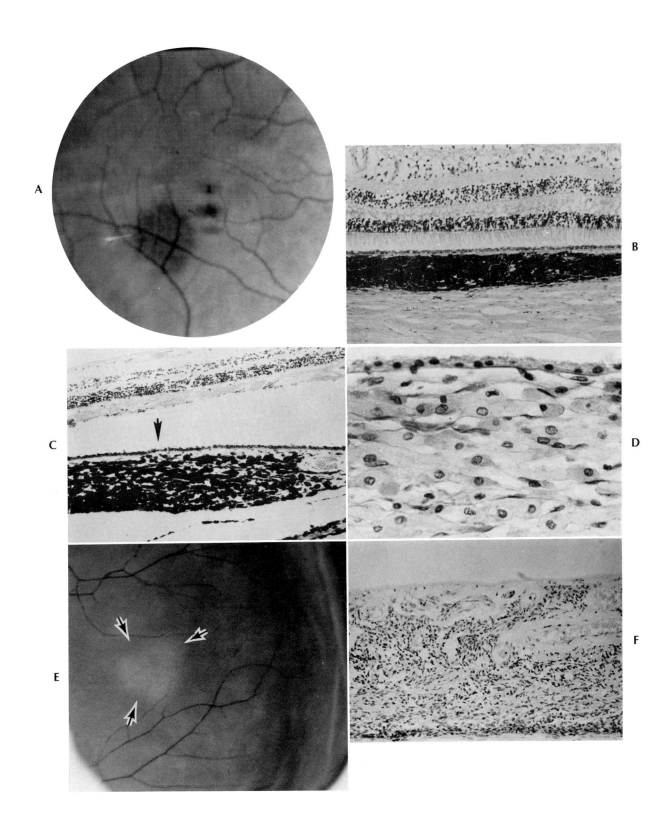

51

Fig. 2-18. Histopathologic changes in the pigment epithelium secondary to choroidal and ciliary body nevi.

A, Discrete drusen *(arrows)*.

B, Calcified drusen *(arrow)*.

C, Diffuse serous elevation of the pigment epithelium.

D, Neovascular ingrowth from the choroid into areas of diffuse pigment epithelial detachment *(arrow)*. Note the distinct tumor compression and replacement of the choriocapillaris that underlies the changes in the pigment epithelium in **A** and **D**.

E, Disciform submacular fibrovascular scar and proliferation of the pigment epithelium overlying a choroidal nevus. This scar presumably resulted from hemorrhage from new vessels that had grown through breaks in Bruch's membrane overlying the choroidal nevus. These changes led to a misdiagnosis of malignant melanoma and enucleation of the eye.

F, Choroidal and ciliary body nevus *(arrow)* that was discovered on a routine eye examination and was misdiagnosed as a melanoma. There were degenerative changes in the overlying pigment epithelium.

(**D** to **E** from Gass[1]; **F** from Gordon.[5])

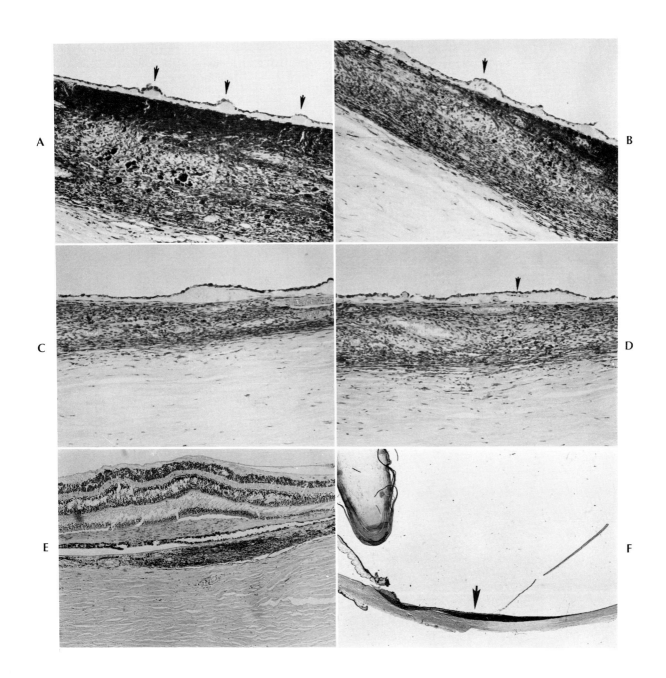

53

Fig. 2-19. Melanocytomas of the optic nerve head.

A, A small melanocytoma of the inferotemporal margin of the optic nerve head extended into the adjacent choroid *(arrows)* in this 54-year-old white woman who was asymptomatic and whose eye examination was otherwise unremarkable.

B, A melanocytoma in a 77-year-old white man has not changed since he was initially photographed at age 66 years (From Zimmerman[6]). Note the feathery margins of the tumor where it extends into the nerve fiber layer superonasally.

C, A slightly elevated melanocytoma involving most of the optic nerve head in this 46-year-old white man.

D to **F,** Flourescein angiography revealed that the tumor obscured from view some of the normal capillary bed of the optic nerve head. There were no abnormal-appearing vessels within the tumor and there was minimal staining in the late photographs. It showed no change over a 9-year period.

G, Histopathologic condition of a large melanocytoma. Clinically this large tumor probably appeared similar to those shown in Fig. 2-20. (AFIP Accession No. 1159938; courtesy Dr. L. E. Zimmerman, Washington, D. C.)

G

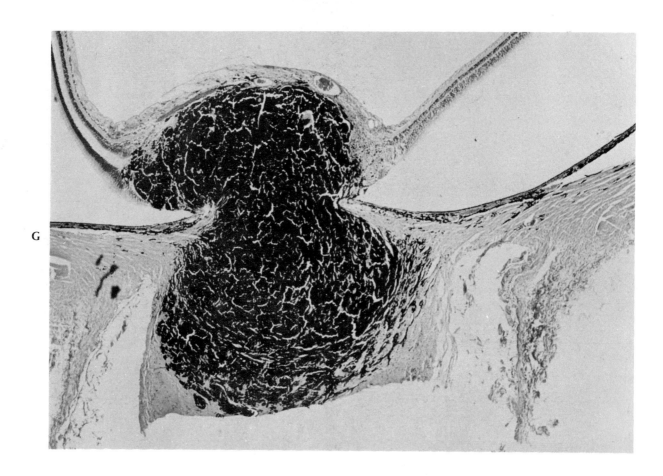

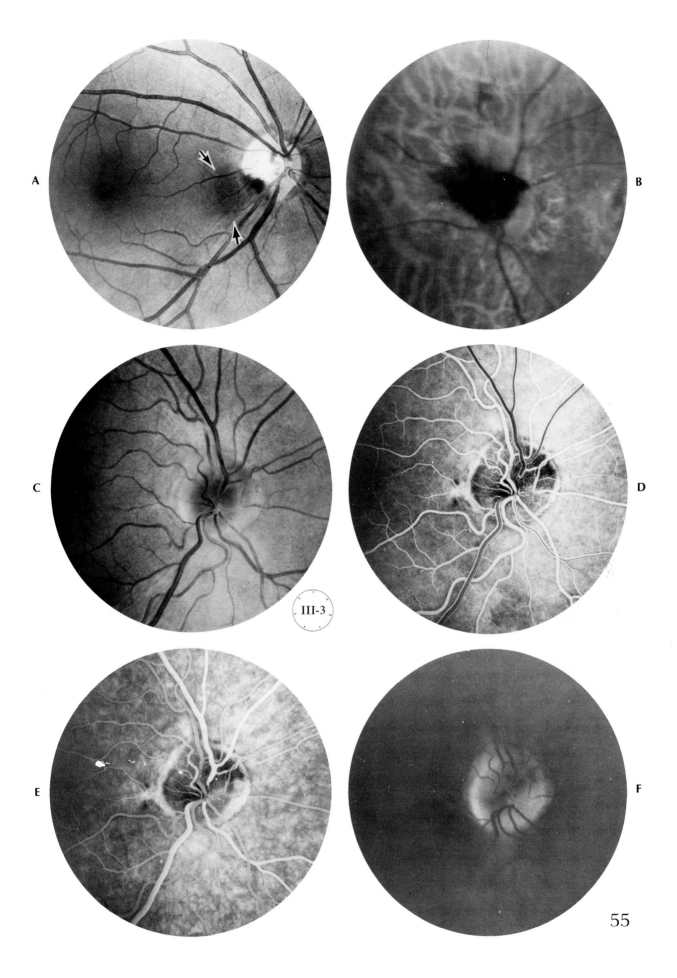

Fig. 2-20. Large melanocytomas of the optic nerve head.

A to **C,** A 21-year-old black woman was examined on January 27, 1969. She gave a 4-month history of slight blurring of vision in the right eye involving the inferior field. Visual acuity in the right eye was 20/20. In the left eye visual acuity was 20/15. Visual field examination revealed a profound unilateral loss of visual field with only the upper temporal field remaining intact in the right eye. The left visual field was normal.

A, The right optic nerve head was enlarged and elevated by a black mass that extended into the peripapillary choroid as well as onto the temporal surface of the optic nerve head where the tumor partly obscured the underlying major retinal vessels from view. There was slight sheathing of the superior retinal view. There were no exudates or hemorrhages.

B and **C,** Angiography revealed hypovascularity of the surface of the tumor and minimal evidence of staining of the main mass of the tumor. Note the tumor vessel *(arrow)* that appears to be present in that portion of the tumor that extends anterior to the major retinal vessels. This patient was followed for a period of 27 months without any change in visual acuity, visual fields, or appearance of the tumor.

D to **F,** A 39-year-old black man was examined on February 19, 1971, with a 1-year history of blurred vision in his left eye. Visual acuity in the right eye was 20/20 and in the left eye was 20/60. Peripheral field examination revealed loss of the inferonasal quadrant and some generalized constriction in the left eye.

D, Funduscopic examination in the left eye revealed a highly elevated pigmented lesion involving the optic nerve head and surrounding choroid. Note the admixture of the orange and black pigment near the tumor surface.

E and **F,** Fluorescein angiography revealed dilated capillaries near the surface of the tumor. There was evidence of leakage of dye from these vessels in the later stages. This patient has been followed without any change for 3 years.

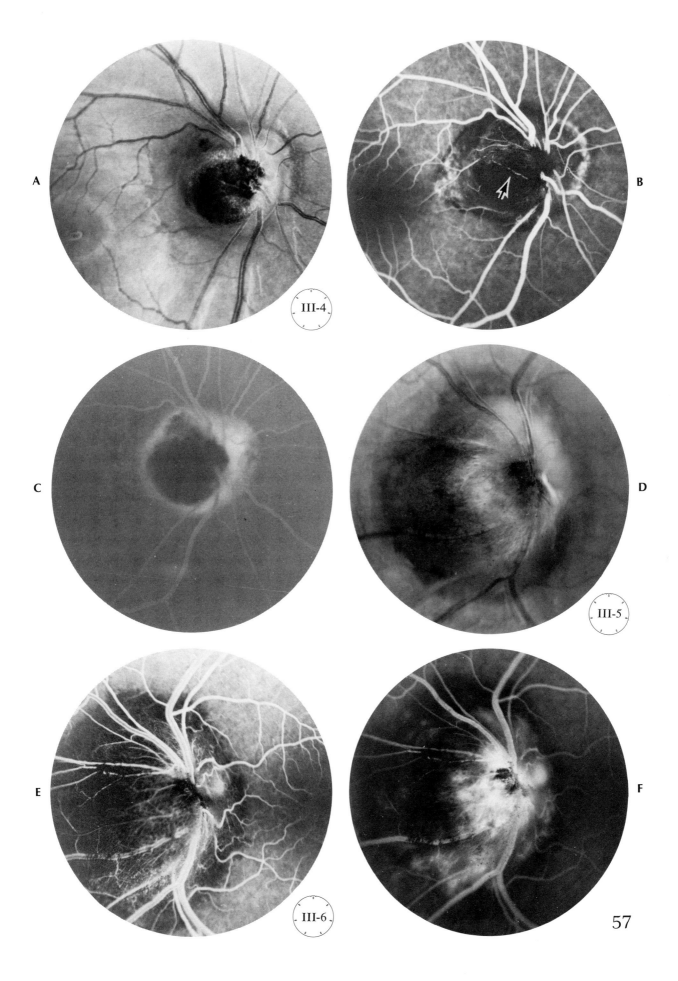

REFERENCES

1. Gass, J. D. M.: Pathogenesis of disciform detachment of the neuroepithelium. VI. Disciform detachment secondary to heredodegenerative, neoplastic and traumatic lesions of the choroid. Am. J. Ophthalmol **63:**689-711, 1967.
2. Gass, J. D. M.: Stereoscopic atlas of macular diseases, St. Louis, 1970, The C. V. Mosby Co., and pp. (a) 90 and (b) 89.
3. Gass, J. D. M.: Fluorescein angiography: An aid in the differential diagnosis of intraocular tumors, Int. Ophthalmol. Clin. **12**(1): 85-120, Spring 1972.
4. Naumann, Yanoff, M., and Zimmerman, L. E.: Histogenesis of malignant melanoma of the uvea, Arch. Ophthalmol. **76:**784-796, 1966.
5. Gordon, E.: Nevus of the choroid and pars plana, Survey Ophthalmol. **8:**507-511, 1963.
6. Zimmerman, L. E.: Melanocytes, melanocytic nevi, and melanocytomas, Invest. Ophthalmol. **4:**11-41, 1965.

SUGGESTED READINGS

Ganley, J. P., and Comstock, G. W.: Benign nevi and malignant melanomas of the choroid, Am. J. Ophthalmol. **76:**19-25, 1973.

Hale, P. N., Allen, R. A., and Straatsma, B. R.: Benign melanomas (nevi) of the choroid and ciliary body, Arch. Ophthalmol. **74:**532-538, 1965.

Hogan, M. M., and Zimmerman, L. E. (editors): Ophthalmic pathology, ed. 2, Philadelphia, 1963, W. B. Saunders Co., p. 413.

Naumann, G., Hellner, K., and Naumann, L. R.: Pigmented nevi of the choroid. Clinical study of secondary changes in the overlying tissues, Trans. Am. Acad. Ophthalmol. Otolaryngol. **75:**110-123, 1971.

Reese, A. B.: Tumors of the eye, New York, 1963, Paul B. Hoeber, Inc., Harper & Row, Publishers, pp. 214-363.

Shields, J. A., and Font, R. L.: Melanocytoma of the choroid clinically simulating a malignant melanoma, Arch. Ophthalmol. **87:**396-400, 1972.

Smith, L. T., and Irvine, A. R.: Diagnostic significance of orange pigment accumulation over choroidal tumors, Am. J. Ophthalmol. **76:**212-222, 1973.

Tamler, E., and Maumenee, A. E.: A clinical study of choroidal nevi, Arch. Ophthalmol. **62:**196-202, 1959.

Tamler, E.: A clinical study of choroidal nevi. A follow-up report, Arch. Ophthalmol. **84:**29-32, 1970.

deVeer, J. A.: Juxtapapillary malignant melanoma of the choroid and so-called malignant melanoma of the optic disc, Arch. Ophthalmol. **51:**147-160, 1954.

Yanoff, M., and Zimmerman, L. E.: Histogenesis of malignant melanomas of the uvea. III. The relationship of congenital ocular melanocytosis and neurofibromatosis to uveal melanomas, Arch. Ophthalmol. **77:**331-336, 1967.

Zimmerman, L. E., and Garron, L. K.: Melanocytoma of the optic disc, Int. Ophthalmol. Clin. **2:**431-440, 1962.

CHAPTER THREE

Uveal malignant melanomas

Malignant melanoma of the choroid and ciliary body may occur at any age but at least half of them are first detected in patients between the ages of 50 and 70 years. There is no sex predilection. They are rare in Negroes. There is only one case on file at the Armed Forces Institute of Pathology for each 165 cases occurring in Caucasians.

The histopathologic classification of uveal melanomas proposed by Callender is widely used by pathologists and has some practical clinical implications. In this classification malignant melanomas of the uveal tract are subdivided into six groups as follows: (1) spindle A (Fig. 3-1, A), (2) spindle B (Fig. 3-1, B), (3) fascicular (Fig. 3-1, C), (4) epithelioid (Fig. 3-1, D and E), (5) mixed, or a combination of epithelioid and spindle A or B cells, and (6) necrotic. In addition to the three basic cell types, deeply pigmented branched melanocytes and nests of large foamy cells (presumed to represent lipoidal degeneration of melanoma cells) may be observed (Fig. 3-1, F). Actuarial data obtained at the Armed Forces Institute of Pathology have revealed that 75 percent of the patients with spindle A, spindle B, or fascicular tumors of the choroid and ciliary body are alive and well 15 years after enucleation of their eyes. Had the tumor classification been based on the examination of serial sections of each tumor to rule out foci of epithelioid cells, the 15-year survival rate for the patients with pure spindle A and spindle B tumors might have been higher. This is in striking contrast to those patients with the more malignant cell types. Fifty percent of all patients with epithelioid cell tumors are dead in 3.4 years and 50 percent of patients with either mixed or necrotic tumors are dead within 9.3 years. In general, the prognosis for melanomas in young patients is better than in older patients.

In the study of the relationship of prognosis to the size, shape, and histologic characteristics of choroidal and ciliary body melanomas in enucleated eyes, Flocks and co-workers[1] found the following: (1) patients with large tumors have a significantly poorer prognosis; the prognosis suddenly becomes worse when the product of the tumor's three dimensions in cubic millimeters is over 1,300; (2) large tumors show a pronounced tendency to contain those cell types of established bad prognosis; (3) large heavily pigmented tumors have a poorer prognosis than do large lightly pigmented tumors; (4) the shape of the tumor is unrelated to prognosis; and (5) rupture of Bruch's membrane is a function of tumor size and patient age and does not affect prognosis if tumors of the same size are considered. Thus, their finding that most small tumors were of either spindle A or spindle B type, together with the Armed Forces Institute of Pathology actuarial data that 75 percent of patients with these two cell types are alive 15 years after enucleation, suggests that the clinician who encounters a patient with a slightly elevated pigmented choroidal tumor that is five disc diameters or smaller in size should proceed cautiously before informing the patient that he has a malignant tumor or before recommending enucleation of the eye.

CHOROIDAL MALIGNANT MELANOMA

Early development. Malignant transformation of a melanocyte, either in the otherwise normal choroid or within a choroidal nevus (see Fig. 2-16) leads to unchecked mitotic activity and the development of a progressively enlarging tumor mass. The rate of mitosis, the degree of pigment production, and the pattern of growth in malignant melanomas are quite variable. A melanoma in its earlier stages of development is most likely to be observed clinically when it arises in or near the macular area where it may cause early symptoms (Figs. 3-2 to 3-6). Usually such a tumor is associated with a serous detachment of the macula. The clinician who discovers a small pigmented choroidal lesion associated with a macular detachment should not, however, conclude that the lesion is a malignant melanoma since, as was demonstrated in the previous chapter, macular detachment may occur overlying a choroidal nevus. Some of the signs that suggest but do not definitely indicate that a relatively small pigmented choroidal tumor is a malignant melanoma are (1) the presence of widespread changes in the overlying pigment epithelium associated with areas of orange pigment deposition on the tumor surface (Figs. 3-2, 3-4, and 3-5), (2) globular elevation of the choroidal lesion, (3) serous retinal detachment, (4) evidence of tumor breaking through Bruch's membrane, (5) biomicroscopic or fluorescein angiographic evidence of large blood vessels within the tumor (Fig. 3-7), (6) fluorescein angiographic evidence of multiple pinpoint leaks over much of the surface of the tumor (Figs. 3-2 and 3-4), and (7) a dense negative scotoma that occupies most of the area of the tumor. Early in its development a malignant melanoma encroaches upon the choriocapillaris and causes varying degrees of damage to the overlying pigment epithelium and receptor cells of the retina. These changes are usually maximum over the central portion of the tumor. The changes in the pigment epithelium include depigmentation (Fig. 3-6), focal areas of destruction and degeneration, and occasionally detachment (Fig. 3-5). Depigmentation of the pigment epithelium may not be readily apparent ophthalmoscopically, particularly when it occurs overlying a pigmented tumor. A frequent ophthalmoscopic manifestation of pigment epithelial damage secondary to early growth of a malignant melanoma is that of patches of finely granular orange pigment on the surface of the tumor (Figs. 3-2, 3-4, 3-5, and 3-17). Occasionally small granules of this pigment are also present in the outer layers of the retina. Histologically, this pigment is attributable to clumps of pigment-laden cells, either macrophages or pigment epithelial cells (Figs. 3-5, *F*, and 3-17, *E*). Some authors have suggested that this pigment is the result primarily of lipofuscin. Although this pigment occurs often over malignant melanomas, it may also occur over localized serous detachments of the pigment epithelium, hemangiomas of the choroid, and metastatic tumors and occasionally over choroidal nevi (Figs. 2-7 to 2-9). Its presence probably is indicative of a moderately severe insult to the pigment epithelial cells. Curiously the orange color of the pigment is identical to that of the normal pigment epithelium, whereas the pigment resulting from reactive proliferation of the pigment epithelial cells typically appears black ophthalmoscopically. This suggests the possibility that these orange patches of pigment may be caused by clumping together of pigment epithelial cells that have simply been dislodged from their attachment to Bruch's membrane by a variety of underlying pathologic processes. Further electron-microscopic and histochemical studies are required, however, to further clarify the nature of this pigment. A rare change involving damage to the pigment epithelium over an early melanoma is illustrated in Fig. 3-6. In this patient there was clumping of pigment to form a stellate figure, simulating that seen in some patients with serous detachment of the pigment epithelium and in so-called butterfly macular dystrophy. Varying degrees of serous retinal detachment usually accompany rapidly developing damage to the overlying pigment epithelium by a choroidal tumor.

Fluorescein angiography is helpful in detecting early changes in the pigment epithelium overlying a newly developing melanoma. Prior to damaging the pigment epithelium, lateral growth of the tumor in the choroid produces an area of relative hypofluorescence angiographically (Fig. 3-3). Once inward growth of the tumor has caused depigmentation, degeneration, destruction, or detachment of the pigment epithelium, varying degrees of hyperfluorescence will be evident angiographically. Depigmentation of the pigment epithelium usually causes areas of hyperfluorescence during the early phases of angiography (Fig. 3-3). This fluorescence is secondary to greater visibility of the dye in the choriocapillaris or near the surface of the tumor. Small focal areas of elevation and destruction of the pigment epithelium cause focal pinpoint areas of intense fluorescence that gradually increase in size during the course of angiography (Figs. 3-2 and 3-4 to 3-6). These small areas of fluorescein staining may simulate angiographically those seen in fine drusen overlying choroidal nevi. The fluorescence in the latter, however, is usually not as intense and shows no tendency to increase in size during the course of angiography. Since malignant melanomas damage the pigment epithelium very early in their development, some degree of abnormal fluorescence is always apparent over at least some part of these tumors by the time the patient presents. The rare occurrence of a diffuse, slightly elevated, highly pigmented melanoma unassociated with significant changes in the overlying pigment epithelium might prove to be the exception to this rule (Fig. 3-8). The orange pigment clumps overlying the surface of melanomas appear hypofluorescent during the early phases of angiography, and they often become enveloped in fluorescein during the later phases of angiography (Figs. 3-2, 3-4, and 3-5). The angiographic demonstration of large blood vessels within a small pigmented choroidal tumor occurs infrequently (Fig. 3-7) but is evidence that the lesion is probably a melanoma rather than a nevus. The irregular pattern of these large vessels in melanomas should be differentiated from the cartwheel- or seafan-shaped subpigment epithelial neovascular membranes, which occur more commonly over nevi than melanomas (see Chapter 2).

It is important to realize that any of the seven signs of an early melanoma listed above, with the exception of numbers four and five, may be present in a patient with serous retinal detachment secondary to a choroidal nevus (see Chapter 2). The diameter of the lesion as well as the presence of some elevation are not always reliable criteria to differentiate a nevus from a melanoma. Caution should be exercised in making a positive diagnosis of malignant melanoma in the presence of a slightly elevated tumor five disc diameters in size or smaller. With few exceptions, patients with such tumors should be followed at frequent intervals with fundus stereophotographs, fluorescein angiography, and visual fields to ascertain definite growth of the lesion prior to recommending enucleation. If the macular detachment persists and the choroidal lesion remains unchanged, low to moderate intensity photocoagulation may be applied to the areas of fluorescein leakage to obtain resolution of the subretinal fluid (Fig. 3-2). Only the leaking areas should be treated and no attempt should be made to destroy the tumor. At each follow-up visit, it is essential to review the previous photographs and visual fields to avoid missing evidence of further growth.

Later development and variations in growth pattern. An expanding choroidal melanoma causes widespread destruction of the overlying pigment epithelium and the outer retinal layers, which histologically appear to melt away (Fig. 3-3, *E*). The retina is often separated from the tumor surface by a layer of either clear or light gray exudate. In slowly growing melanomas a gray or partly pigmented plaque of proliferated and metaplastic pigment epithelium may develop between the tumor and the retina. There is frequently serous detachment of the surrounding retina. Clear subretinal exudate may extend inferiorly and be in continuity with an area of bullous retinal detachment. The subretinal fluid usually shifts freely with the positioning of the patient. As greater areas of pigment epithelium are destroyed by the tumor, angiography shows larger and more widespread areas of diffusion of dye from the tumor surface into the subretinal space (Figs. 3-3, 3-9, and 3-10).

Extensive cystoid retinal degeneration and edema occur less frequently overlying choroidal melanomas (Fig. 3-4) than over choroidal hemangiomas. When they occur, they are probably indicative of a more slowly growing melanoma. Cystoid retinal changes are usually visible biomicroscopically and are evident angiographically as a multiloculated fluorescent pattern seen during the late stages of angiography (Fig. 3-4). Angiographic evidence of alteration of the retinal vascular permeability overlying the melanoma may occasionally be demonstrated (Figs. 3-9 and 3-16).

As a melanoma grows, large blood vessels in the tumor near its anterior surface may become visible, particularly if the tumor is relatively hypopigmented (Figs. 3-6, 3-7, 3-10, and 3-11). They are often more apparent angiographically than ophthalmoscopically. These blood vessels may be confused with normal choroidal blood vessels. Although they are frequently visible in large hypopigmented choroidal melanomas, they may also occur in choroidal hemangiomas, a variety of organized disciform lesions, and less often in metastatic tumors to the choroid (Fig. 5-5).

Inward growth of a melanoma stretches, attenuates, and may finally invade and break through the overlying Bruch's membrane in one or more focal areas (Figs. 3-6 and 3-11 to 3-15). This often occurs near the center of the lesion. As the subretinal portion of the tumor grows, a mushroom configuration results. Angiographically the portion of the tumor that has broken through Bruch's membrane typically appears relatively hypofluorescent because the head of the pigmented tumor is pressed against the posterior surface of the detached retina and there may be little extracellular exudate available for pooling of the dye. This area is in contrast to the heavily stained subretinal exudate surrounding the neck of the tumor (Fig. 3-11). This contrast is less if the subretinal portion of the tumor is amelanotic (Fig. 3-12).

The tumor may invade and may even perforate the overlying retina (Figs. 3-13 to 3-15). Sites of tumor invasion into the retina usually appear hypofluorescent angiographically because of the relative absence of exudate in these areas as compared to the surrounding areas where subretinal exudate is present (Fig. 3-15). Melanomas that have extended through the retina present as a smooth-surfaced, domelike mass (Figs. 3-13, and 3-14, *A*) or as an irregularly surfaced cauliflower mass (Fig. 3-14, *F*) in the vitreous. In either case they appear relatively hypofluorescent because dye diffusing from the anterior surface of the tumor spreads into the vitreous in concentrations that are relatively low in contrast to the dye trapped in the subretinal space around the base of the lesion (Figs. 3-13 to 3-15).

The blood vessels within that portion of a melanoma that has either extended through Bruch's membrane into the subretinal space or through the retina into the vitreous are often dilated. This dilatation has been attributed to the constricting effect of Bruch's membrane around the tumor neck. These blood vessels are usually visible ophthalmoscopically in hypopigmented tumors (Figs. 3-6 and 3-12), but they may be hidden from view in the more highly pigmented melanomas. In the latter case angiography may detect those vessels near the tumor surface. This detection may be important in differentiating a deeply pigmented melanoma from a mound of blood (Figs. 3-13 and 3-14).

Choroidal melanomas may occasionally be the cause of subretinal bleeding either from the choriocapillaris overlying the tumor or as is more frequently the case, from the blood vessels on the surface of the tumor that has replaced the choriocapillaris (Fig. 3-11). Melanomas that have invaded the overlying retina may be responsible for bleeding into the retina or vitreous (Figs. 3-13 and 3-14). Hemorrhage secondary to melanomas is most likely to occur when the tumor arises near the posterior pole of the eye. Although a good general rule is that small mass lesions in the posterior pole associated with hemorrhage are probably not malignant melanomas, one must remember that the presence of bleeding does not exclude the diagnosis of a melanoma. Examination of the macular region of the opposite eye is most important in ruling out the ordinary causes of hemorrhagic disciform detachments in such cases. Fluorescein angiography is often helpful in differentiating the various stages of serous and hemorrhagic disciform detachment of the pigment epithelium and retina from a choroidal melanoma. (see Chapter 7).

As choroidal and ciliary body melanomas become very large, they may outgrow their blood supply. The necrosis that results is often associated with secondary intraocular inflammation. The patient may present with a clinical picture simulating that of severe uveitis or infectious endophthalmitis. Focal areas of tumor atrophy and scarring presumably caused by spontaneous tumor necrosis may occur in smaller melanomas, and this may be unassociated with any evidence of intraocular inflammation. Ophthalmoscopically these focal areas are manifest as depressed gray-white areas within the tumor (Fig. 3-16).

Extraocular spread of malignant melanoma of the uveal tract occurs primarily by the intravascular route. It may, however, spread outside the eye directly by way of scleral channels containing the ciliary arteries, ciliary nerves, and the vortex veins. In general, direct extrascleral extension of a choroidal melanoma occurs primarily in the larger, more malignant cell tumors. The incidence of extrascleral extension is also high in diffusely infiltrating, slightly elevated choroidal melanomas. Rarely, extrascleral extension occurs from a relatively small choroidal melanoma (Fig. 3-17). The optic nerve head is relatively resistent to invasion by a choroidal melanoma. Noticeable distortion and displacement of the optic nerve head by a peripapillary choroidal melanoma may cause the false ophthalmoscopic impression that the optic nerve head has been invaded (Figs. 3-4, 3-8, and 3-18). Rarely a melanoma may invade the optic nerve head and extend into the meninges (Fig. 3-17).

Rapidly growing malignant melanomas of the choroid may occasionally displace the neighboring choroid, pigment epithelium, and retina laterally and produce linear chorioretinal folds (Fig. 3-19). The early phases of angiography shows a characteristic pattern of alternate hyperfluorescent and hypofluorescent bands in such cases. Similar chorioretinal folds may occur adjacent to other subretinal masses caused by scleral buckling for a retinal detachment, granulomatous scleritis (Fig. 7-11), and a retrobulbar tumor.

Differential diagnosis. Lesions that may be mistaken for malignant melanoma of the choroid include metastatic carcinoma (Chapter 5), hemangioma of the choroid (Chapter 4), choroidal nevi (Chapter 2), melanocytomas of the optic disc (Chapter 2), serous and hemorrhagic disciform detachment of the pigment epithelium and retina (Chapter 7), pigment epithelial and retinal hamartomas (Chapter 8), serous retinal detachment secondary to choroiditis and scleritis (Chapter 7), rhegmatogenous retinal detachment (Chapter 7), retinoschisis (Chapter 7), serous detachment of the choroid and ciliary body (Chapter 7), organized exudative detachment secondary to retinal vascular disease (Chapter 9), and exophytic capillary angioma of the retina (Chapter 10).

MALIGNANT MELANOMA OF THE CILIARY BODY

Malignant melanoma of the ciliary body often involves to some degree either the choroid or the iris or both. Ciliary body melanomas are less common than choroidal melanomas but are more common that iris melanomas. Because of their location, they are often large when first discovered. They frequently are globular in shape (Fig. 3-20) and have a relatively smooth inner surface. In some cases, however, their surface may be quite irregular (Fig. 3-21). They are often discovered on routine ophthalmoscopic examination. Retinal detachment occurs late and usually only after the lesion has extended posteriorly to involve the choroid. Patients with anterior extension of the tumor may present with blurred vision secondary to lens distortion and cataract, heterochromia of the iris, pigmented or non-pigmented iris masses, ocular pain, iridocyclitis, redness, and glaucoma. The tumor may diffusely involve the pars plicata for 360°. These tumors, referred to as ring melanomas, are usually minimally elevated and are often associated with glaucoma and evidence of iridocyclitis. Ciliary body melanomas may extend through the anterior emissary scleral canals and simulate a conjunctival melanoma. There may be dilatation of the episcleral and conjunctival vessels overlying the melanoma. Transillumination may be helpful in identifying the presence and extent of a pigmented ciliary body melanoma. It is particularly useful in differentiating it from a serous detachment of the ciliary body and choroid and from an intercalary staphyloma. Biomicroscopy with and without a three-mirror fundus lens is important in differentiating ciliary body melanomas from other nonsolid tumors. The presence of degeneration and destruction of the overlying ciliary epithelium, the presence of pigment beneath the surface of the tumor, and the presence of blood vessels within the tumor are biomicroscopic findings suggesting a ciliary body melanoma (Fig. 3-20). Fluorescein angiography may be helpful in identifying blood vessels near the tumor surface. A prominent fluorescent vitreous haze often develops along the vitreous surface of a ciliary body melanoma (Figs. 3-20 and 3-21). This finding differentiates it from a cyst of the ciliary epithelium. Radioactive phosphorus studies are helpful in distinguishing melanoma of the ciliary body from nonsolid masses but are of less value in distinguishing these tumors from other solid cellular tumors of the ciliary body.

Some of the lesions that should be considered in the differential diagnosis of a ciliary body melanoma include ciliary body nevus, pseudoadenomatous hyperplasia of the ciliary epithelium, cysts of the ciliary epithelium, medulloepitheliomas, metastatic carcinoma, leukemia, reactive lymphoid hyperplasia, sarcoidosis, and rheumatoid scleral uveitis.

IRIS MELANOMAS (See Chapter 15)

AIDS TO DIAGNOSIS OF MALIGNANT MELANOMAS OF THE CHOROID AND CILIARY BODY

The binocular indirect ophthalmoscope is the most important single aid to accurate diagnosis of intraocular tumors. The wide field of view, the stereopsis, and the bright illumination possible with this instrument make it far superior to the direct ophthalmoscope for determining gross anatomic relationships, in differentiating solid from nonsolid tumors, and in detecting fine color differences that may be critical to accurate diagnosis. The ophthalmoscopic findings, whether obtained by the indirect or direct method, should always be supplemented by those provided by the stereoscopic and magnified view of the tumor with the binocular slit-lamp. The clinical history together with the opthalmoscopic and biomicroscopic findings should provide the primary basis for diagnosis.

Other special techniques of examination, such as transillumination, radioactive phosphorus–uptake studies, fluorescein angiography, and ultrasonography may provide additional information, but the findings of these examinations should be used cautiously and only as a means of confirming those made with the ophthalmoscope and slit-lamp. If the latter findings are inconclusive in an eye with potential useful vision, the clinician should choose a conservative course of patient management rather than relying on the results of one or several special tests to make a diagnosis that requires radical treatment.

Transillumination is of particular value in confirming the presence of pigmented tumors of the choroid and ciliary body. It is done best in a completely darkened room after topical application of an anesthetic. The effect of lesions on transcleral transillumination applied to the site of the lesion may be studied indirectly by looking for defects in the normal red pupillary reflex or directly by transpupillary viewing of the lesion. Another technique of detection of anterior lesions involves the use of either transcleral or transpupillary illumination of the inside of the eye while one observes the outer wall of the eye. In patients with average pigmentation, a darkened band corresponding with the ciliary body is normally present. This defect in scleral transillumination is less posteriorly in the region of the pars plana than it is anteriorly in the region of the pars plicata. Pigmented lesions that extend into the pars plana or posteriorly will be outlined as a defect in transillumination. Dark areas beneath the bulbar conjunctiva attributable to focal scleral ectasis or intercalary staphyloma may simulate extrascleral extension of a ciliary body melanoma. The former transilluminate, the latter does not. Serous detachment of the choroid and ciliary body and serous detachment of the pigment epithelium may be mistaken for solid pigmented tumors of the choroid and ciliary body. Unlike the latter, however, they transilluminate vividly. Although it is not possible to directly transilluminate masses in the postequatorial portion of the fundus outside the operating room, it is possible to view them in retroillumination. The transilluminator is placed as far posteriorly as possible on the sclera while the tumor is observed through the unlighted ophthalmoscope. If the mass contains melanin or blood, it appears as a dark area surrounded by a halo of light at its margin. Nonpigmented tumors, whether solid or cystic, are relatively inapparent when viewed by retroillumination. Transillumination and retroillumination are of limited value in differentiating pigmented melanomas from (1) lesions containing blood, (2) lesions containing proliferated pigment epithelium, and (3) heavily pigmented pigment epithelial cysts. They are also of no value in differentiating the various types of nonpigmented lesions.

There has been a recent revival of interest in the radioactive phosphorus–uptake test as a means of diagnosing malignant melanomas. Precise placement of the probe over the center of the tumor utilizing indirect ophthalmoscopy is essential for accurate readings. The test has a number of limitations that require that it be used only as a confirmatory test to verify clinical observations. Although there is good correlation between a positive test and a histopathologic diagnosis of melanoma, some false-positive and false-negative results do occur. Since the test usually requires introduction of a probe into the orbit, relatively few nonmalignant lesions have been examined in comparison to the large number of patients with obvious melanomas. The test cannot differentiate a melanoma from other neoplastic tumors and at least in some cases from inflammatory cell masses. There is no evidence that it can differentiate a rapidly growing epithelioid cell melanoma from a very slow growing spindle A melanoma. Despite its limitations, it may provide valuable information in some patients with atypical lesions (Fig. 3-6). Further investigation in its use is indicated now that improved equipment and techniques are available.

Ultrasonography is a relatively new technique valuable in detecting and differentiating solid intraocular masses from nonsolid masses. It is of particular value in eyes where the fundus is not clearly visible. Its value in differentiating melanomas from other solid tumors has not been clearly established.

Surgical biopsy of intraocular tumors is technically possible but is not recommended because of the danger of extraocular spread should the tumor prove to be a melanoma.

TREATMENT OF CHOROIDAL AND CILIARY BODY MELANOMAS

Prior to proceeding with therapy of an intraocular melanoma the patient should have a thorough general medical history and physical examination. The patient should have routine blood counts, urinalysis, a test for urine melanin, and a chest x-ray examination. A liver scan may also be helpful in detecting evidence of liver metastases.

The standard treatment for malignant melanomas of the choroid and ciliary body is enucleation of the eye. No other form of treatment guarantees the eradication of the primary tumor. Although spread of a melanoma by way of the optic nerve is rare, a good portion of the optic nerve should be included with the enucleation. A careful search for evidence of extraocular extensions should be made at the time of enucleation. If there is any evidence of a tumor remaining in the orbit, additional orbital tissue should be removed at that time and a subsequent orbital exenteration may be advisable. More conservative means of therapy, including x-ray irradiation, chemotherapy, photocoagulation, diathermy, cryotherapy, and simple observation may be employed in the following special circumstances: (1) the melanoma involves the only eye with useful vision, (2) the patient's age and general health are such that the risks of conservative management are justified, or (3) there is some doubt concerning the correct diagnosis. In the last case observation and occasional use of photocoagulation treatment to eradicate serous detachment of the macula are preferable to all other means of treatment. High dosages of x-ray irradiation therapy delivered by means of episcleral cobalt applicators may successfully destroy or retard growth of a small malignant melanoma of the choroid in some patients. In other patients, this therapy has little or no effect on the tumor (Fig. 3-15). The use of episcleral cobalt therapy should be considered only in patients with melanomas that are less than 12 to 13 millimeters in diameter at their base, that are confined to an area of at least four to six disc diameters from either the optic disc or macula, and that do not extend anterior to the posterior half of the pars plana. Secondary retinal vascular exudative and proliferative changes are major complications that may arise in patients treated with x-ray irradiation therapy.

Photocoagulation, cryotherapy, diathermy, and local excision of choroidal and ciliary body melanomas are of questionable value in eradicating truly malignant melanomas.

Large tumors of the peripheral choroid and ciliary body discovered on routine examination of an eye with normal visual acuity and in the absence of retinal detachment may in some cases be extremely slow growing tumors. In elderly patients or in patients with serious medical diseases it may be prudent to follow them at frequent intervals rather than resorting to enucleation.

Fig. 3-1. Cytologic classification of malignant melanomas of the uveal tract.

A, Spindle A melanoma. Many of the cells show a chromatin stripe extending the length of the nucleus. Note the absence of nucleoli.

B, Spindle B melanoma. Note the nucleoli present within the plump spindle cells.

C, Fascicular melanoma. This low-power photomicrograph reveals the palisade arrangement of nuclei that is characteristic of this type of tumor composed primarily of spindle B and lesser numbers of spindle A cells.

D, Epithelioid cell melanoma. The oval-round and polygonal cells of varying sizes have large nuclei with prominent nucleoli.

E, Epithelioid cell melanoma showing many giant cells some of which are multinucleated.

F, Lipoidal degeneration in malignant melanomas. Note the nests of balloon cells present in this mixed cell type of melanoma.

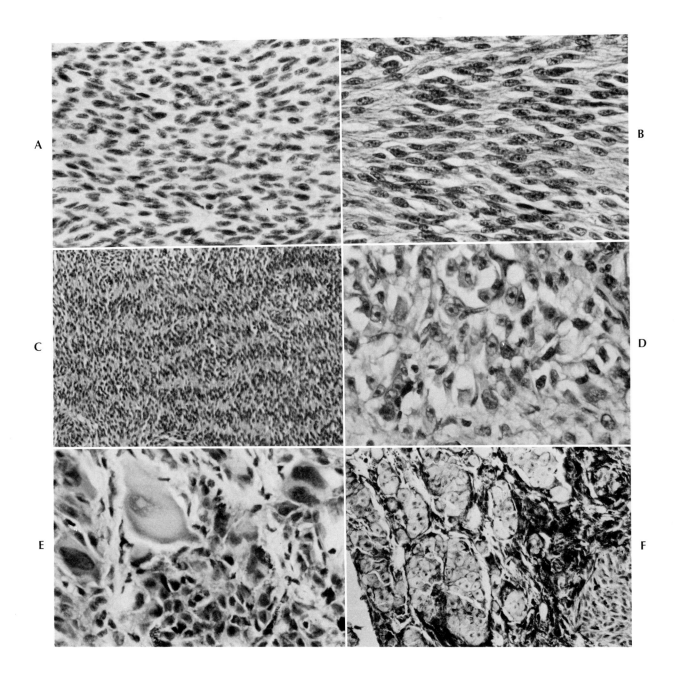

69

Fig. 3-2. Growth of a small choroidal malignant melanoma: A 75-year-old white man was first examined on October 22, 1969, because of a 1-month history of blurred vision in his right eye; 2½ years previously a small choroidal nevus was noted in the right eye; visual acuity in the right eye was 20/50 and in the left eye was 20/20.

A, A relatively small elevated two-by-three-disc-diameter-size pigmented lesion lies just superior to the macula and is associated with a serous retinal detachment extending into the macular area. Note the small yellowish drusen (*1*) near the superior margin of the tumor and the irregular deposition of finely granular orange pigment (*2*) overlying the tumor surface. Some of the pigment granules lie within the substance of the retina. The color of the pigment is identical to the orange color of the normal pigment epithelium surrounding the tumor. The degree of elevation of the lesion and the amount of overlying orange pigment are features that suggest that this lesion is indeed an early malignant melanoma arising in a choroidal nevus.

B, *Arrows* indicate serous retinal detachment extending into the macular area.

C, Early angiogram reveals multiple pinpoint areas of intense fluorescence and early diffusion of the dye from the surface of the tumor. A less intense mottled fluorescence is caused by loss of pigment from the pigment epithelium. Note that the orange pigment appears hypofluorescent.

D, Late angiogram reveals evidence of staining of the thin layer of subretinal exudate overlying the central portion of the tumor. Note the orange pigment is enveloped by the subretinal dye. The amount of dye diffusing into the subretinal exudate inferior to the tumor is inadequate in this patient to make it appear fluorescent. The multiple punctate areas of staining over the periphery of this tumor superficially resembling that seen in drusen overlying a nevus are unrelated to the presence of drusen (compare with **A**) and is a feature seen more commonly over malignant melanomas. The punctate dots of staining are presumably related to multiple small localized areas of damage to the retinal pigment epithelium by the underlying tumor.

E, The initial clinical impression was a probably early choroidal melanoma, but because the lesion had been present for 2½ years and because of the small size of the lesion the patient was followed. On October 22, 1969, xenon photocoagulation was used to treat the surface of the lesion. The subretinal fluid cleared and the vision improved to 20/25 within several months.

F, The patient was followed at frequent intervals with photographs, and the lesion showed no definite evidence of growth until he returned on November 23, 1970. The tumor had enlarged greatly and the eye was enucleated. Histopathologically it was a spindle B melanoma of the choroid.

(**A** to **E** from Gass.[2])

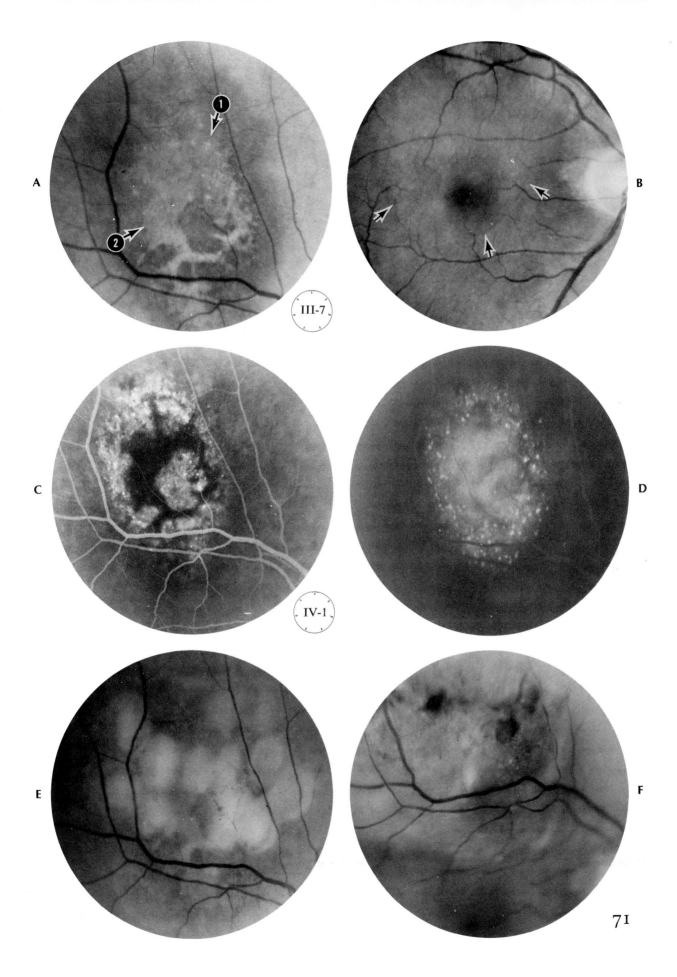

III-7

IV-1

71

Fig. 3-3. Slightly elevated highly pigmented choroidal melanoma causing circinate maculopathy. A 42-year-old white woman gave a 2-day history of poor vision in the left eye. Her vision was 20/70. She had a central scotoma. Because of the relatively small size of the lesion, a number of consultants recommended that she be followed.

A and **B,** Slightly elevated black choroidal melanoma surrounded the lower half of the optic disc and extended into the central macular area. Note the macular star.

C, Early angiography revealed abnormal hyperfluorescence secondary to damage to the retinal pigment epithelium. Note that the temporal and inferior edge of the hyperfluorescent area does not extend as far as the margin of the tumor. Compare with **A** and **B**. See **E** for histopathologic condition of the region indicated by the letter x, and see **F** for the region indicated by letter y.

D, There was staining of the subretinal exudate over the central portions of the tumor (*black arrows*). *Black and white arrows* indicate the inferior margin of the tumor.

E, The eye was enucleated and revealed a malignant melanoma. This section was taken from an area corresponding with the hyperfluorescence in the nasal periphery of the macula (see x in **C**). Note the destructive changes in the pigment epithelium and the outer retinal cells and the underlying thin layer of subretinal eosinophilic exudate, which stained during the course of angiography.

F, Histopathologic condition of the tumor in the macula where the tumor did not fluoresce (see y in **C**). Note that the pigment epithelium and retina are intact.

(**A** to **D** from Norton[3]; **E** and **F** from Gass.[4])

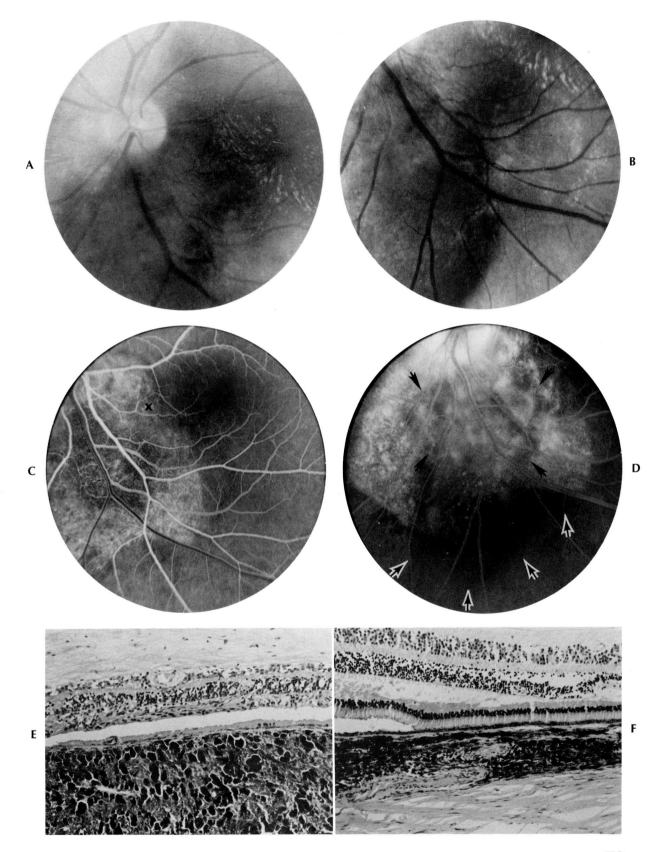

Fig. 3-4. Slowly growing choroidal melanoma. A 55-year-old white female nurse was aware of some disturbance of her central vision in the right eye 6 years before she was initially examined. Her vision in the right eye was 20/70 and in the left eye was 20/20.

A, A relatively small pigmented choroidal tumor associated with serous macular detachment and numerous patches of orange pigment (*arrows*) was present at the superotemporal margin of the optic disc in the right eye.

B and **C,** Angiograms revealed irregular fluorescence caused by loss of pigment from the pigment epithelium and multiple pinpoint areas of dye leakage from the surface of the tumor. Note that the areas of orange pigment appeared hypofluorescent (*arrows*). The presence of the orange pigment and the finding of multiple pinpoint dots of fluorescein staining unrelated to drusen suggested that this lesion was probably a malignant melanoma. Because of the relatively small size of the lesion and the history of decreased vision of 6-year duration, the patient was followed at frequent intervals. When she returned 11 months after her original examination, there was some photographic evidence of slight increase in the size of the lesion.

D, When she returned 19 months after initial examination, however, the tumor had definitely enlarged and appeared to be encroaching upon the optic nerve head.

E, A late angiogram showed diffused staining of the subretinal exudate and a multiloculated pattern of staining (*arrow*) indicative of cystoid edema or degeneration, or both, of the retina overlying the tumor.

F, The right eye was enucleated and histopathologic examination revealed polycystic degenerative changes of the retina overlying a malignant melanoma, spindle A and spindle B types, which had extensively damaged the pigment epithelium but had not invaded the optic nerve head despite the clinical appearance of the lesion depicted in **B**. She was alive and well 8 years later.

74

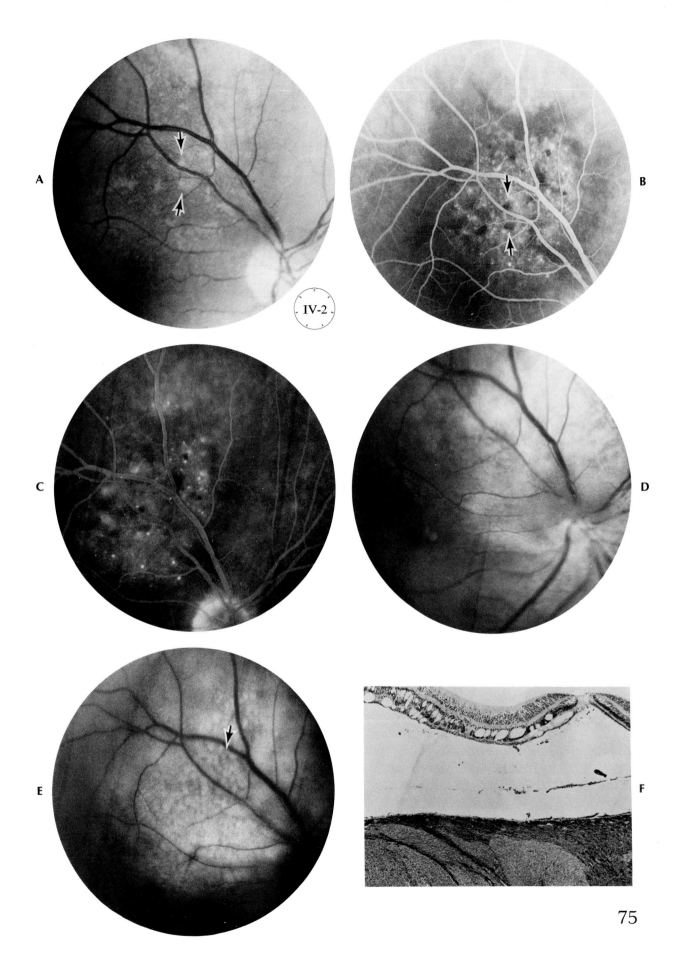

Fig. 3-5. Serous detachment of the pigment epithelium overlying a choroidal melanoma. A 70-year-old white woman complained of defective vision first discovered in her left eye in November 1966. The fundus was not examined at that time. When she was seen 1 year later, visual acuity in the left eye was measured at 20/80 and at that time a pigmented tumor was noted. By January 16, 1968, the visual acuity in the left eye had decreased to 20/300.

A, A well-circumscribed, pigmented tumor was present in the left macular area. The feathery edges of the lesion, the presence of orange pigment patches, and the absence of a rim of blood at the margins of the lesion were important features that clearly differentiated this lesion from a submacular hematoma. There was a localized serous detachment of the overlying pigment epithelium *(arrows)* and a rim of subretinal exudate surrounding it. The dome shape of this lesion served to differentiate it from a localized collar-button herniation of tumor through a break in Bruch's membrane.

B and **C,** Angiography revealed early fluorescein staining of the subretinal pigment epithelial exudate *(arrows),* pinpoint foci of dye leakage, and hypofluorescence in the region of the orange pigment.

D, Late angiogram.

E, The eye was enucleated on February 19, 1968. Note the focal area of pigment epithelial detachment *(black arrows),* and clumps of pigment cells *(black and white arrows)* in the subretinal space overlying a spindle B choroidal melanoma.

F, High-power view of clumps of pigment-laden cells either pigment epithelial cells or macrophages, which correspond to the orange pigment clumps noted in **A**.

(**A** to **C** and **E** to **F** from Gass.[5])

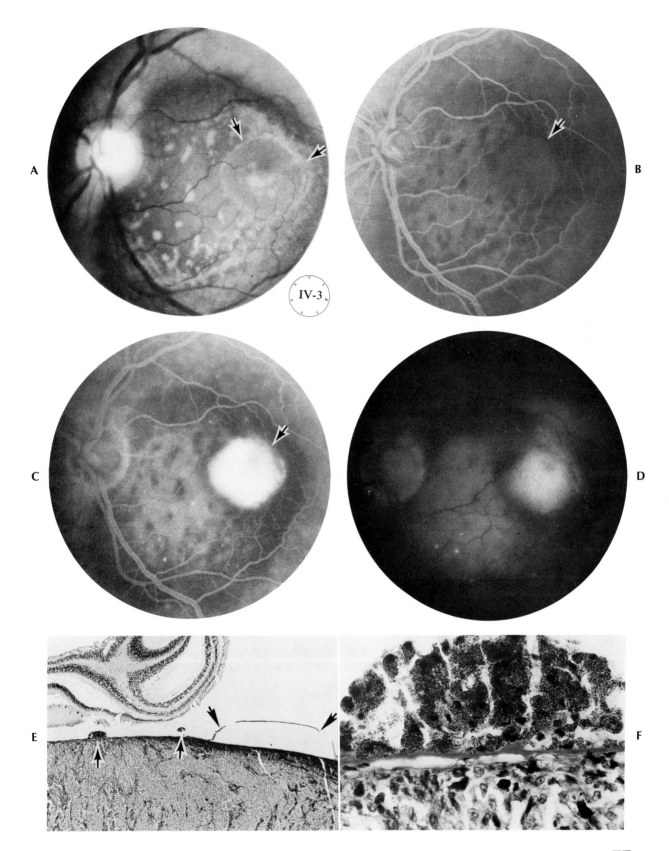

Fig. 3-6. Unusual choroidal melanoma simulating an exudative detachment of the pigment epithelium in a teen-ager. A healthy 14-year-old white girl was asymptomatic until March 1973, when she noted blurred vision in the left eye. Her local ophthalmologist found a lesion in the left macula. One year previously an examination by the same physician was normal. She was referred to another ophthalmologist for evaluation. Her visual acuity in the right eye was 20/20 and in the left eye was 20/50.

A, Ophthalmoscopic examination of the left eye in June 1973 revealed a well-defined smooth oval subretinal mass in the left macular area. The margins of the tumor were pigmented and there was a dark-gray figure covering the nonpigmented portion of the lesion. The right fundus was normal.

B and **C,** Fluorescein angiography revealed prominent hyperfluorescence corresponding with the nonpigmented portions of the tumor during the arterial phase of angiography. Except for the development of multiple small pinpoint areas of fluorescence, the pattern of fluorescence remained constant for 2 minutes after dye injection. Unfortunately no later photographs were recorded. Prompt appearance of fluorescence in the arterial phase and the failure of the pattern of fluorescence to change during the brief course of angiography were findings atypical for a melanoma. Multiple pinpoint areas of intense fluorescence were compatible with an early melanoma. The angiographic findings and the presence of the overlying pigment figure suggested the possibility of an unusual exudative detachment of the pigment epithelium. The high intensity of the fluorescence in the arterial phase, however, was atypical for a serous detachment of the pigment epithelium. A radioactive phosphorus (P-32) uptake test was positive. The patient was followed, however, because of the atypical appearance of the lesion, its small size, and the age of the patient. In November 1973, the lesion was unchanged. A repeat P-32 test was strongly positive. The patient was referred to the Bascom Palmer Eye Institute on December 27, 1973. The patient's visual acuity in the left eye was 20/50.

D, Ophthalmoscopic examination revealed no change in the diameter of the lesion but there was evidence of a well-defined nodular area of highly vascularized amelanotic tumor that appeared to have broken through Bruch's membrane (*arrows*).

E, Fluorescein angiography confirmed the vascularity of the tumor and showed many pinpoint areas of intense fluorescence and staining during the later phases of angiography. On January 7, 1974, the eye was enucleated.

F, Histopathologic examination revealed a hypopigmented spindle A and spindle B malignant melanoma of the choroid with extension through Bruch's membrane. The dark pigment figure in the tumor surface was caused by clumping of pigment laden cells (*arrow*) identical to that depicted in Figs. 3-5, *F,* and 3-17, *E.* This case illustrates that even small melanomas in the macular area may yield a positive P-32 test when it is properly performed. It further illustrates the problems which may arise in the interpretation of fluorescein angiography, particularly when an incomplete study is done.

(Courtesy Dr. W. Hagler, Atlanta, Ga.)

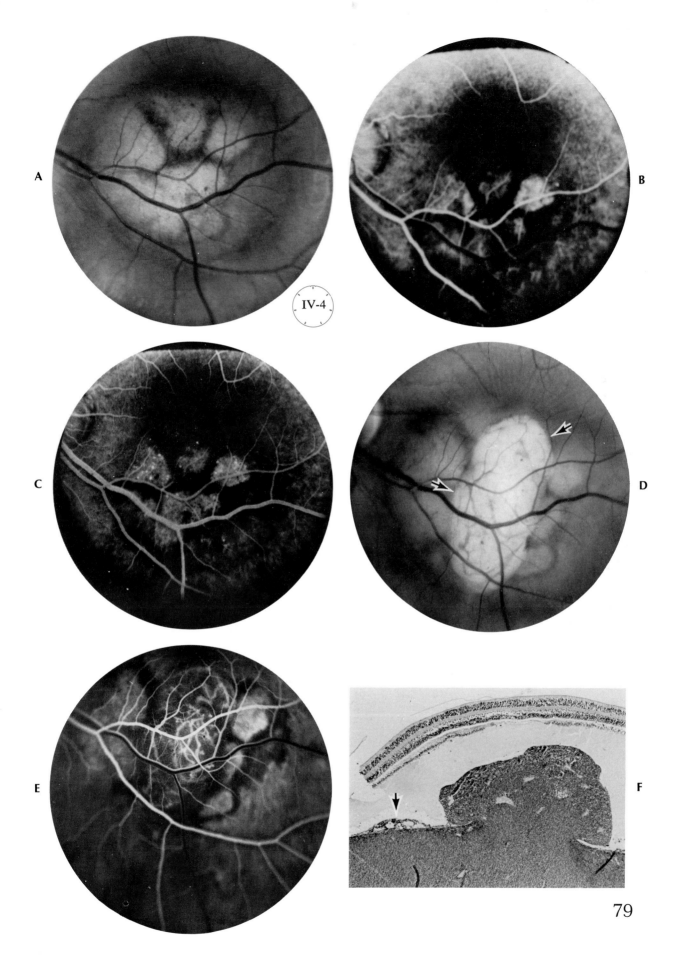

Fig. 3-7. Rapid growth of a small malignant melanoma. A 51-year-old white woman presented with a 2-month history of photopsia in the temporal field of vision in her right eye. Her visual acuity was 20/25 in both eyes.

A, Funduscopic examination of the right eye revealed a four-disc-diameter-size elevated pigmented tumor of the choroid near the nasal margin of the optic disc. Granular flecks of orange pigment were scattered on its surface. Note the orange pigment ring *(black arrow)*. A fine vascular network was visible beneath the retina over the central portion of the tumor. Irregular deposits of yellow exudate *(black and white arrows)* were present near this vascular network. There was no retinal detachment. An absolute field defect corresponding with the tumor was present.

B, Early angiography revealed the presence of a subretinal network of blood vessels *(arrows)* near the surface of the choroidal tumor.

C, Fluorescein angiography showed the development of multiple pinpoint areas of fluorescein staining. Note that the orange pigment appears hypofluorescent and the blood vessels near the tumor surface are no longer visible.

D, One-hour angiogram showing diffuse staining of the surface of the tumor. The history of recent onset of photopsia, the absolute visual field defect, the presence of large amounts of orange pigment on the tumor surface, and the angiographic findings of blood vessels within the pigmented tumor and multiple pinpoint areas of intense staining were all features suggesting that this was a malignant melanoma and not a choroidal nevus. Because of the size of the lesion and the normal visual acuity, however, the patient was followed.

E, Six weeks later the tumor had enlarged. Note the increase in size of the pigmented ring *(arrow)* (compare with **A**).

F, The eye was enucleated. Histopathologic diagnosis was malignant melanoma of the choroid, mixed-cell type. Blood vessels *(arrows)* were present near the surface of the tumor. Clumps of pigment-laden macrophages were present beneath the retina.

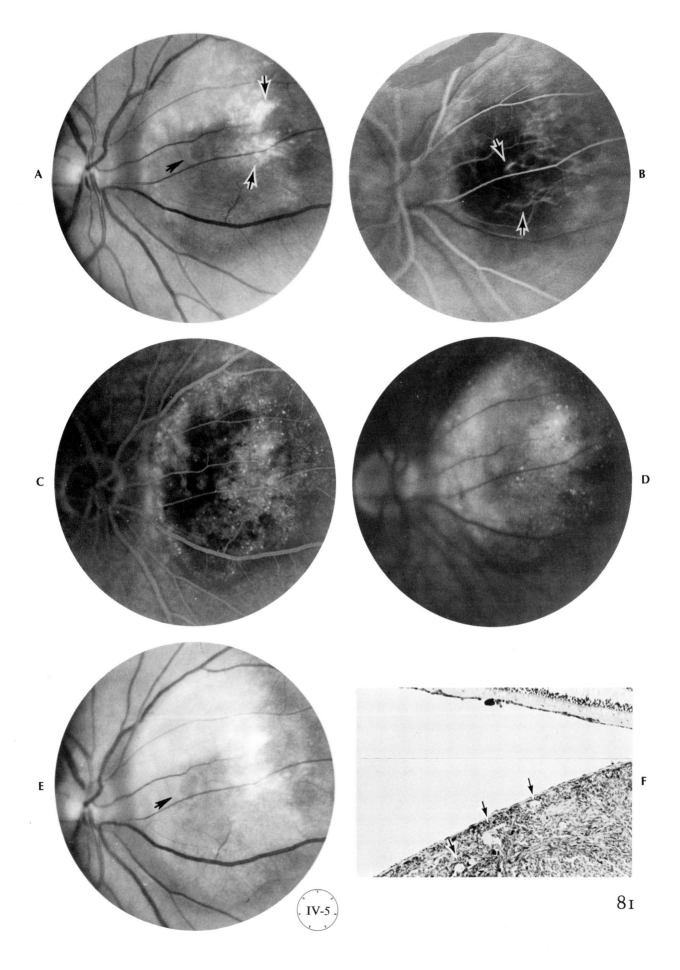

81

Fig. 3-8. Slightly elevated diffusely infiltrating choroidal melanoma simulating angiographically a subretinal hemorrhage. A 66-year-old white man was seen initially on August 16, 1966, complaining of recent loss of vision in his right eye. He had been followed by his local physician since 1963. Annual examinations in 1963 and 1964 revealed no fundus abnormality. In 1965, a pigmented lesion was noted temporal to the right optic disc. A year later this had enlarged and the patient's vision had decreased from 20/60 to 20/100.

A, There was minimal evidence of subretinal exudation overlying a heavily pigmented melanoma that appeared to be infiltrating the temporal portion of the optic nerve head. There was shifting subretinal fluid in the far periphery inferiorly. The nerve head encroachment, the feathery edges of the lesion, and the absence of a red margin were important features differentiating this lesion from a hematoma beneath the pigment epithelium and retina.

B to **D,** Note the relative absence of early hyperfluorescence but late staining overlying this tumor. The appearance of the early phases of the angiogram was more suggestive of subretinal blood than a melanoma. Late staining, however, was atypical for subretinal or subpigment epithelial hematomas.

E, The patient developed further detachment of the retina and the eye was enucleated on October 25, 1966. Histopathologic examination revealed a diffuse spindle B malignant melanoma of the choroid that extended from the optic disc into the far periphery of the eye temporally. The inner aspect of the tumor was heavily pigmented, particularly in the macula and peripapillary region *(arrows),* but the bulk of the tumor was hypopigmented. At the time of enucleation the retina was detached over the entire posterior pole of the eye.

F, Note that the juxtapapillary melanoma compressed but did not invade the optic nerve head despite the clinical appearance in **A**.

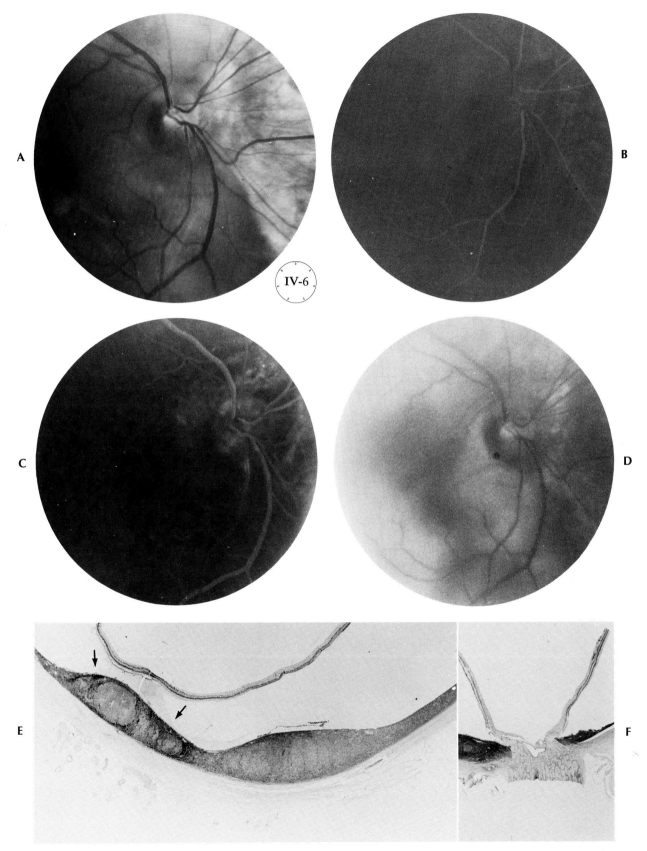

Fig. 3-9. Retinal vascular changes overlying a malignant melanoma of the choroid. A slightly pigmented choroidal tumor with overlying retinal degenerative changes was discovered in the peripheral fundus of a 28-year-old man who had normal visual acuity in each eye.

A, In the right eye, just nasal to the optic disc, there was a four-disc-diameter-size elevated hypopigmented tumor with exudative detachment and some cystoid changes of the overlying retina.

B and **C,** The early phases of angiography revealed dilated retinal capillaries and evidence of leakage of dye from these capillaries overlying the tumor *(arrows)*. Note the extensive early hyperfluorescence over much of the tumor and the hypofluorescent geographic area over the central portion of the tumor.

D, Late angiogram revealed extensive staining of the subretinal exudate and some evidence of cystoid retinal edema *(arrow)*.

E, The eye was enucleated and histopathologic examination revealed a choroidal melanoma of the spindle cell B type. A large retinal cyst *(arrow)* was present.

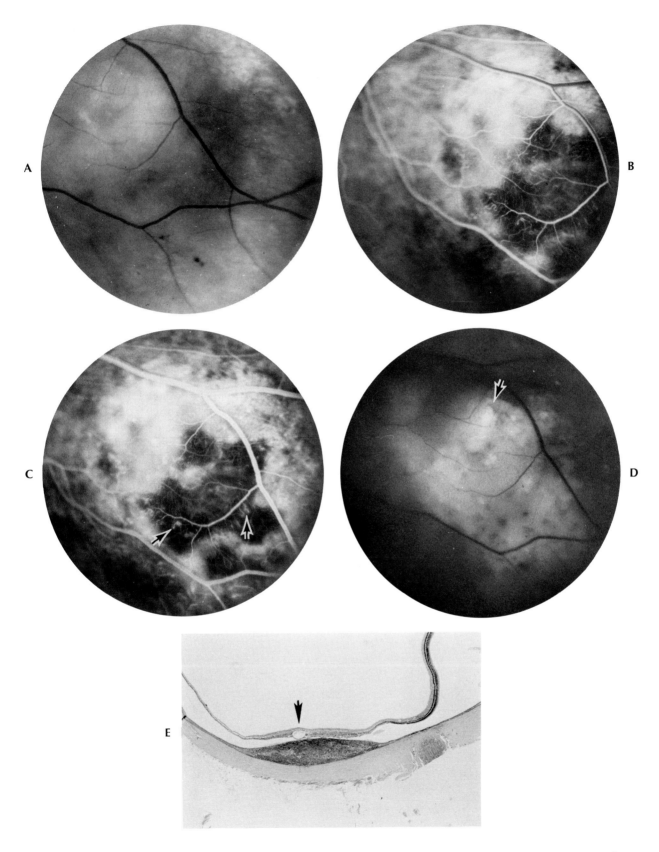

Fig. 3-10. Choroidal melanoma simulating clinically and angiographically a choroidal hemangioma in a teen-aged patient. This 17-year-old white girl developed infectious mononucleosis in 1966. At that time she noted slight blurring of vision in her right eye. She was examined by her local ophthalmologist in September 1966. A six-disc-diameter-size elevated lesion involving the choroid was noted superiorly. This was interpreted as an inflammatory lesion. A uveitis survey was negative. Fluorescein angiography showed several areas of leakage and these were treated lightly with photocoagulation on March 15, 1967. The vision in the right eye deteriorated to 20/70. On July 17, 1967, she was first seen at the Bascom Palmer Eye Institute. Her vision in the right eye was 20/70.

A, There was a slightly elevated hypopigmented, seven-to-eight-disc-diameter-size choroidal tumor associated with some serous detachment of the overlying retina. Note the areas of circinate retinopathy and the gray areas in the otherwise orange color tumor. Comparison of these photographs with those made by her local physician prior to photocoagulation revealed no significant change in its appearance except for the focal areas of hyperpigmentation *(arrows),* which are believed to be secondary to the photocoagulation.

B, The prearterial phase angiogram revealed within the tumor, vascular channels that filled with dye before perfusion of the retinal circulation. This is an angiographic feature typical of a choroidal hemangioma but not pathognomonic.

C, Arteriovenous phase showing a mottled pattern of fluorescence.

D, One-hour angiogram revealed a faint diffuse staining of the subretinal exudate and a multiloculated pattern of more intense staining *(arrows)* indicative of cystoid retinal edema or degeneration, or both. The orange color, the early perfusion of the blood vessels within the tumor, and the angiographic evidence of cystoid edema and degeneration overlying the tumor were features that suggested the diagnosis of hemangioma of the choroid. The patient was followed and showed no change over a period of several years.

E, By January 1970, the lesion appeared to be larger. P-32 uptake studies were positive and the eye was enucleated. Histopathologic examination revealed a spindle A melanoma.

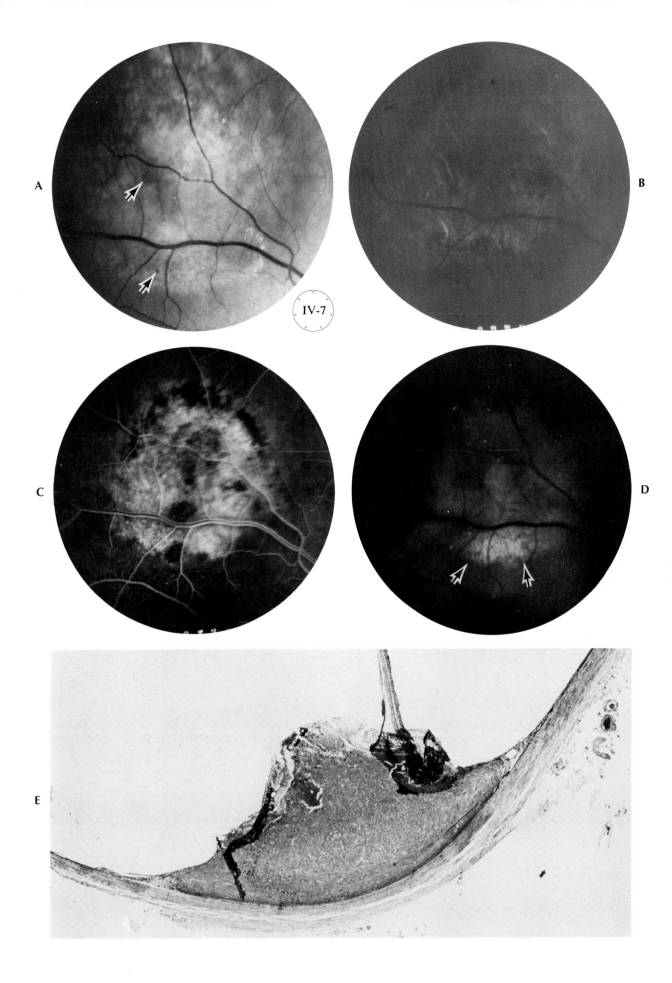

Fig. 3-11. Rapid growth of a choroidal melanoma through a break in Bruch's membrane. A 72-year-old white man was seen on November 4, 1966, complaining of recent loss of vision in his left eye. A large choroidal melanoma was present. Enucleation was advised. The patient was reluctant to submit to surgery and he was followed for a period of 11 days during which time the tumor exhibited growth through a break in Bruch's membrane.

A, November 4, 1966. There was a serous retinal detachment overlying a choroidal melanoma. Note the orange pigment patches over the superior surface of the tumor. *Arrow* indicates the site of future tumor break through Bruch's membrane.

B and **C,** Angiography reveals staining of the subretinal exudate.

D, November 8, 1966. A small amount of subretinal blood *(arrow)* was present at the site of early tumor break through Bruch's membrane.

E and **F,** Angiography revealed evidence of the subretinal blood.

G, November 15, 1966. A large tumor nodule *(arrows)* has extended through Bruch's membrane and was against the posterior surface of the retina. Note the subretinal blood and serous exudate surrounding the collar-button tumor.

H and **I,** Angiography reveals staining of the exudate surrounding the tumor as well as a few pockets of subretinal serous fluid overlying the tumor nodule *(arrows)*.

J, The eye was enucleated on November 16, 1966, and histopathologic examination confirmed the presence of a tumor nodule breaking through Bruch's membrane *(arrows)*.

K, High-power view showing breaks in Bruch's membrane *(arrows)* and serosanguinous subretinal exudate surrounding the margin of the subretinal tumor nodule. The pathologic diagnosis was mixed-cell type of malignant melanoma of the choroid.

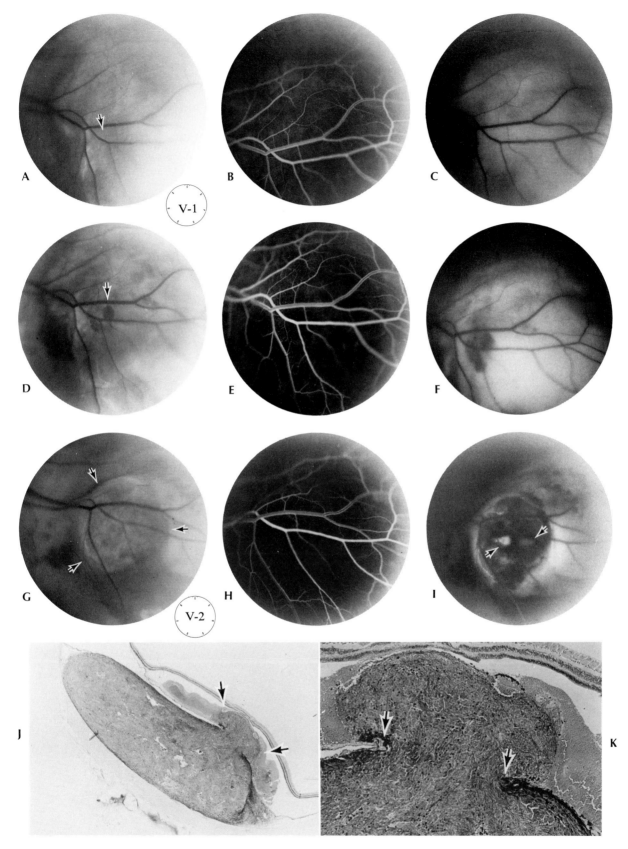

Fig. 3-12. Amelanotic melanoma breaking through Bruch's membrane. A 28-year-old white woman presented with a 3-month history of photopsia in the right eye. Visual acuity was 20/15 in both eyes.

A, There was a nonpigmented tumor of the choroid superior to the optic disc. Note the collar-button extension of the tumor through Bruch's membrane and the engorgement of the tumor vessels. There was a small amount of subretinal blood inferior to the tumor.

B to **D,** Angiography revealed perfusion of dilated vessels within the tumor nodule, leakage of dye from the tumor vessels, and staining of the surface of the tumor and subretinal exudate.

E, There was no evidence of a primary tumor elsewhere and the eye was enucleated. The histopathologic examination confirmed the presence of the amelanotic melanoma breaking through Bruch's membrane (*arrows*).

F, High-power view showing large blood vessels (*arrows*) near the tumor surface. The pathologic diagnosis was spindle A and spindle B melanoma of the choroid. The clinical recognition of tumor extension through Bruch's membrane in this patient was evidence in favor of this amelanotic lesion's being a malignant melanoma rather than a metastatic tumor, which rarely breaks through Bruch's membrane in a collar-button fashion.

(From Flindall et al.[6])

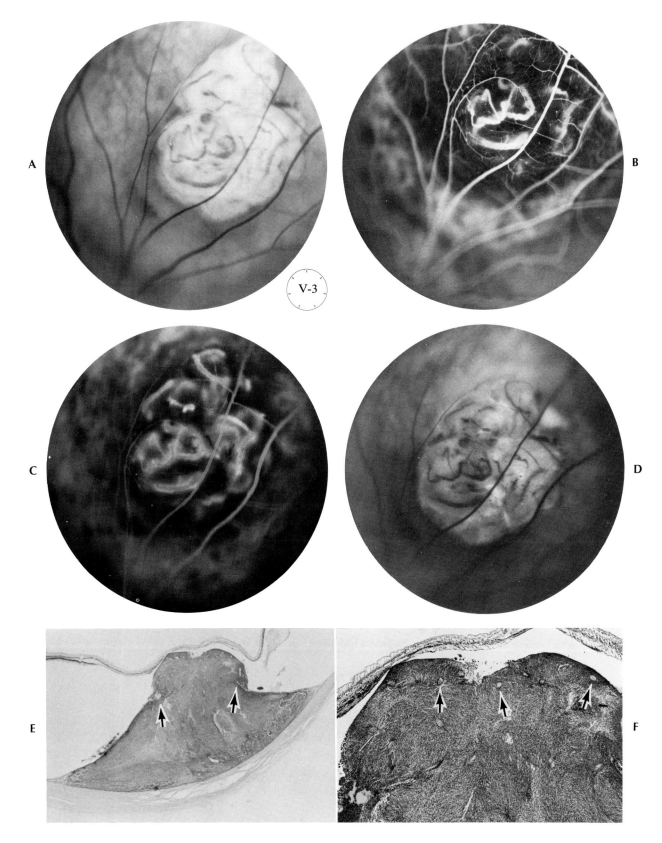

Fig. 3-13. Subretinal and vitreous hemorrhage secondary to a choroidal melanoma breaking through Bruch's membrane and retina. A 60-year-old white man gave a 3-week history of a cloud over the temporal half of the right eye. His vision was 20/20.

A and **B,** On May 29, 1967, there was a pigmented choroidal tumor surrounding the superotemporal aspect of the optic disc. A brown collar-button tumor nodule had invaded and broken through Bruch's membrane and the retina into the vitreous. Some observers misinterpreted this nodule as a mound of blood. Note the granular surface of the tumor, the intraretinal and preretinal blood, and surrounding intraretinal yellowish exudate and subretinal serous exudates.

C and **D,** Angiography revealed a few fine vessels (*arrows*) near the surface of the tumor nodule and staining of the surrounding intraretinal and subretinal exudate. The demonstration of these fine vessels clearly differentiated this dark nodular mass from a mound of preretinal blood. The tumor nodule did not stain because the dye escaping from the tumor surface diffused into the vitreous in concentrations too low to be visualized.

E, The eye was enucleated on July 20, 1967, and histopathologic examination revealed a large highly pigmented malignant melanoma that had broken through Bruch's membrane and the retina. Note the subretinal fluid and the extensive cystic retinal degeneration surrounding the base of the tumor nodule. Serosanguinous exudate was present in some of the large cysts.

F, High-power view showing tumor extension through the retina. The histopathologic diagnosis was malignant melanoma of the choroid, mixed-cell type.

(**A** to **D** from Gass.[4])

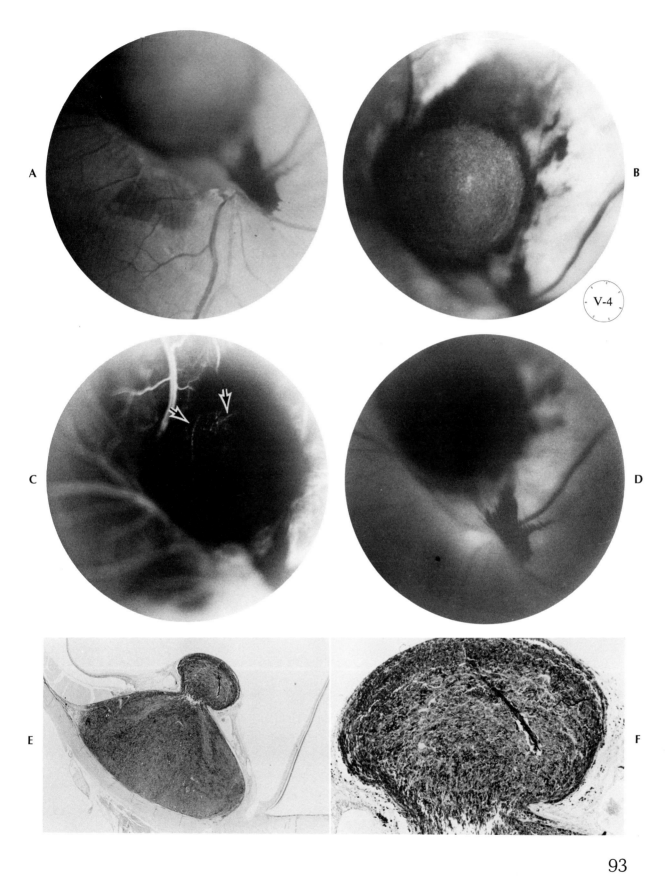

Fig. 3-14. "Mulberry" intravitreal malignant melanoma initially misdiagnosed as a hematoma of the retinal pigment epithelium. A 65-year-old white woman developed blurred vision in her right eye in May 1971.

A, She was evaluated at several eye centers in June 1971. At that time funduscopic examination of the right eye revealed an elevated black mass arising from the optic nerve head and adjacent choroid. There was some blood in the vitreous. The dark mass in front of the optic disc was interpreted as blood that had escaped from beneath the pigment epithelium and had detached the hyaloid membrane in front of the optic disc. Ultrasonography was interpreted as showing probable blood in the posterior pole of the right eye.

B, Fluorescein angiogram showed evidence of a mass in front of the optic disc and obscuration of the background choroidal fluorescence surrounding the optic disc. Note the evidence of small vessels present near the surface of the tumor *(arrows)*. This was good angiographic evidence that this was a solid vascular tumor and not a mass of blood. She was followed by her local physician over the next year at frequent intervals. There was gradual enlargement of the tumor. In June 1972, she was first examined at the Bascom Palmer Eye Institute. Her visual acuity in the right eye was 20/25, and in the left eye she could count fingers at 6 feet.

C, Funduscopic examination revealed a very large, mulberry-like, chocolate brown mass protruding from the posterior pole into the vitreous. It completely obscured the posterior pole from view. There was old vitreous blood inferiorly. There were no blood vessels visible on the tumor surface.

D and **E,** The early phases of fluorescein angiography showed no evidence of fluorescence in the tumor. Later phases of angiography, however, showed a gradual diffusion of dye into the valleys separating the nodules on the surface of the tumor. The clinical impression at this time was that this was a malignant melanoma of the choroid.

F, The eye was enucleated and histopathologic examination revealed a large pigmented malignant melanoma arising from the peripapillary choroid and extending through Bruch's membrane and retina into the vitreous. Note the irregular surface of the tumor, which corresponded to its clinical appearance.

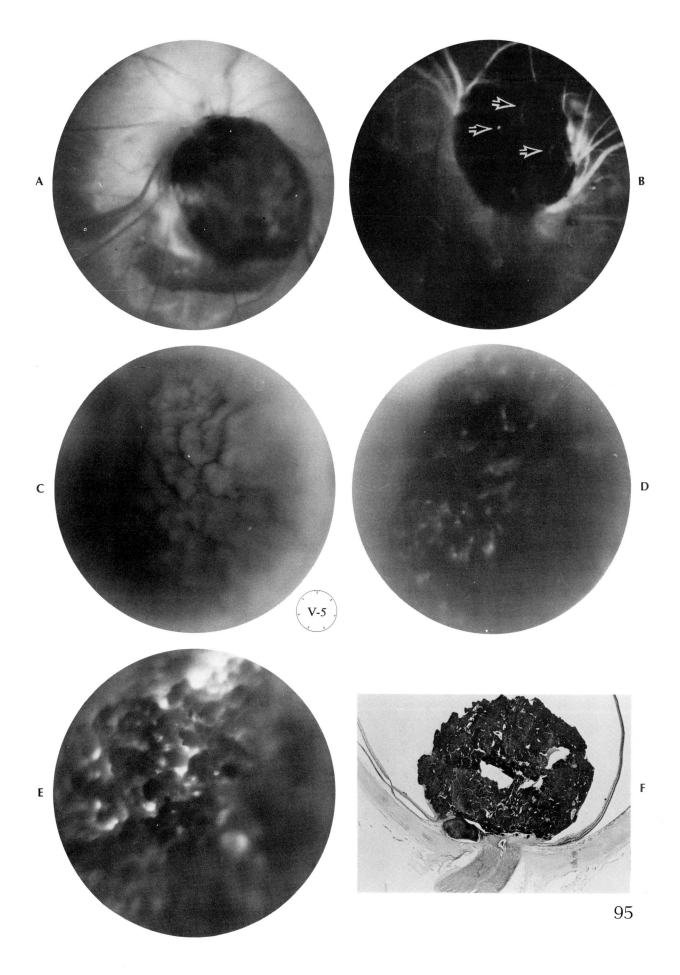

Fig. 3-15. Unsuccessful cobalt plaque therapy for a choroidal melanoma with multinodular growth into and through the retina. A 64-year-old white woman complained of blurred vision in her right eye of 1-month duration. Her vision in the left eye had always been poor because of a chorioretinal scar diagnosed as congenital toxoplasmosis. Her vision in the right eye was 20/25 and the left eye was 20/400.

A, A large pigmented choroidal mass was present in the temporal periphery of the right eye. Multiple dark brown nodules protruded from its anterior surface and extended into and through the overlying retina.

B to **D,** Angiography revealed leakage of dye from the tumor surface and staining of the subretinal exudate but no staining of the tumor nodules. Because of the macular scar in the left eye, treatment of the tumor with an episcleral cobalt plaque was elected.

E, The tumor continued to grow, however, over the following 4 months.

F, The eye was enucleated and histopathologic examination revealed virtually no evidence of necrosis secondary to irradiation. There were multiple areas of tumor invasion into and through the overlying retina *(arrows)*.

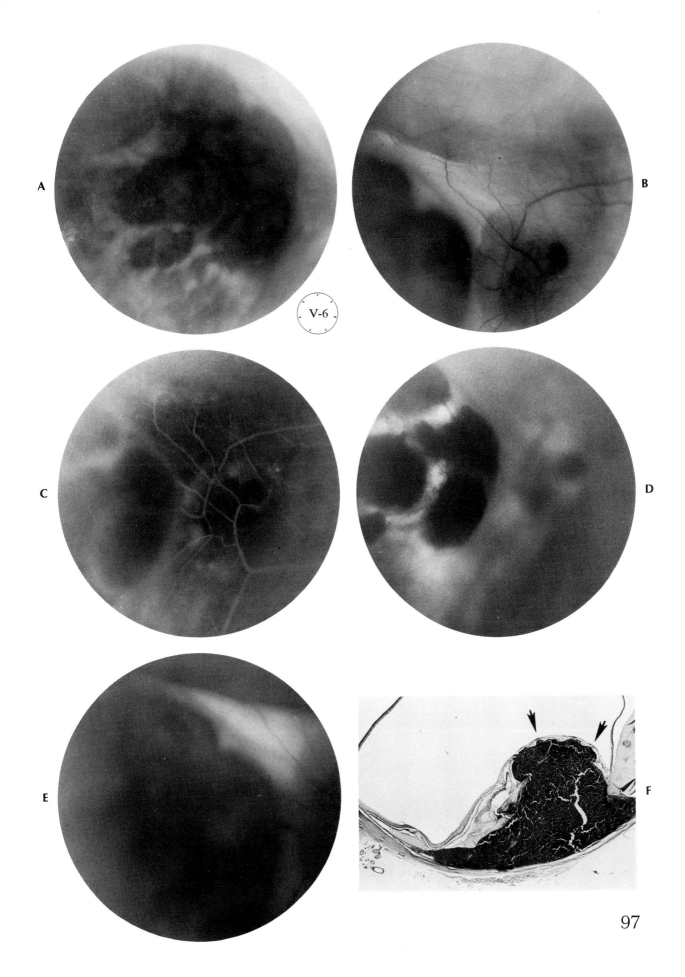

Fig. 3-16. Focal tumor scar and retinal cyst after spontaneous necrosis in a choroidal melanoma. A 64-year-old woman noted photopsia in her right eye in November 1971. Her visual acuity in the right eye was 20/400 and in the left eye was 20/30. She had a large pigmented melanoma in the inferonasal quadrant of the right eye. There was a bullous detachment of the retina involving the inferior half of the fundus.

A, There was a depressed white scar *(arrows)* near the center of a rather large highly pigmented choroidal tumor. A retinal cyst was present over the scar.

B, There was early leakage of dye from the capillaries in the anterior wall of the retinal cyst as well as from the tissues surrounding the cyst.

C and **D,** The fluid within the overlying retinal cyst and the surrounding subretinal exudate stained intensely with dye.

E, Histopathologic examination revealed a focal scar *(arrows)* containing pigment-laden macrophages in the center of a large malignant melanoma of the choroid. A large retinal cyst was present overlying the tumor scar. This scar is presumed to be the end result of a localized area of spontaneous tumor necrosis.

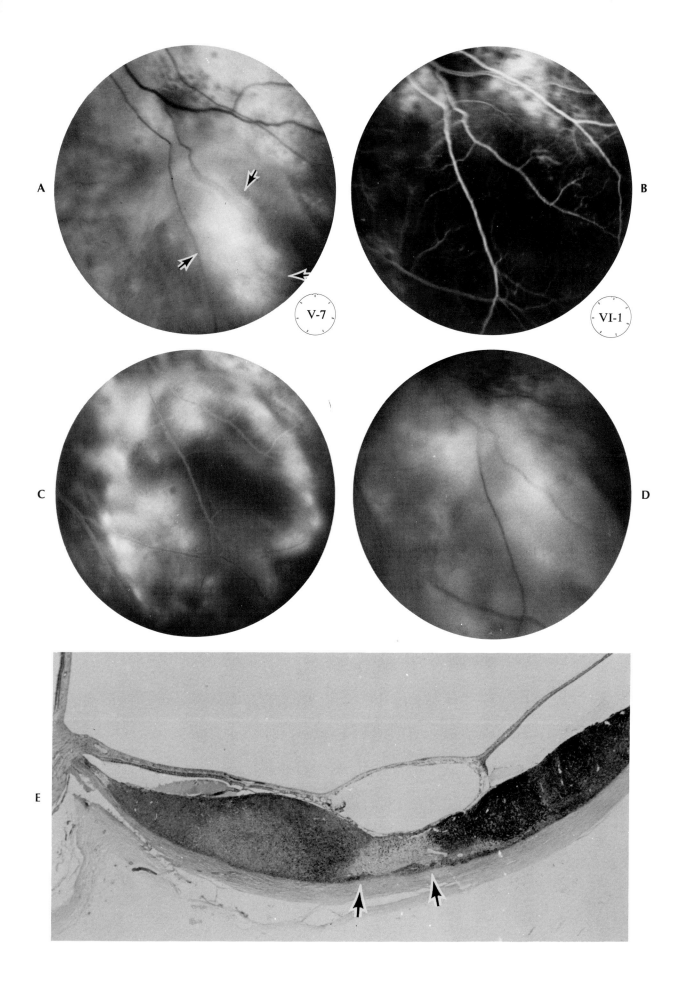

Fig. 3-17. Retrobulbar extension of a small amelanotic choroidal melanoma suspected of being an inflammatory lesion or a metastatic tumor. A woman noted blurred vision in her right eye.

A, On May 22, 1970, a small nonpigmented tumor was present in the choroid at the inferior margin of the optic disc. Note the similar pattern of orange pigment *(arrows)* overlying the tumor and the dark pigment in the macular region, which does not appear to be elevated. The pattern of pigment disturbance in the macula suggests that the underlying choroid is diffusely infiltrated with tumor.

B, By July 6, 1970, the lesion had enlarged and had encroached upon the optic disc. The patient had developed a serous detachment of the macula.

C, Angiography revealed extensive leakage of dye from the tumor surface as well as from the dilated peripapillary retinal capillary network. Because of the continued growth of the tumor and the failure to find an extraocular primary site, the eye was enucleated.

D, On histopathologic examination an epithelioid cell type amelanotic melanoma of the peripapillary choroid extended through the posterior scleral canals *(smaller arrow)* and along the edge of the optic nerve into the meninges and retrobulbar tissues. Clumps of pigment-laden cells were present on the surface of the tumor *(larger arrow)*. Note the cystoid retinal edema between the disc and the macula in the area where angiography depicted evidence of increased retinal capillary permeability, **C.**

E, High-power view of subretinal pigment epithelial clumps shown in **D**. These pigment-laden cells were either pigment epithelial cells or macrophages.

(Courtesy Dr. M. D. Davis, Madison, Wis.)

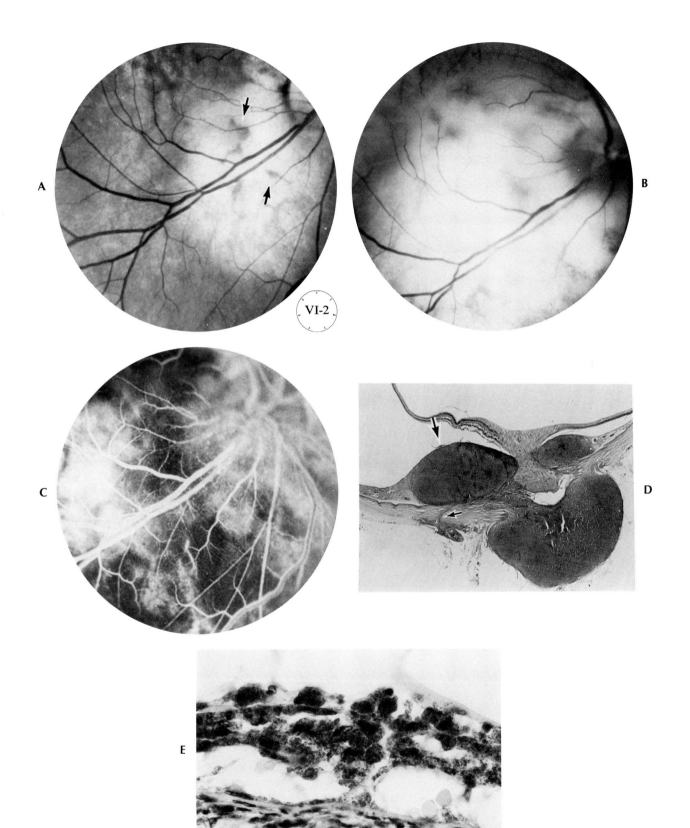

Fig. 3-18. Choroidal melanoma arising in a Caucasian patient with ocular melanocytosis. A 47-year-old white man was seen by his local ophthalmologist on May 21, 1963, because of blurred vision in his right eye. A tumor was present on the nasal side of the optic disc. His visual acuity in the right eye was 20/25. He had a dense field defect involving almost the entire temporal half of the visual field in the right eye. The irides appeared somewhat atrophic, but there was no heterochromia. He had strikingly slate-blue melanosis of the subconjunctival tissue in the right eye. There was a Horner's syndrome on the right and a large strawberry birthmark on the right side of his neck.

A, Note the deep episcleral pigmentation characteristic of melanosis oculi.

B, A relatively small hypopigmented mass was present in the choroid nasal to the optic disc and appeared to have replaced the optic nerve head.

C, Histopathologic examination revealed the presence of a relatively hypopigmented melanoma of the choroid that surrounded and compressed but did not invade the optic nerve head.

D, The choroid throughout the eye was thickened by the presence of abnormal numbers of normal choroidal melanocytes *(arrows)*.

E, Bleached section of the choroid revealed the increased population of normal oval to round melanocytes characteristic of melanosis oculi.

F, Note the large number of melanocytes in the iris stroma and along its anterior surface. Melanosis oculi and oculodermal melanocytosis (nevus of Ota) occur most commonly in non-Caucasians. Malignant melanoma of the uveal tract occurs as a complication of melanosis oculi and nevus of Ota only in Caucasians.

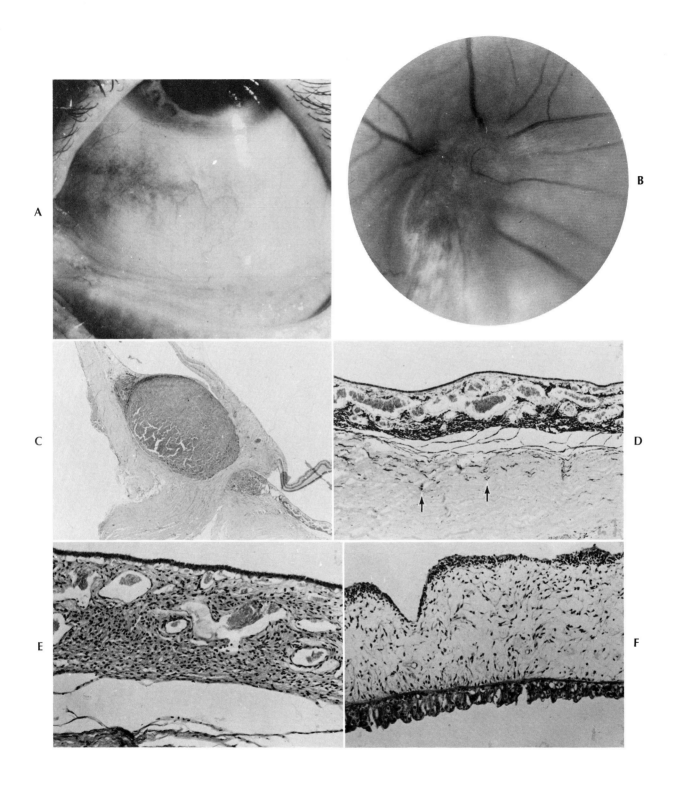

Fig. 3-19. Choroidal folds caused by choroidal melanoma. A 74-year-old white woman gave a 6-month history of a shadow in the temporal field of vision in the right eye. Her visual acuity was 20/40.

A, Horizontal chorioretinal folds were present at the inferior margin of a large choroidal melanoma *(arrows)*. Note the alternate pattern of orange and gray lines extending through the macula. The orange lines correspond with the crest of the folds and the gray lines with the valleys of the fold.

B, Angiography revealed increased choroidal hyperfluorescence corresponding with the crests of the folds. This pattern of fluorescence is caused by the difference in the effective thickness of the pigment epithelium at the crests of the folds where the incident blue light passes at right angles through the pigment epithelium and the troughs of the folds where it must pass obliquely through the pigment epithelium. An additional factor is the thinness of the pigment epithelium at the crests of the folds and compression of the pigment epithelium in the valleys of the folds.

C, The eye was enucleated and revealed the presence of a malignant melanoma of the choroid *(large arrow)*. Inferior to the tumor the choroid was engorged and its inner surface along with the overlying pigment epithelium was thrown into a series of folds *(small arrows)*. The retina in this section is artifactitiously detached. (From Norton.[7])

D, Another section where both the retina and pigment epithelium were artifactitiously detached from the underlying folded choroid shows minimal folding of the retina in comparison to that seen in the pigment epithelium. Two years after enucleation of the right eye, the patient developed a nodular tumor between her eyebrows. This was removed elsewhere and was reported as showing malignant cells believed to be a basal cell carcinoma. Three years after enucleation of the eye, she developed an enlarged liver. Exploratory laparotomy revealed a tumor that was diagnosed as a malignant hepatoma. She received x-ray irradiation treatment for this. It was only on later review of the histopathologic condition of the liver that it was realized that the tumor was a metastatic malignant melanoma rather than a hepatoma.

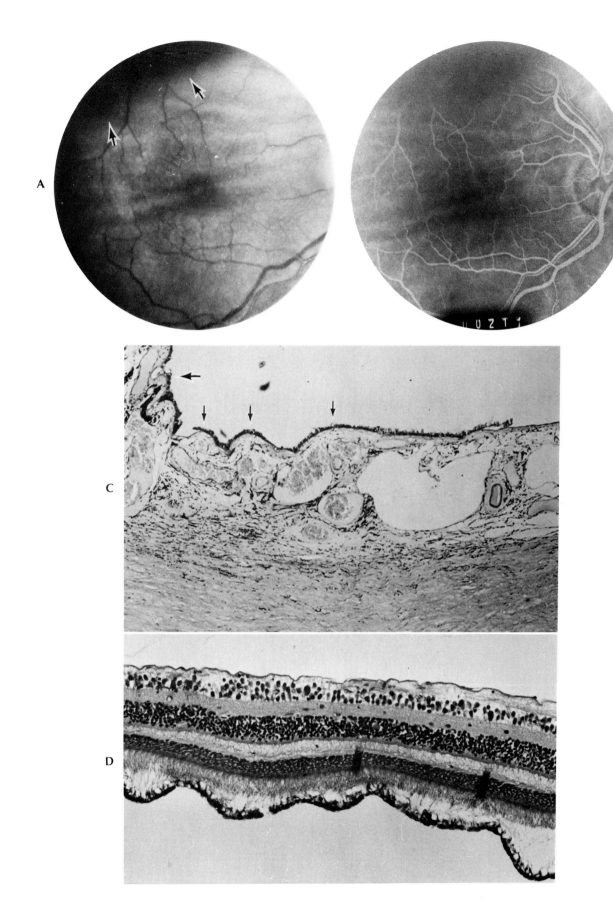

Fig. 3-20. Hypopigmented ciliary body and choroidal melanoma. A 62-year-old white woman noted blurred vision in one eye of a 3-month duration. She had had a radical mastectomy for breast carcinoma 8 years previously.

A and **B,** Biomicroscopy and ophthalmoscopy revealed a large partly pigmented mass protruding from the ciliary body and peripheral choroid. Blood vessels were visible near the surface of the nonpigmented portion of the tumor *(arrows)*. There were inflammatory cells in the vitreous and anterior chamber. Cystoid macular edema was present. The opposite eye was normal.

C, Angiography revealed perfusion of blood vessels within the pigmented *(arrow)* as well as nonpigmented portions of the tumor.

D, The late angiogram revealed fluorescein dye along the inner surface of the tumor.

E, The eye was enucleated and histopathologic examination revealed a spindle B cell melanoma of the ciliary body and choroid. Note the tumor extension into the anterior chamber angle and the detachment of the thinned ciliary epithelium *(arrows)*. The intense fluorescence seen in **D** was probably caused by dye trapped beneath the detached ciliary epithelium.

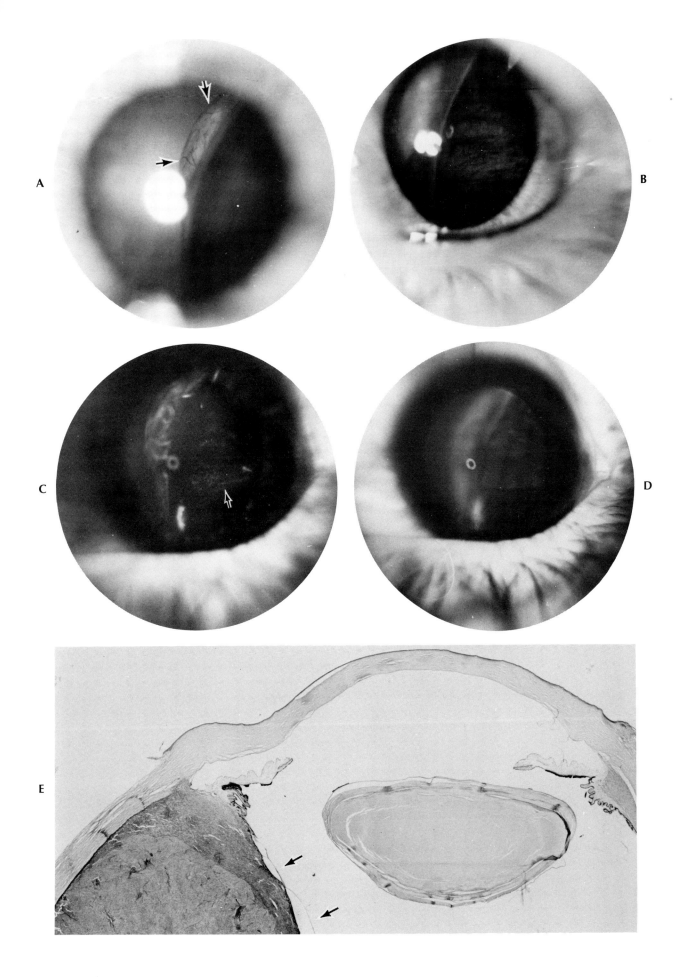

Fig. 3-21. Melanoma of the peripheral iris and ciliary body. A middle-aged white man was referred because of an iris lesion.

A, A pigmented iris tumor extended into the angle between 8:30 and 10:30 o'clock.

B, On dilated funduscopic examination, the iris lesion was in continuity with a pigmented ciliary body mass that had an irregular surface. No blood vessels were evident near the tumor surface.

C and **D,** Fluorescein dye diffused out of the ciliary body tumor and produced a fluorescent haze along its surface. A pigmented ciliary body cyst in the same location would have a smooth surface and would not show fluorescein along its inner surface.

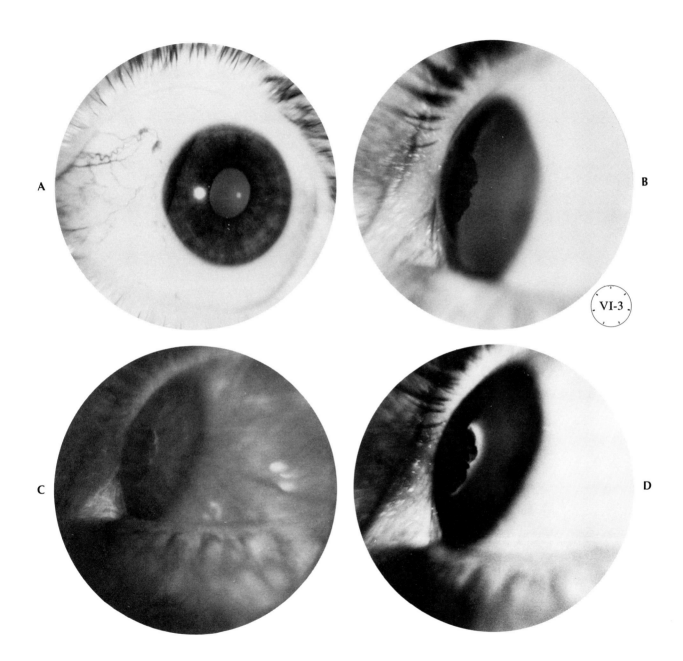

REFERENCES

1. Flocks, M., Gerende, J. H., and Zimmerman, L. E.: The size and shape of malignant melanomas of the choroid and histologic characteristics. A statistical study of 210 tumors, Trans. Am. Acad. Ophthalmol. Otolaryngol. **59:**740-758, 1955.
2. Gass, J. D. M.: Photocoagulation of macular lesions, Trans. Am. Acad. Ophthalmol. Otolaryngol. **75:**599-608, 1971.
3. Norton, E. W. D., Smith, J. L., Curtin, V. T., and Justice, J., Jr.: Fluorescein fundus photography: An aid in differential diagnosis of posterior ocular lesions, Trans. Am. Acad. Ophthalmol. Otolaryngol. **68:**755-765, 1964.
4. Gass, J. D. M.: Fluorescein angiography: An aid in the differential diagnosis of intraocular tumors, Int. Ophthalmol. Clinic. **12**(1):85-120, Spring 1972.
5. Gass, J. D. M.: Stereoscopic atlas of macular diseases, St. Louis, 1970, The C. V. Mosby Co., p. 91.
6. Flindall, R. J., and Gass, J. D. M.: A histopathologic fluorescein angiographic correlated study of malignant melanomas of the choroid, Can. J. Ophthalmol. **6:**258-267, 1971.
7. Norton, E. W. D.: A characteristic fluorescein angiographic pattern in choroid folds, Proc. Roy. Soc. Med. **62:**119-128, 1969.

SUGGESTED READINGS

Apple, D. J., Goldberg, M. F., Wyhinny, G., and Levi, S.: Argon laser photocoagulation of choroidal malignant melanoma, Arch. Ophthalmol. **90:**97-101, 1973.

Bedford, M. A., Bedotto, C., and MacFaul, P. A.: Radiation retinopathy after the application of a cobalt plaque, Brit. J. Ophthalmol. **54:**505-509, 1970.

Boniuk, M., and Zimmerman, L. E.: Occurrence and behavior of choroidal melanomas in eyes subject to operation for retinal detachment, Trans. Am. Ophthalmol. **66:**642-658, 1962.

Callender, G. R.: Malignant melanotic tumors of the eye: A study of histologic types in III cases, Trans. Am. Acad. Ophthalmol. Otolaryngol. **36:**131-142, 1931.

Daicken, B.: Melanosis retinae et papillae durch transretinal in den Glaskörper eingebrochenes malignes adherant Melanom, Ophthalmologica **166:**460-471, 1963.

Davidorf, F. H., Newman, G. H., Havener, W. H., and Makley, T.: Conservative management of malignant melanoma. II. Transcleral diathermy as a method of treatment for malignant melanomas of the choroid, Arch. Ophthalmol. **83:**273-280, 1970.

deVeer, J. A.: Juxtapapillary malignant melanoma of the choroid and so-called malignant melanoma of the optic disc, A.M.A. Arch. Ophthalmol. **51:**147-160, 1954.

deVeer, J. A.: Melanotic tumors of the optic nerve head, A.M.A. Arch. Ophthalmol. **65:**536-541, 1961.

Edwards, W. C., Layden, W. E., and Macdonald, R., Jr.: Fluorescein angiography of malignant melanoma of the choroid, Am. J. Ophthalmol. **68:**797-808, 1969.

Ganley, J. P., and Comstock, G. W.: Benign nevi and malignant melanoma of the choroid, Am. J. Ophthalmol. **76:**19-25, 1973.

Hagler, W. S., Jarrett, W. H., and Humphrey, W. T.: The radioactive phosphorus uptake test in diagnosis of uveal melanoma, Arch. Ophthalmol. **83:**548-557, 1970.

Halasa, A.: Malignant melanoma in a case of bilateral nevus of Ota, Arch. Ophthalmol. **84:**176-178, 1970.

Hayreh, S. S.: Choroidal melanomata. Fluorescence angiographic and histopathological study, Brit. J. Ophthalmol. **54:**145-160, 1970.

Hogan, M. J.: Clinical aspects, management and prognosis of melanomas of the uvea and optic nerve. In Boniuk, M. (editor): International symposium on ocular tumors, Houston, Texas, 1962: Ocular and adnexal tumors, St. Louis, 1964, The C. V. Mosby Co., pp. 203-302.

Insolf, H. L., Wallow, M. D., and Ts'o, M. O. M.: Proliferation of the retinal pigment epithelium over malignant choroidal tumors: A light and electron microscopic study, Am. J. Ophthalmol. **73:**914-925, 1972.

Jensen, O. A.: Malignant melanomas of the uvea in Denmark, 1943-1952, Acta Ophthalmol., suppl. 75, 1963.

Kirk, H. Q., and Petty, R. W.: Malignant melanoma of the choroid: A correlation of clinical and histological findings, A.M.A. Arch. Ophthalmol. **56:**843-860, 1965.

Litricin, O.: Unsuspected uveal melanomas, Am. J. Ophthalmol. **76:**734-738, 1973.

Lloyd, R. I.: Retroillumination, Am. J. Ophthalmol. **26:**799-801, 1943.

Lund, O.: Changes in choroidal tumors after light coagulation (and diathermy coagulation), Arch. Ophthalmol. **75:**458-466, 1966.

Makley, T. A., and Teed, R. W.: Unsuspected intraocular malignant melanomas, Arch. Ophthalmol. **60:**475-478, 1958.

Newman, G. H., Davidorf, F. H., Havener, W. H., and Makley, T. A. Jr.: Conservative management of malignant melanoma. I. Irradiation as a method of treatment for malignant melanoma of the choroid, Arch. Ophthalmol. **83:**21-26, 1970.

Nordmann, J., and Brini, A.: Von Recklinghausen's disease and melanoma of the uvea, Brit. J. Ophthalmol. **54:**641-647, 1970.

Oosterhuis, J. A., and Van Waveren, C. W.: Fluorescein photography in malignant melanoma, Ophthalmologica **156:**101-116, 1968.

Ossoinig, K., and Till, P.: Methods and results of ultrasonography in diagnosing intraocular tumors. In Gittner, K., et al. (editors): International congress of ultrasonography in ophthalmology, 4th, Philadelphia, 1968: Ophthalmic Ultrasound, St. Louis, 1969, The C. V. Mosby Co., pp. 294-300.

Paul, E. V., Parnell, B. L., and Fraker, M.: Prognosis of malignant melanomas of the choroid and ciliary body, Int. Ophthalmol. Clin. **2:**387-402, 1962.

Pettit, T. H., Barton, A., Foos, R. Y., and Christensen, R. E.: Fluorescein angiography of choroidal melanomas, Arch. Ophthalmol. **83:**27-38, 1970.

Reese, A. B.: Tumors of the eye, New York, 1963, Paul B. Hoeber, Inc., Harper & Row, Publishers, Chapter 7, pp. 214-363.

Reese, A. B., Archila, E. A., Jones, I. S., and Cooper, W. C.: Necrosis of malignant melanoma of the choroid, Am. J. Ophthalmol. **69:**91-104, 1970.

Reese, A. B., and Howard, G. M.: Flat uveal melanomas, Am. J. Ophthalmol. **64:**1021-1028, 1967.

Samuels, B.: Anatomic and clinical manifestations of necrosis in 84 cases of choroidal sarcoma, Arch. Ophthalmol. **11:**998-1027, 1934.

Smith, L. T., and Irvine, A. R.: Diagnostic significance of orange pigment accumulation over choroidal tumors, Am. J. Ophthalmol. **76:**212-216, 1973.

Stallard, H. B.: Malignant melanoma of the choroid treated with radioactive applicators, Trans. Ophthalmol. Soc. U. K. **79:**373-392, 1959.

Stallard, H. B.: Malignant melanoblastoma of the choroid, Mod. Probl. Ophthalmol. **7:**16-38, 1968.

Stallard, H. B.: Malignant melanoma of the choroid treated with radioactive applicators, In Boniuk, M. (editor): Ocular and adnexal tumors, St. Louis, 1964, The C. V. Mosby Co., pp. 322-333.

Starr, H. J., and Zimmerman, L. E.: Extrascleral extension and orbital recurrence of malignant melanomas of the choroid and ciliary body, Int. Ophthalmol. Clin. **2:**369-385, 1962.

Terner, I. S., Leopold, I. H., and Eisenberg, I. J.: The radioactive phosphorus (P^{32}) uptake test in ophthalmology: a review of the literature and analysis of results in 262 cases of ocular and adnexal pathology, Arch. Ophthalmol. **55:**52-83, 1956.

Vannas, M.: On the diagnosis of intraocular tumors and foreign bodies by means of anterior pupillary transillumination, Acta Ophthalmol. **26:**125-134, 1948.

Vogel, M. H.: Treatment of malignant choroidal melanomas with photocoagulation, Am. J. Ophthalmol. **74:**1-11, 1972.

Westerveld-Brandon, E. R., and Zeeman, W. P. C.: The prognosis of melanoblastomata of the choroid, Ophthalmologica **134:**20-29, 1957.

Wolter, J. R., Schut, A. L., and Martonyi, C. L.: Hemangioma-like clinical appearance of a collar-button melanoma caused by the strangulation effect of Bruch's membrane, Am. J. Ophthalmol. **76:**730-733, 1973.

Zimmerman, L. E.: Changing concepts concerning the malignancy of ocular tumors, Arch. Ophthalmol. **78:**166-173, 1967.

Zimmerman, L. E.: Problems in the diagnosis of malignant melanomas of the choroid and ciliary body, Am. J. Ophthalmol. **75:**917-929, 1973.

CHAPTER FOUR

Cavernous hemangioma of the choroid

Cavernous hemangioma of the choroid is a benign developmental tumor or hamartoma that typically occurs either as a localized tumefaction, usually in patients without other vascular malformations, or as a diffuse thickening of the choroid in patients with the Sturge-Weber syndrome.

LOCALIZED CAVERNOUS HEMANGIOMA OF THE CHOROID

Localized cavernous hemangiomas of the choroid are rarely detected prior to the third decade of life. Their rate of growth is probably maximum during the normal growth period of the individual. By adulthood the hemangioma may cause secondary degenerative and proliferative changes in the overlying pigment epithelium and cystic degeneration of the retina. Unless the tumor is large and is located directly in the macular area, the patient is usually asymptomatic until middle or later life when he develops serous retinal detachment, which spreads from the edge of the tumor into the macular area (Figs. 4-1 to 4-3). Less often, these tumors may be discovered as an incidental finding (Fig. 4-4) or may cause distortion of central vision merely by their presence in the macula prior to causing significant alterations in the overlying pigment epithelium and retina (Fig. 4-5).

A total of 22 patients with localized cavernous hemangiomas unassociated with other evidence of Sturge-Weber syndrome have been studied at the Bascom Palmer Eye Institute. Fifteen occurred in males and seven in females. All were Caucasians. The average age of the patients was 51 years (range 25 to 73 years). The tumor was present in the left eye of 12 patients and in the right eye of 10 patients. Many of the patients were referred with the diagnosis of central serous retinopathy, choroiditis, disciform degeneration, metastatic carcinoma, malignant melanoma, or rhegmatogenous detachment. The hemangiomas were typically round or oval, slightly elevated, orange-red tumors with an indistinct border. They measured between two and ten disc diameters in size. Varying amounts of splotchy yellow material was present on the surface of most of the lesions. Most of the tumors were centered in the paramacular area, but many extended into the edge of the central macular area. Only one tumor was centered near the fovea. Only two tumors were confined to the nasal half of the eye and both were located superonasally. Five tumors were located immediately superior to the optic disc. All others were located temporally to the optic disc in the macula or paramacular area. In 13 patients the tumor was associated with a localized serous retinal detachment surrounding the margins of the tumor. In only two patients was a large area of bullous retinal detachment present. One of these patients had been misdiagnosed as having a rhegmatogenous detachment. Complete separation of the tumor from the overlying retina by a serous detachment occurred in only one of the 22 patients. Three patients had clinical evidence of previous retinal detachment. One patient had a large apron-shaped area of depigmentation of the pigment epithelium extending from the lower edge of the tumor down the nasal side of the fundus (Fig. 4-4). This was associated with a bone spicule pattern of migration of pigment into the overlying retina. Three patients had minimal evidence of changes in the overlying pigment epithelium and had no evidence of either cystic retinal degeneration or retinal detachment. In each case the tumor had been discovered during a routine eye examination. One of these patients with a large tumor, extending to the edge of his fovea, gave a history of reduced vision in that eye all of his life (Fig. 4-5). Seven of the patients presented with localized serous detachment of the macula of recent onset, and all recovered good central vision after photocoagulation of the tumor surface (Fig. 4-3). Eight patients had evidence of permanent macular damage including cystic retinal degeneration and edema (Figs. 4-1 and 4-2), circinate retinopathy, distinct pigment epithelial derangement, and in one case a macular pucker.

Because the color of a choroidal hemangioma so closely resembles that of the surrounding normal fundus and because most hemangiomas are only slightly elevated, they are easily overlooked by any means of examination other than the binocular indirect ophthalmoscope. Although indirect ophthalmoscopy is the best means of detecting and diagnosing a choroidal hemangioma, biomicroscopy provides useful information concerning the pigment epithelial and retinal changes overlying the tumor. The retina is typically thickened and cystic. Large cystic areas or schisis may be present. The yellowish mottled material that accompanies these cystic changes appears to lie in the depth of the degenerated retina or beneath the retina.

Choroidal hemangiomas are transilluminated easily. Some may show a faint circular zone of defect in transillumination at the tumor margin. This corresponds to a similar zone of hypofluorescence seen angiographically (see below). A few hemangiomas may blanch on manual compression of the eye.

Hemangiomas associated with overlying cystic changes demonstrate field defects corresponding with the site of the tumor and the surrounding detachment. Nerve fiber bundle defects secondary to choroidal hemangiomas have been reported but are unusual.

The characteristic angiographic findings in choroidal hemangioma are (1) a coarse vascular pattern of fluorescence corresponding to the location of the tumor in the pre-arterial and arterial phase of angiography, (2) widespread and irregular areas of fluorescence secondary to diffusion of dye from the surface of the tumor during the course of angiography, and (3) a diffuse multiloculated pattern of fluorescein accumulation in the outer retina characteristic of polycystic degeneration and edema during the later stages of angiography (Figs. 4-1 to 4-3). A circular zone of hypofluorescence is often present at the tumor margins during the early and middle stages of angiography (Figs. 4-1, C, 4-2, C, and 4-3, D). The cause of the hypofluorescent ring is unknown, but it may be the proliferative changes in the pigment epithelium often found overlying hemangiomas in eyes enucleated with the mistaken diagnosis of melanoma (Fig. 4-6, G). In some cases angiography may demonstrate evidence of retinal capillary permeability alterations overlying the hemangioma (Fig. 4-2). In patients with choroidal hemangiomas without extensive secondary changes in the overlying pigment epithelium and retina, angiography reveals an exaggerated choroidal fluorescence in the area of the tumor during the first few minutes of the study. This fades rapidly into a near normal angiographic pattern thereafter (Fig. 4-5).

Histopathologically, a cavernous hemangioma of the choroid is made up of large, dilated, thin-walled vessels that blend almost imperceptibly into the normal choroidal tissue near the margins of the tumor (Fig. 4-6). Most of the available specimens that have been obtained after the misdiagnosis of malignant melanoma show extensive changes in the overlying pigment epithelium, including proliferation and metaplasia of the pigment epithelium and cystic degeneration of the overlying retina (Fig. 4-6, E to G). Extensive proliferation of the overlying pigment epithelium, though unusual in my clinical experience, might cause these tumors to have at least a partly pigmented appearance and closely resemble a melanoma.

Localized cavernous hemangiomas of the choroid located in the extrafoveal area associated with serous detachment of the retina may be treated successfully with xenon or argon photocoagulation directed to that portion of the tumor surface where fluorescein angiography shows evidence of diffusion of dye from the surface of the tumor (Figs. 4-1, *E*, and 4-3, *E*). Photocoagulation should be sufficiently intense to create some whitening in the outer retinal layers. It is successful in virtually all cases in collapsing the cystic retina onto the surface of the tumor and in causing complete resolution of all subretinal fluid. It does not alter the size of the tumor. Since these tumors are presumed to be hamartomas, very little change in the size of these tumors is expected after adulthood. In cases where the edge of the tumor extends into the foveal area, photocoagulation should be done no closer than the edge of the avascular zone of the foveal area. In such cases resolution of the serous macular detachment may occur despite incomplete treatment of the surface of the lesion. Treatment is unnecessary in patients with the incidental finding of cavernous hemangioma unassociated with retinal detachment or evidence of previous detachment. They should, however, be examined at yearly intervals. Treatment of patients with evidence of severe permanent macular damage is optional. Photocoagulation of the extrafoveal portions of the tumor might be considered to prevent further retinal damage caused by prolonged serous retinal detachment.

Although not pathognomonic for cavernous hemangioma of the choroid, the early pattern of fluorescence caused by the large vascular spaces in the tumor, and the late pattern of dye staining as a result of cystic degeneration of the overlying retina are infrequently found in association with other tumors (Figs. 3-5 and 3-16). The P-32 radioactive uptake study is usually but not always negative in cavernous hemangioma. Ultrasonography has been reported to be helpful in differentiating choroidal hemangiomas from melanomas. In the last analysis, however, the reddish orange color of choroidal hemangiomas as viewed with the binocular indirect ophthalmoscope is the most important differential diagnostic sign that differentiates it from the white or creamy color of metastatic carcinoma and amelanotic melanomas.

In rare instances, localized cavernous hemangiomas of the choroid may be large and highly elevated and may be associated with massive detachment of the retina early in life. In such instances, particularly when the fundus cannot be well visualized, patients may be misdiagnosed as retinoblastoma (Fig. 4-6, *H*). I have examined one patient with Sturge-Weber syndrome who had a large localized rather than diffuse hemangioma underlying a secondary retinal detachment (Fig. 4-9).

DIFFUSE CHOROIDAL HEMANGIOMA IN THE STURGE-WEBER SYNDROME

Diffuse cavernous hemangioma, or hypertrophy of the choroid (Figs. 4-7, *A* and *B*, and 4-8), usually occurs in one eye of patients with other manifestations of the Sturge-Weber syndrome including (1) ipsilateral cutaneous angioma, or nevus flammeus (Fig. 4-7, *C* and *D*), (2) ipsilateral angioma of the meninges and brain (Fig. 4-7, *F*), (3) ipsilateral intracranial calcification (Fig. 4-7, *E*), (4) ipsilateral developmental glaucoma (Figs. 4-8 and 4-10), and (5) contralateral Jacksonian seizures.

The cutaneous lesion although usually apparent at birth may become more apparent with age. It may escape notice in the more deeply pigmented patient (Fig. 4-7, *D*). It typically involves roughly the area of distribution of the first and second division of the trigeminal nerve on one side and is often associated with hemihypertrophy of the face. The lower face is involved less often (Fig. 4-7, C). The lesion may extend across the midline (Fig. 4-7, C). The trunk and extremities may be involved. The lesion is usually flat but may become elevated. The angioma of the lid may be continuous with dilated vascular channels in the conjunctiva and episclera. The incidence of glaucoma accompanying the lid involvement is higher in the Sturge-Weber syndrome than in von Recklinghausen's disease. The glaucoma may be evident early in life or may develop later. The eye on the side of the facial angioma may be enlarged (Fig. 4-7, C). This may be secondary to glaucoma or may be a manifestation only of the generalized hemihypertrophy of the facial tissues. Gonioscopy of patients with glaucoma reveals anterior chamber alterations identical to those seen in developmental glaucoma unrelated to other abnormalities.

The diffuse choroidal hemangioma may be easily overlooked on cursory ophthalmoscopy (Figs. 4-7, B, and 4-8, A). Comparison of both fundi, however, usually reveals a deep red color in the posterior fundus on the side of the facial angioma. Details of the normal choroidal vasculature are obscured in the eye with the hemangioma (Fig. 4-7, B). The optic disc may be cupped (Fig. 4-8, A). In a few patients, evidence of increased pigmentation of the fundus on the side of the angioma may be present. Cases showing combined evidence of melanocytosis and angiomatosis of the fundus and brain have been reported.

Diffuse choroidal hemangioma may be complicated in later life by degeneration of the overlying pigment epithelium, cystic retinal degeneration, and secondary retinal detachment. In one boy with nevus flammeus without evidence of intracranial involvement or glaucoma, I have observed a secondary retinal detachment overlying a large localized choroidal hemangioma confined to the inferior half of the fundus (Fig. 4-9). The large angioma was associated with a small focal area of degeneration of the overlying pigment epithelium and retina. Photocoagulation of this focal area, which showed evidence of dye leakage with fluorescein angiography, was successful in reattaching the retina.

The histopathology of the choroidal lesion in Sturge-Weber syndrome (Fig. 4-10, A) is identical to that in localized cavernous hemangiomas of the choroid. The anterior chamber angle in patients with glaucoma shows histopathologic evidence of incomplete cleavage of the anterior chamber angle (Fig. 4-10, B) identical to that found in congenital glaucoma without associated lesions.

A pial racemose angioma may be present in the parieto-occipital area on the same side as the facial angioma (Fig. 4-7, F). These may calcify and be associated with calcification of the neighboring cerebral vessels, atrophy of the neighboring cortex, and, occasionally, maldevelopment of the brain on the involved side. The lesions are usually accompanied by Jacksonian type of seizures on the contralateral side. The seizures may become generalized and may be followed by hemiparesis, hemiplegia, and hemianopia. Varying degrees of mental deficiency are common. The intracranial lesion has a characteristic x-ray picture (Fig. 4-7, E) consisting of sinuous, double-contoured lines corresponding to calcification of vessels.

Unlike the other phakomatoses, there is little evidence that the Sturge-Weber syndrome is a hereditary condition. The pattern of angiomatous involvement apparently results as a mesodermal malformation involving that portion of the primordial vascular system destined to supply the face, meninges, and choroid.

Fig. 4-1. Cystic macular degeneration and detachment secondary to a choroidal hemangioma. A 54-year-old woman was seen on March 23, 1971, with a 3-week history of right esotropia. While covering the left eye, she noted that the vision in her right eye was blurred. Her visual acuity in the right eye was finger counting and in the left eye was 20/25.

A, On funduscopic examination there was a four-by-six-disc-diameter-size reddish tumor involving the choroid on the temporal side of the macular area. It was surrounded by a serous retinal detachment. The tumor extended into the central macular region. There were extensive cystic changes of the overlying retina as well as in the macular region.

B, The early arterial angiogram revealed many fluorescent vascular channels within the choroidal tumor.

C, There was extensive leakage of dye from the surface of the tumor. Note the hypofluorescent ring at the tumor margins (*arrows*).

D, One-hour angiogram revealed a multiloculated pattern of fluorescence indicative of cystic changes in the overlying retina as well as diffuse staining of the subretinal fluid on either side of the tumor. The dark stellate figure in the macular area is indicative of extensive cystoid macular edema (*arrow*).

E, Almost certainly this patient had had a long-standing retinal detachment and cystic degeneration that extended into the macular area. Xenon photocoagulation was used to get rid of the subretinal exudate to prevent further paracentral field loss. It was not anticipated that good visual acuity would be restored.

F, On November 18, 1971, the subretinal exudate had resolved. Large cysts (*arrow*) persisted in the macular area and her visual acuity was unchanged.

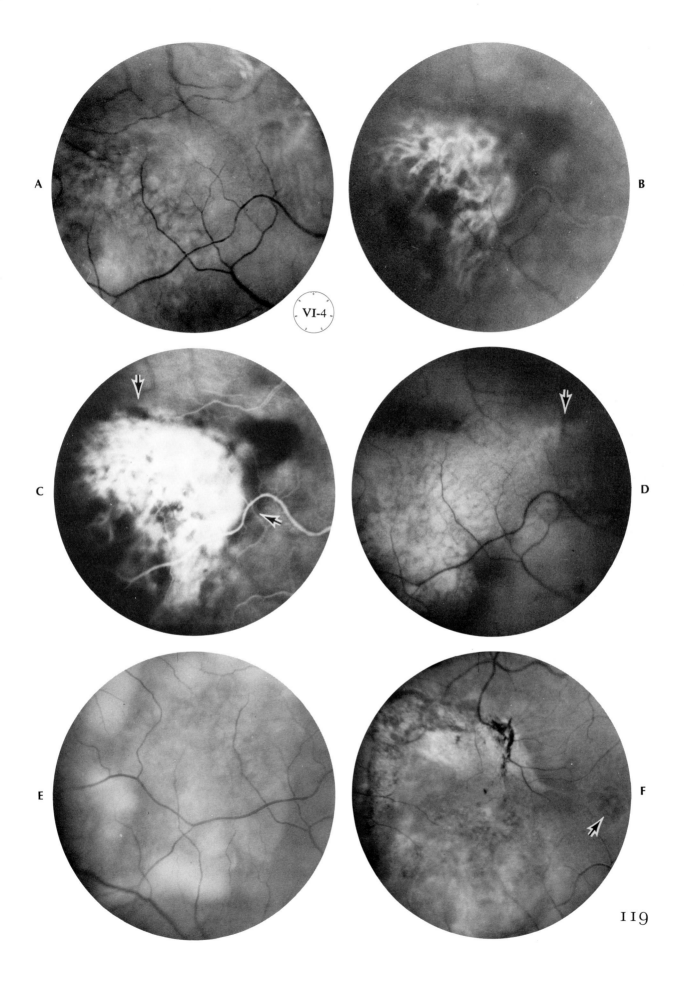

Fig. 4-2. Cystoid macular edema and serous detachment of the macula secondary to a choroidal hemangioma. A 40-year-old white man had a 2-year history of poor vision in the left eye. His visual acuity in the right eye was 20/20 and in the left eye was 20/200.

A, A localized hemangioma of the choroid was present superior to the macula. There was a serous detachment of the retina and cystoid macular edema. The thickening of the overlying retina was attributable primarily to extensive cystic degeneration and edema of the retina. Note the irregular deposit of yellowish material on the surface of the tumor.

B, Arterial phase revealed prominent fluorescence of the cavernous channels within the tumor.

C, There was early leakage of dye from the surface of the tumor as well as leakage of dye from the retinal vessels surrounding the tumor *(arrows)*. Note the hypofluorescent zone at the tumor margin.

D, One-hour angiogram revealed extensive pooling of dye within the cystoid spaces of the retina. Note the dark stellate figure outlined by dye indicative of cystoid macular edema *(arrow)*.

(From Gass[1].)

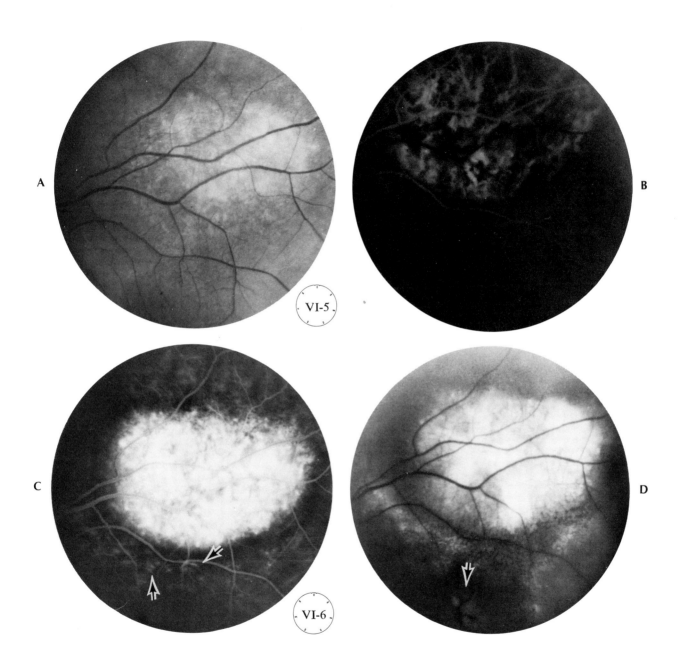

Fig. 4-3. Serous detachment of the macula secondary to a choroidal hemangioma. A 49-year-old physician gave a 2-day history of a positive scotoma in his left eye. Visual acuity in the right eye was 20/25, and in the left eye was 20/50.

A and **B,** He had a serous detachment of the retina in the macular region of the left eye. A round, elevated, red tumor of the choroid *(arrows)* was present just temporal to the macula and was associated with extensive cystoid changes in the overlying retina.

C, Fluorescein angiography revealed extensive leakage of dye from the surface of the tumor. Note that the tumor is over two disc diameters away from the fovea *(arrow)*. There was a hypofluorescent ring at the tumor margin.

D, One-hour angiogram showing multiloculated fluorescent pattern indicative of cystoid retinal edema and degeneration. **E,** Xenon photocoagulation was applied to the surface of the tumor.

F, Three weeks after photocoagulation the retinal detachment had resolved and the visual acuity was 20/20 and J-1. Four years after treatment the acuity and the tumor size were unchanged.

(**A** to **C** and **E** from Gass.[2])

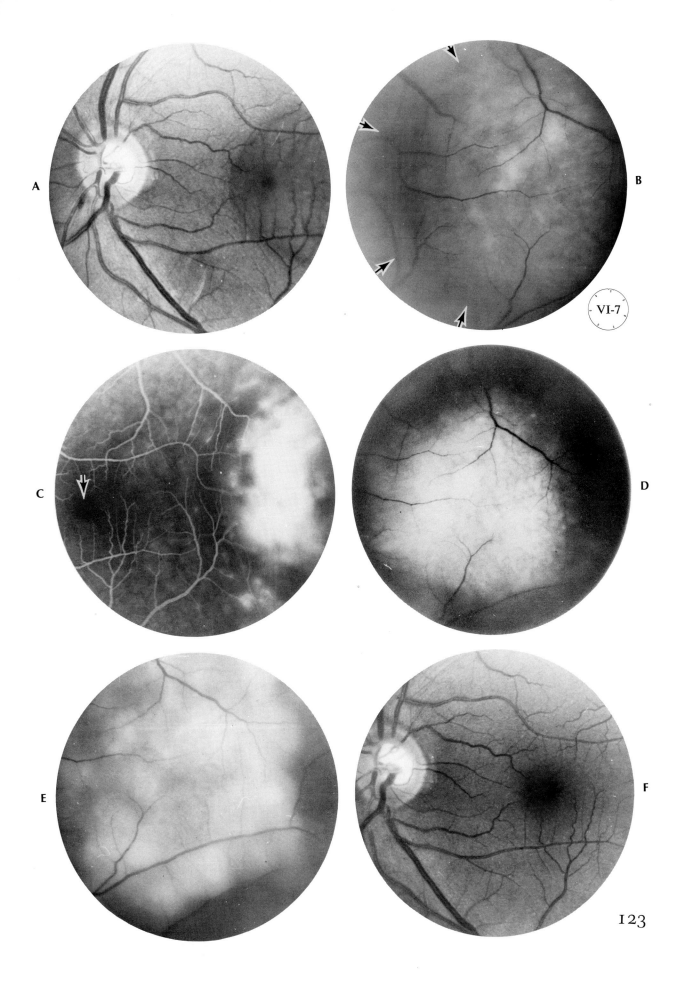

Fig. 4-4. Pigmentary migration into the retina secondary to long-standing retinal detachment associated with a choroidal hemangioma. A 46-year-old white woman noted rapid loss of the superior field of vision in her right eye 6 years previously. This gradually improved over a period of 6 months. She was asymptomatic thereafter. On a routine eye examination 5½ years later a mass was discovered in the right eye. Her visual acuity was 20/25 in both eyes. The left fundus was normal.

A and **B,** Just superior to the right optic disc there was an elevated reddish choroidal tumor (its nasal margins are indicated by *small arrows*). On the nasal margins of the tumor there was a broad zone of depigmentation of the pigment epithelium (the nasal margin of this zone is indicated by the *large arrows*) that extended nasal to the optic disc and inferiorly almost as far as the equator. There was bone spicule migration of pigment into the retina within the superior portion of this zone. There was mottled yellowish material lying on the surface of the tumor.

C to **E,** Fluorescein angiography revealed diffusion of dye from the tumor surface and evidence of loss of pigment in a large area *(arrows)* extending inferior to the tumor.

F, Note the nonfluorescent ring *(arrows)* near the tumor margin. This is probably caused by proliferative changes in the pigment epithelium. Note the pigment surrounding the retinal vein at the upper margin of the tumor. This patient probably had a long-standing secondary detachment that extended inferior to the hemangioma. Spontaneous reattachment of the retina in such cases may be followed by migration of pigment into the overlying retina (see Fig. 2-15).

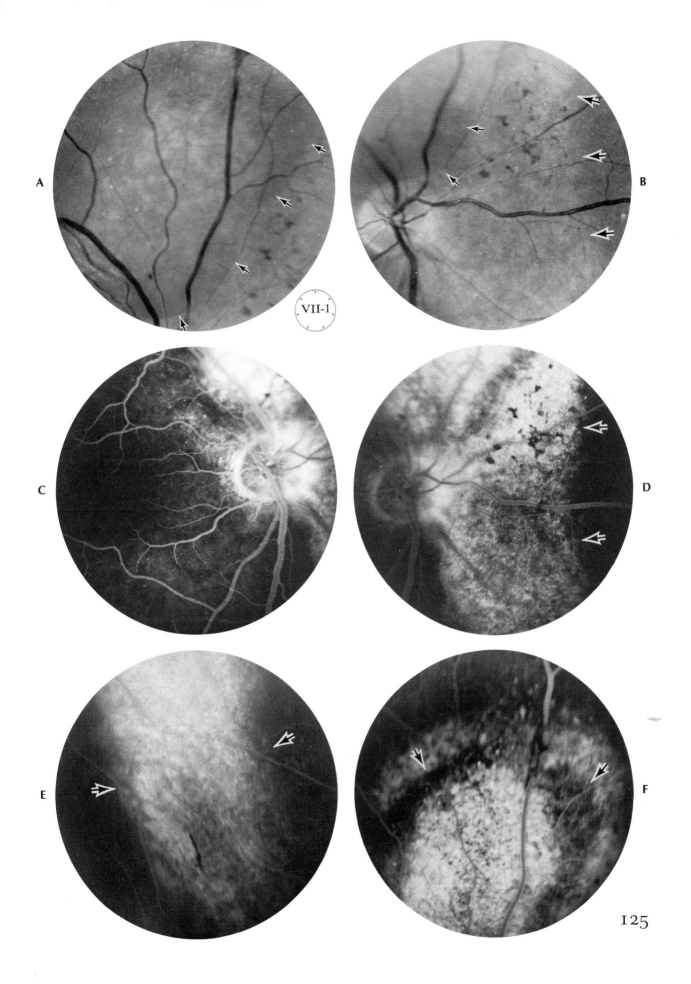

Fig. 4-5. Choroidal hemangioma unassociated with extensive damage to the retinal pigment epithelium or cystic degeneration of the retina. A 39-year-old white man was examined because of failure to pass his recent driver's test. He stated that the vision in his left eye had always been fuzzy compared with the right eye. His visual acuity in the right eye was 20/20 and in the left eye was 20/70.

A and **B,** A large red, round, tumefaction of the choroid extended from the macula out to the equator temporally. The tumor's edge bisected the fovea. There was no evidence of serous detachment. The overlying pigment epithelium and retina appeared normal.

C and **D,** The early phases of angiography revealed mottled hyperfluorescence as well as evidence of large vascular channels in the area of the tumor. Note the many large relatively hypofluorescent blood vessels surrounded by fluorescein staining of the extravascular tissues within the tumor.

E, The fluorescence gradually faded from view and the later stages of angiography appeared relatively normal.

F, Ultrasonography revealed evidence of a solid choroidal tumor *(arrows)*. This patient is unusual in that this fairly large, highly elevated, vascular tumor has caused little or no degenerative or exudative changes in the overlying pigment epithelium and retina. Thirty months later the visual function and the tumor were unchanged.

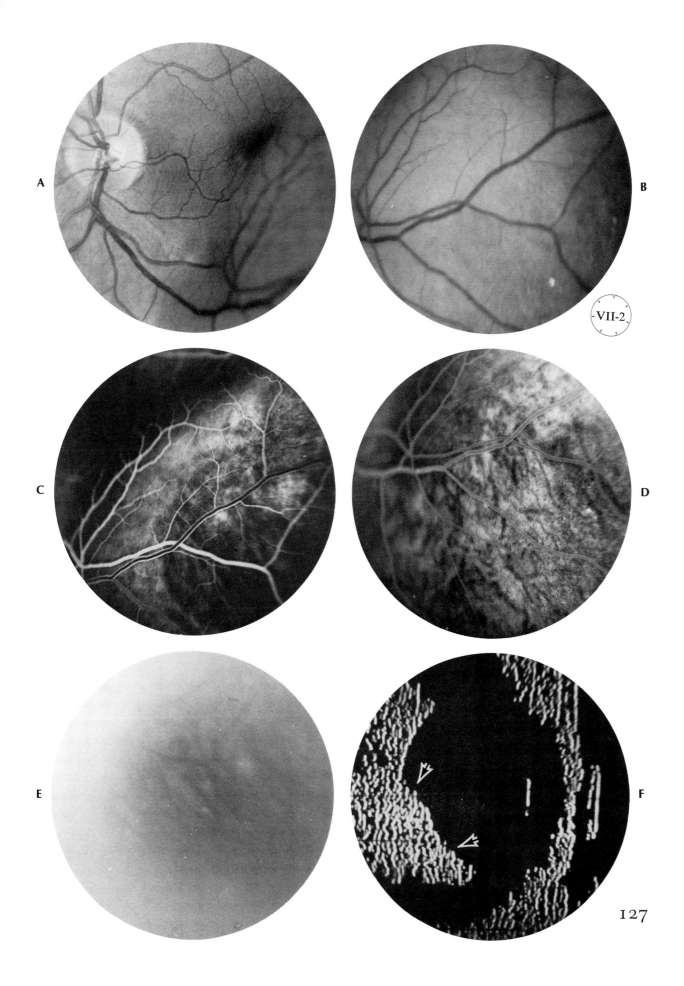

Fig. 4-6. Histopathologic findings in choroidal hemangiomas in four eyes enucleated with the mistaken diagnosis of malignant intraocular tumors.

A, This 66-year-old white woman was seen because of loss of vision secondary to a retinal detachment. She had a large elevated, reddish tumor (*arrows*) at the superonasal margin of the right optic disc. The lesion was diagnosed as a possible malignant melanoma and the eye was enucleated. (From Norton et al.[3])

B, Histopathologic examination of the lesion shown in **A** revealed a cavernous hemangioma of the choroid underlying an area of cystic degeneration of the overlying retina. The retina was artifactitiously detached. (From Norton et al.[3])

C and **D,** High-power view of the lesion depicted in **B** showing cystic retinal degenerative changes, scattered pigment-laden cells in the retina (*arrows*), and extensive degenerative changes in the pigment epithelium overlying the cavernous hemangioma.

E, This choroidal hemangioma was misdiagnosed clinically as a melanoma. Note the extensive cystic degeneration of the retina, which is thickened and is adherent to the underlying hemangioma by means of a plaque of fibrous metaplasia and proliferation of the pigment epithelium. Clinically this tumor may have presented as a partly pigmented mass simulating a melanoma.

F and **G,** Histopathologic findings in this cavernous hemangioma, which was misdiagnosed as a melanoma, revealed extensive thickening of the retina in the macular area. Note the thick plaque of metaplastic pigment epithelium overlying the extramacular portion of the tumor (*arrow*). Plaques of tissue such as this may be responsible for the hypofluorescent halo seen angiographically at the margins of hemangiomas.

H, An 8-year-old black girl was struck in the right eye with a basketball. Her eye was red for a few days. Two months later she developed a mature cataract in the right eye. She was the product of a full-term normal pregnancy and delivery. The past medical history was unremarkable except for a single episode of febrile seizure. On examination the visual

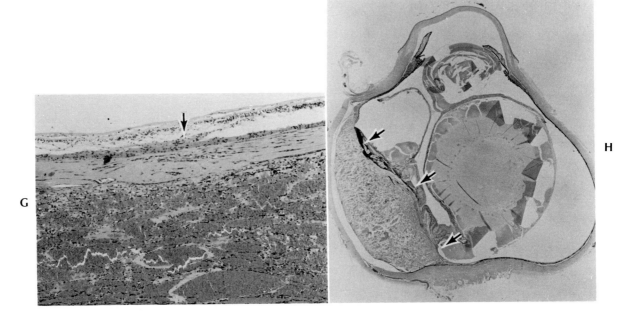

acuity in the right eye was questionable light perception, and the left eye was 20/30. The eye was enucleated because of possible retinoblastoma. The pathologic examination revealed a large cavernous hemangioma of the choroid (*arrows*) extending from the optic disc nasally to the pars plana. This was associated with a massive retinal detachment and a cataract.

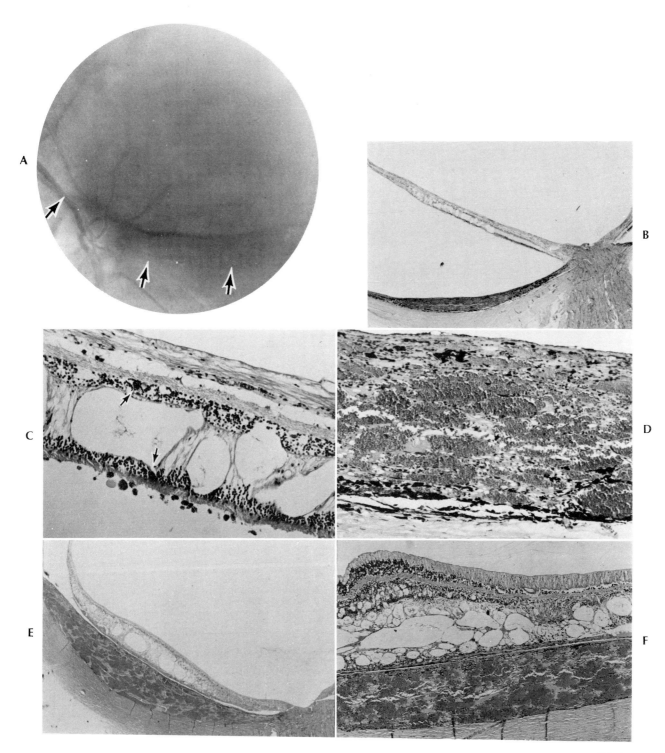

Fig. 4-7. Sturge-Weber syndrome.

A and **B.** Right and left eyes respectively of a child with the Sturge-Weber syndrome with nevus flammeus involving the left side of the face. The large choroidal vessels in the normal fundus of the right eye were easily seen. The left fundus appeared red and no vascular details of the choroid were visible.

C, This 3-year-old white child with Sturge-Weber syndrome was seen for evaluation of possible glaucoma in the left eye. Note the nevus flammeus involving the left side of the upper face and both sides of the lower face. There was noticeable hypertrophy of the left side of the face and tongue. Heterochromia iridis was present. The intraocular pressures in both eyes were normal. The fundus of the right eye was blond and the fundus of the left eye showed a prominent reddish hue, but otherwise was unremarkable.

D, Sturge-Weber syndrome in a 17-year-old black girl. Note the nevus flammeus over the right side of the forehead. Both eyes were normal and of equal size. There was glaucomatous cupping and evidence of a diffuse angioma of the choroid in the right eye (see Fig. 4-8).

E, Skull x-ray of a patient with Sturge-Weber syndrome showing the typical railroad-track calcification of the vascular anomaly of the brain.

F, Vascular anomaly of the brain associated with Sturge-Weber syndrome.

(**A** and **B** from Smith[4]; **C** from Gass[5a]; **E** from Gass[5b]; and **F** from Alexander et al.[6])

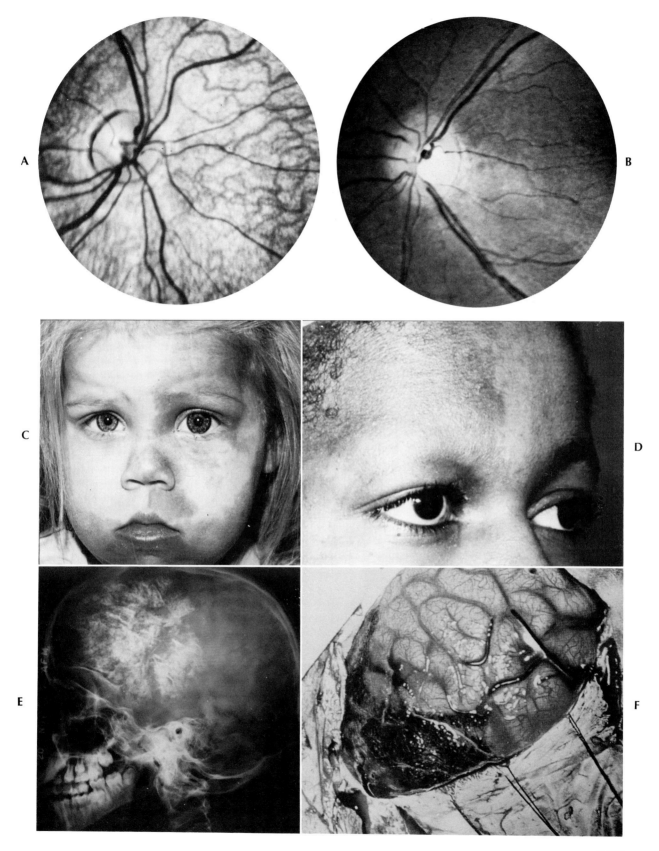

Fig. 4-8. Diffuse choroidal hemangioma in Sturge-Weber syndrome. A 17-year-old black female with Sturge-Weber syndrome and nevus flammeus involving the right forehead and right upper lid (Fig. 4-7, *D*) was examined because of glaucoma in her right eye. She gave a history of seizures since early childhood. Visual acuity in both eyes was 20/20.

A, There was diffuse thickening of the choroid associated with irregular hyperpigmentation of the pigment epithelium, particularly in the area surrounding the optic disc and over the inferior half of the fundus. There was deep cupping of the optic nerve head.

B to **D,** The arterial phases of angiography showed a prominent choroidal flush involving the upper half of the fundus. This rapidly disappeared and the later phases of angiography were normal except for the hypovascularity of the atrophic optic disc.

E, Left fundus of the same patient. Note the color difference between the normal left fundus and the right fundus in **A**.

F, Normal angiogram in the left eye.

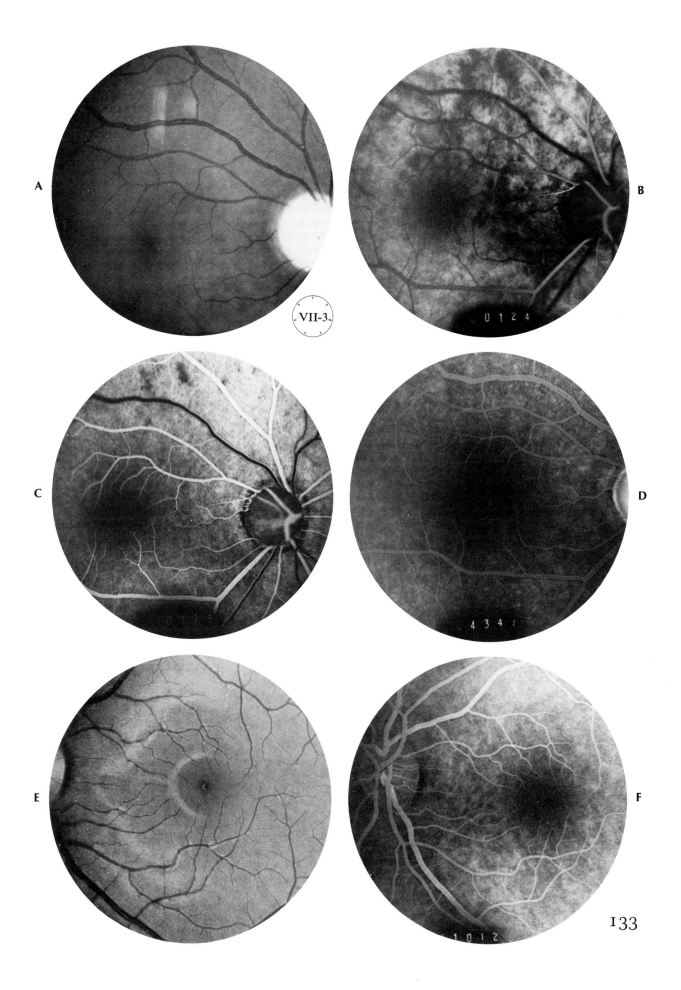

A

B

C

D

E

F

VII-3

I33

Fig. 4-9. Localized choroidal hemangioma in Sturge-Weber syndrome.

A, A 9-year-old white boy with nevus flammeus of the right side of his face was initially examined at age 7, at which time visual acuity in the right eye was 20/40 and in the left eye was 20/20. His local ophthalmologist noted no abnormality at that time. In November 1971, the visual acuity decreased further. His local physician noted a mass in the inferior fundus for the first time. His intraocular pressure was normal and there was no cupping of the optic discs. The patient was seen initially at the Bascom Palmer Eye Institute in January 1972, with an elevated, reddish tumor involving most of the inferior half of the fundus. It extended up to and bisected the macula. There was serous detachment of the retina overlying the tumor except in one area temporal to the macula where a four-by-six-disc-diameter-size, oval, gray-white exudative membrane was present between the tumor and overlying retina. The retinal detachment did not extend into the superior fundus. The patient was lost to follow-up until March 1973, when he returned with only light perception in the right eye.

B, At that time he had a total bullous detachment of the retina except in the gray-white area (indicated in *black* in the fundus drawing at *arrow*) where the retina was adherent to the tumor (*stippled area* in the fundus drawing).

C, The gray-white subretinal membrane (*arrows*) was unchanged. The pigment epithelium appeared to be normal elsewhere over the surface of the tumor.

D, Fluorescein angiography revealed diffusion of dye from the surface of the tumor into the gray-white subretinal membrane temporal to the macula. There was no evidence of abnormal choroidal fluorescence elsewhere.

E, Heavy xenon photocoagulation was used to treat the area of the subretinal membrane.

F, In May 1973, the retina was completely flat and the visual acuity had returned to 20/400. Note the faint traction lines radiating through the central macular area (*arrow*) toward the area of photocoagulation temporal to the macula.

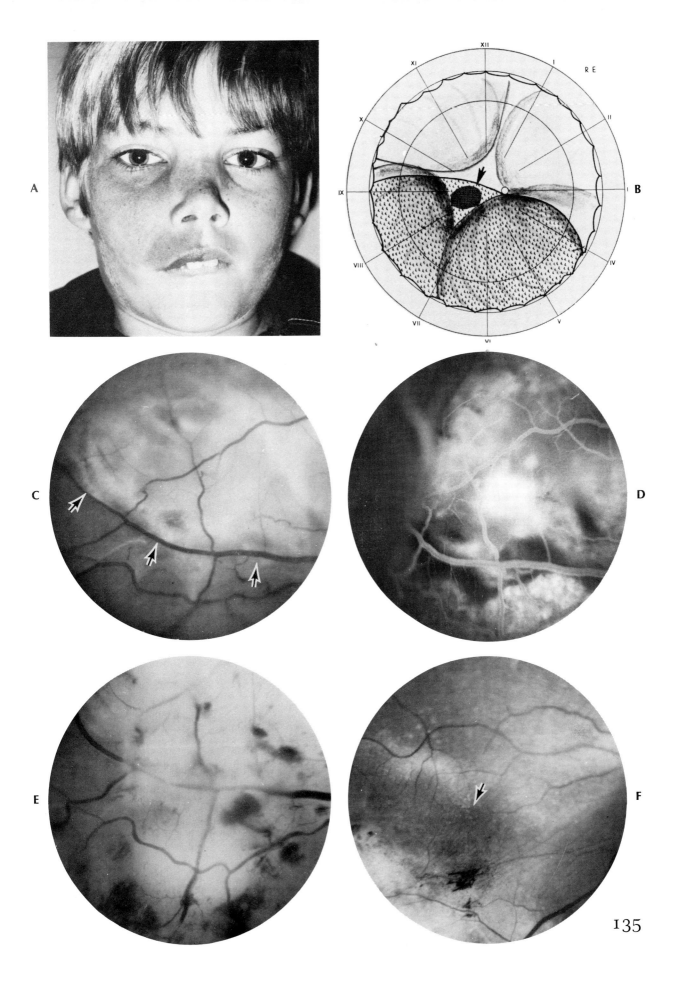

135

Fig. 4-10. Histopathologic condition of diffuse choroidal angioma in the Sturge-Weber syndrome.

A, Note the diffuse thickening of the choroid and the advanced glaucomatous cupping in this patient with the Sturge-Weber syndrome. Note that the pigment epithelium and the overlying retina are normal. The retinal detachment is artifactitious.

B, The anterior chamber angle of the same patient illustrated in **A** shows a relatively normal trabecular meshwork except for incomplete cleavage of the angle. There is no evidence of angiomatous involvement of the ciliary body.

(**A** from Gass[5c]; **B** from Gass.[5d])

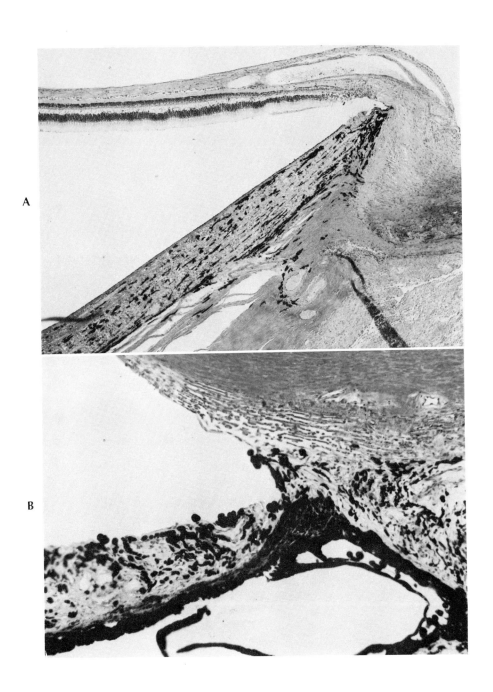

REFERENCES

1. Gass, J. D. M.: Stereoscopic atlas of macular diseases, St. Louis, 1970, The C. V. Mosby Co., p. 85.
2. Gass, J. D. M.: Photocoagulation of macular lesions, Trans. Am. Acad. Ophthalmol. Otolaryngol. **75:**580-608, 1971.
3. Norton, E. W. D., Smith, J. L., Curtin, V. T., and Justice, J., Jr.: Fluorescein fundus photography: An aid in the differential diagnosis of posterior ocular lesions. Trans. Am. Acad. Ophthalmol. Otolaryngol. **68:**755-765, 1964.
4. Susac, J. O., Smith, J. L., Scelfo, R. J.: The "tomato catsup" fundus in Sturge-Weber syndrome. Arch. Opthalmol. **92:**69-70, 1974.
5. Gass, J. D. M.: The phakomatoses. In Lawton Smith, J. (editor): Neuro-ophthalmology. Vol. II. Symposium of the University of Miami and the Bascom Palmer Eye Institute. St. Louis, 1965, The C. V. Mosby Co., (a) p. 254, (b) p. 258, (c) p. 256, and (d) p. 255.
6. Alexander, G. L., and Norman, R. M.: The Sturge-Weber syndrome, Bristol, 1060, John Wright & Sons, Ltd., p. 95.

SUGGESTED READINGS

Ballantyne, A. J.: Buphthalmos with facial nevus and allied conditions, Brit. J. Ophthalmol. **14:**481-495, 1930.
Gass, J. D. M.: Pathogenesis of disciform detachment of the neuroepithelium. VI. Disciform detachment secondary to heredodegenerative, neoplastic and traumatic lesions of the choroid, Am. J. Ophthalmol. **63:**689-711, 1967.
Jones, I. S., and Cleasby, G. W.: Hemangioma of the choroid: A clinicopathologic analysis, Am. J. Ophthalmol. **48:**612-628, 1959.
Joy, H. H.: Nevus flammeus associated with glaucoma, Am. J. Ophthalmol. **33:**1401-1409, 1950.
MacLean, A. L., and Maumenee, A. E.: Hemangioma of the choroid, Am. J. Ophthalmol. **50:**3-11, 1960.
Norton, E. W. D., and Gutman, F.: Fluorescein angiography and hemangiomas of the choroid, Arch. Ophthalmol. **78:**121-125, 1967.
Smith, J. L., David, N. J., Hart, L. M., Levenson, D. S., and Tillett, C. W.: Hemangioma of the choroid. Fluorescein photography and photocoagulation, Arch. Ophthalmol. **69:**51-54, 1963.
Stokes, J. J.: The ocular manifestations of the Sturge-Weber syndrome, Southern Med. J. **50:**82-89, 1957.

Metastatic tumors of the uveal tract

Although metastatic tumors of the uveal tract usually occur in patients with a previous history of a primary malignancy, ocular symptoms may occasionally be the presenting complaints of a patient with an unrecognized malignancy. Metastatic tumors may occur in the eye years after the primary tumor was removed. Metastatic tumors of the uveal tract are more common in females and are more common in adults. The age of peak incidence is between 40 and 50 years. They occur more frequently in the left eye. The lesion occurs bilaterally in approximately 20 to 25 percent of patients. They may occur in patients without clinical evidence of pulmonary metastasis. The lesion may occur anywhere in the uveal tract, but most occur in the posterior choroid on the temporal side. Most of the tumors grow in a relatively flat and diffuse manner in the choroid. Some, however, may be globular and elevated and may duplicate in every way the variety of growth patterns seen in malignant melanomas. The female breast is the most common primary site. In males the lung is the most common primary site. Other primary sites of metastatic tumor seen at the Bascom Palmer Eye Institute include the prostate, thyroid, intestine, testes, skin (melanoma), and pancreas.

CHOROIDAL METASTASIS

Localized tumefactions of the choroid secondary to metastatic carcinoma (Figs. 5-1 to 5-6) and melanoma (Fig. 5-8) may be confused with other tumors arising in the choroid. These tumors are typically amelanotic, white or cream-colored, slightly elevated lesions with ill-defined margins. Patients usually become symptomatic only after developing serous detachment of the retina, frequently in the macular area. Approximately one fourth of the patients will show multiple choroidal lesions in one or both eyes. Similar lesions may involve the anterior uveal tract (Fig. 5-8). The pigment epithelium and retina overlying the flat lesions may be uninvolved (Fig. 5-1, A). Fluorescein angiography in such cases show little or no abnormality in the area of the tumor. Growth is usually, but not always, rapid and is accompanied by secondary changes in the overlying pigment epithelium and serous retinal detachment. Pigment epithelial changes include depigmentation, degeneration, mobilization, and destruction of the pigment epithelium (Fig. 5-1, D). Fluorescein angiography in such cases shows hyperfluorescence in the areas of depigmentation of the pigment epithelium and late fluorescence from staining of the exudate that collects beneath either the pigment epithelium or retina. Blotchy clumps of dark gray or orange pigment may be deposited on the tumor surface (Fig. 5-4). These pigment changes may be misinterpreted as evidence of pigment production by the tumor. Biomicroscopy is invaluable in differentiating this superficial pigment from that within the substance of a melanoma. Cloudy subretinal exudate may obscure details of the underlying tumor (Fig. 5-3, A). Angiography in such cases will reveal multiple areas of diffusion of dye from the surface of the tumor into the subretinal exudate. Metastatic tumors often infiltrate laterally without becoming elevated. Globular growth of metastatic tumors (Figs. 5-4 and 5-6) occurs less frequently. In such tumors large dilated blood vessels within the tumor may be visible ophthalmoscopically and angiographically (Fig. 5-4, A). These tumor vessels are more commonly seen in malignant melanomas than in metastatic tumors of the choroid. Hemorrhagic detachment of the pigment epithelium and retina overlying metastatic tumors, though uncommon, does occur (Fig. 5-6) and may lead to the mistaken diagnosis of a degenerative lesion or a malignant melanoma. Although metastatic tumors may become quite elevated, they rarely break through Bruch's membrane. When they are globular in form, metastatic tumors are more difficult and at times impossible to differentiate from amelanotic melanomas of the choroid. No special techniques of examination including fluorescein angiography, P-32 radioactive uptake studies, and ultrasonography are of proved value in differentiating an amelanotic melanoma of the choroid from a metastatic tumor. Pain is a feature that may occur occasionally in patients with metastatic choroidal tumors but is rare in malignant melanoma. The creamy white color and absence of cystoid degeneration of the overlying retina serve to differentiate metastatic tumors from a choroidal hemangioma that is orange-red color and usually associated with overlying cystic degeneration of the retina. The multiple flat yellow-white lesions occurring in young patient with acute posterior multifocal placoid pigment epitheliopathy may occasionally be mistaken for metastatic carcinoma. Fluorescein angiography, however, usually reveals these pigment epithelial lesions to be much more discretely hypofluorescent during the early phases of angiography than is the case in metastatic carcinoma. The absence of subretinal exudation and the rapid resolution of the lesions in the matter of several weeks is another important feature in differentiating these lesions from metastatic carcinoma.

Metastatic carcinoma of the choroid may also invade and replace the optic nerve head (Fig. 5-7). When this occurs, the patient usually has profound loss of visual function.

Any patient suspected of having a metastatic tumor to the choroid must be carefully evaluated for the presence of a primary lesion. Careful breast examination in women and chest x-ray examination in men are of particular importance, since these are the two most common primary sites for metastatic carcinoma to the eye. Blood counts and bone marrow examination may also help in detecting leukemia, which may mimic in every way metastatic carcinoma, although it more typically presents as a more diffuse choroidal involvement rather than a localized tumefaction (see Chapter 6).

Although the life expectancy of a patient with metastatic carcinoma of the choroid is seldom greater than 2 years, these patients should be considered for therapy if they retain useful vision function and if their general health is otherwise good. The choroidal lesions may respond favorably to antimetabolite, hormonal, or x-ray irradiation therapy (Figs. 5-3 and 5-6). Photocoagulation may be considered in patients with relatively small lesions.

CILIARY BODY AND IRIS METASTASIS

Metastatic tumors to the anterior uveal tract (Figs. 5-8, *F*, and 15-6) occur much less frequently than in the choroid. They are usually difficult to differentiate from amelanotic melanomas.

RETINAL METASTASIS

Metastatic tumors of the retina are rare and none have been seen at the Bascom Palmer Eye Institute.

Fig. 5-1. Small metastatic carcinomas of the choroid. A 47-year-old white woman had multiple foci of metastatic carcinoma of the breast to the choroid in both eyes.

A, This lesion was unassociated with changes in the overlying pigment epithelium or retina.

B and **C,** Angiography showed slight hypofluorescence in the area of space-occupying lesion in the choroid (*arrows*).

D, A 56-year-old woman had known metastatic breast carcinoma. She had a localized slightly raised metastatic lesion in the choroid of the right eye. There was loss of pigment from the overlying pigment epithelium, and a localized serous detachment of the retina.

E and **F,** Angiography revealed early hyperfluorescence caused by changes in the pigment epithelium and multiple areas of diffusion of dye from the surface of the tumor into the subretinal fluid (*arrows*). The pinpoint areas of fluorescein staining are similar to that seen in malignant melanomas of the choroid (see Figs. 3-2, 3-4, 3-6, and 3-7).

(**A** to **C** from Gass.[1])

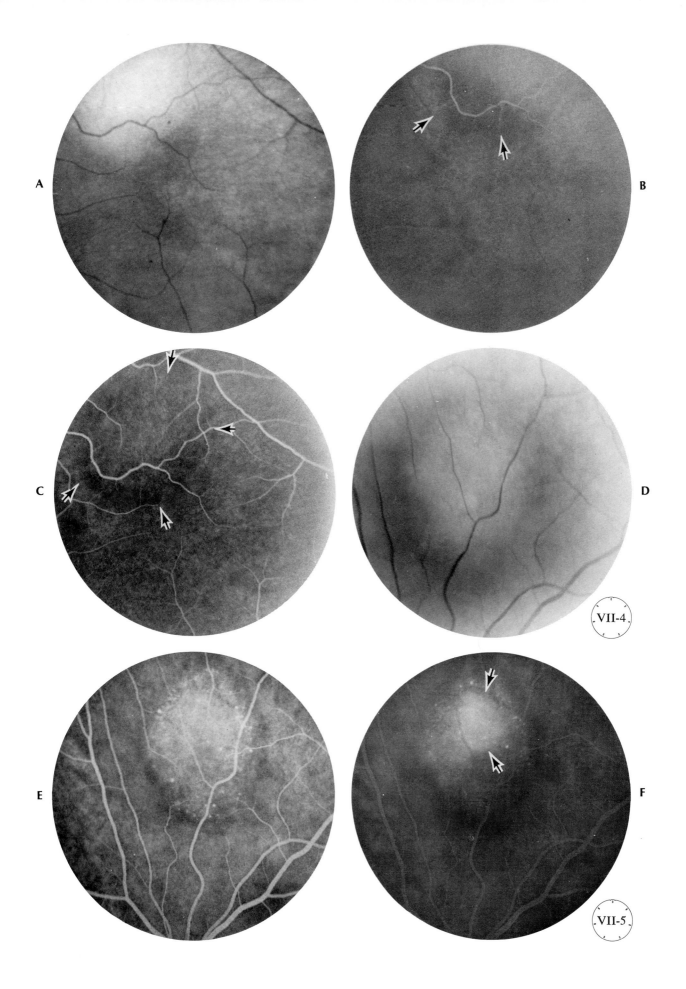

VII-4

VII-5

Fig. 5-2. Metastatic lung carcinoma to the choroid. A 54-year-old white woman noted a positive scotoma in her right eye on January 9, 1972. One month previously she had developed congestive heart failure and cardiomegaly and was digitalized. Visual acuity in the right eye was 20/30 and in the left eye was 20/20.

A and **B,** Funduscopic examination of the right eye revealed four small white slightly elevated choroidal lesions in the posterior pole of the right eye. There were five similar lesions present in the left eye.

C, Fluorescein angiography revealed an area of hyperfluorescence *(arrow)* overlying the tumor in the macular area. The later angiogram revealed evidence of faint staining in this same area. The patient died on March 17, 1972. At autopsy she had a small lesion in the lower lobe of the left lung. In addition, she had multiple metastatic lesions in the heart. The pathologic diagnosis was alveolar cell carcinoma of the lung.

D, The histopathologic examination of the macular lesion in the right eye revealed a focal area of infiltration of the choroid by adenocarcinoma. There was artifactitious detachment of the pigment epithelium except in the area overlying the central portion of the tumor *(arrows).*

E, High-power view of the retinal pigment epithelium overlying the tumor. There was pronounced elongation of the retinal pigment epithelial cells. Note the pigment epithelial granules are concentrated in the anterior extension of the pigment epithelial cells. The nuclei are visible in the basal part of the cell.

F, Relatively normal pigment epithelium at the site of junction where the pigment epithelium was artifactitiously detached (see **D**).

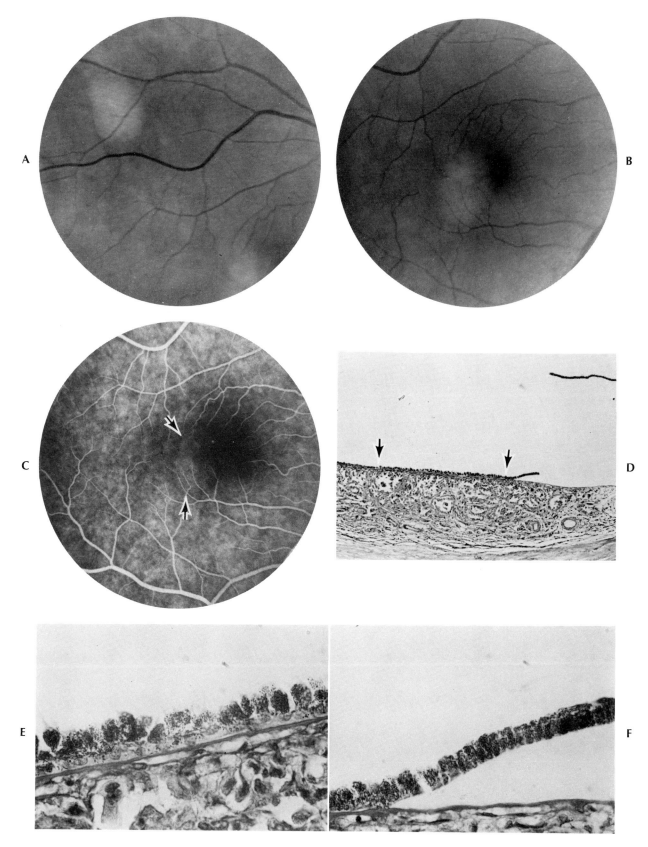

Fig. 5-3. Partial resolution of metastatic breast carcinoma to the choroid after cobalt therapy. A 56-year-old white woman was first examined on July 26, 1965. She had a 2-week history of blurred vision in the right eye. Two years previously she had a mastectomy for breast carcinoma. Visual acuity in the right eye was finger counting at 5 feet.

A, There was an elevated white choroidal mass superior to the right optic disc. Cloudy subretinal exudate covered the surface of the tumor and extended inferior to the macula. Two other small choroidal nodules were present elsewhere in the right eye and a single lesion was present in the left eye.

B to **E,** Angiography revealed a broad area of diffusion of the dye from the tumor surface into the overlying subretinal exudate. The pattern of staining in this case was similar to that seen in a large serous detachment of the pigment epithelium. The patient had cobalt therapy to the right eye in August 1965 and soon thereafter noted improvement in her visual acuity.

F, On October 5, 1965, her visual acuity was 20/30. The choroidal lesion was flat and the subretinal exudate had resolved. Note the distinct changes in the pigment epithelium at the site of the tumor. Repeat angiography demonstrated loss of the pigment from the pigment epithelium and multiple areas of fluorescence caused by clumping of the pigment epithelium. There are oblique dark lines *(arrows)* transversing the area of pigment epithelial change. These are probably caused by chorioretinal folding secondary to the rapid resolution of the choroidal tumor and perhaps to some shrinkage of the underlying sclera.

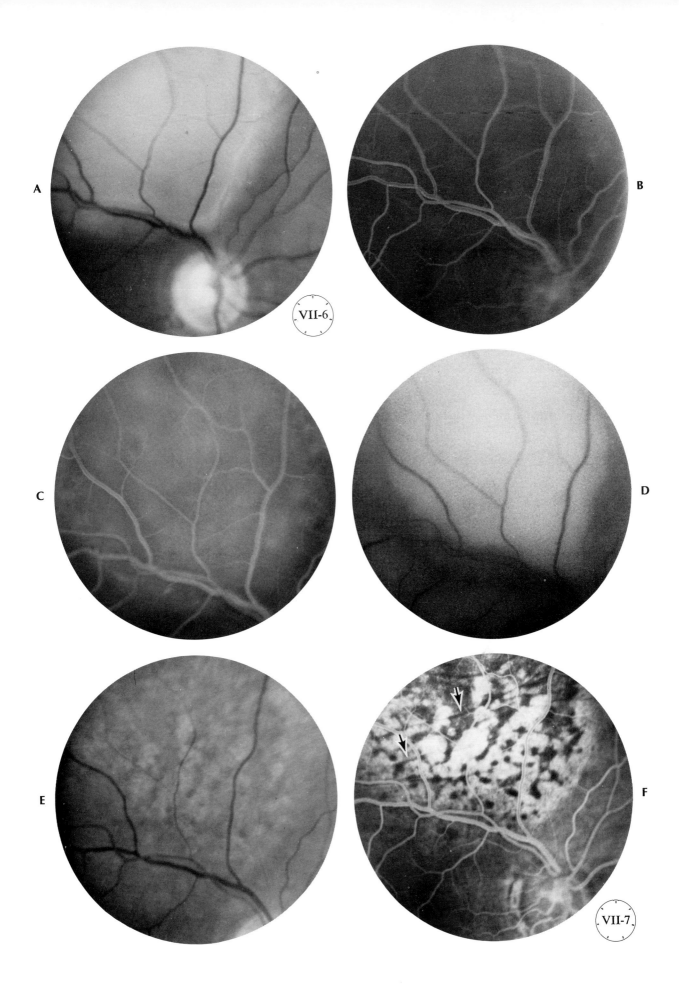

Fig. 5-4. Large choroidal tumor attributable to metastatic breast carcinoma. A 59-year-old white woman with breast carcinoma developed loss of vision in the right eye.

A and **B,** A large, highly elevated, nonpigmented tumor was present in the choroid nasally in the right eye. Note the reticulated pattern of pigment on the tumor surface and the prominent vessels within the tumor *(arrows).*

C, Prearterial phase.

D, Arterial phase revealed perfusion of large blood vessels *(arrows)* near the tumor surface. The angiographic demonstration of large blood vessels in the choroidal is a feature that has been referred to as "double circulation" and is more often demonstrated in melanomas than in metastatic tumors.

E and **F,** Late angiogram showed extensive staining of the subretinal fluid overlying the surface of the tumor.

(From Gass.[1])

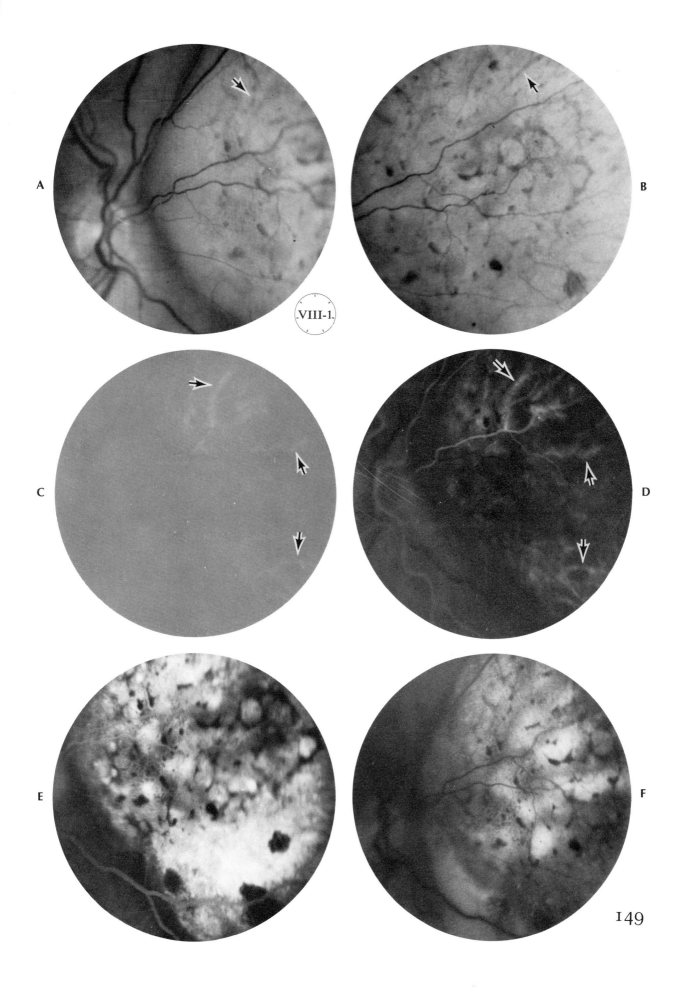

Fig. 5-5. Macular detachment secondary to metastatic thyroid carcinoma to the choroid. On May 24, 1972, a 54-year-old white man noted photopsia and a paracentral scotoma in his right eye. His visual acuity was 20/15 bilaterally.

A, A slightly elevated nonpigmented choroidal tumor with some overlying serous retinal detachment was present in the superotemporal macula area.

B and **C,** Angiography revealed multiple areas of dye diffusion from the tumor into the overlying subretinal exudate.

D, In September 1972, his visual acuity in the right eye was 20/70. The tumor and the area of detachment had spread into the central macular region. In October 1972, a metastatic bone survey showed normal results. In November 1972, the patient was reevaluated and a metastatic bone survey revealed five nodules in the lung and focal metastatic lesions in the ribs, vertebrae, and pelvis. A biopsy of a rib lesion revealed a papillary adenocarcinoma believed to have arisen in the thyroid gland. A thyroid scan showed multinodular hot and cold areas within the tumor. He received cyclophosphamide and x-ray irradiation treatment to areas of metastatic involvement including 2,800 R to the right eye in the period of December 6 to 26, 1972. He died on January 16, 1973, because of aortic insufficiency.

E and **F,** Histopathologic examination of the right eye revealed a metastatic papillary adenocarcinoma of the choroid. There were extensive areas of tumor necrosis, probably secondary to the antimetabolite and x-ray therapy. Note the extensive degenerative changes in the pigment epithelium overlying the tumor.

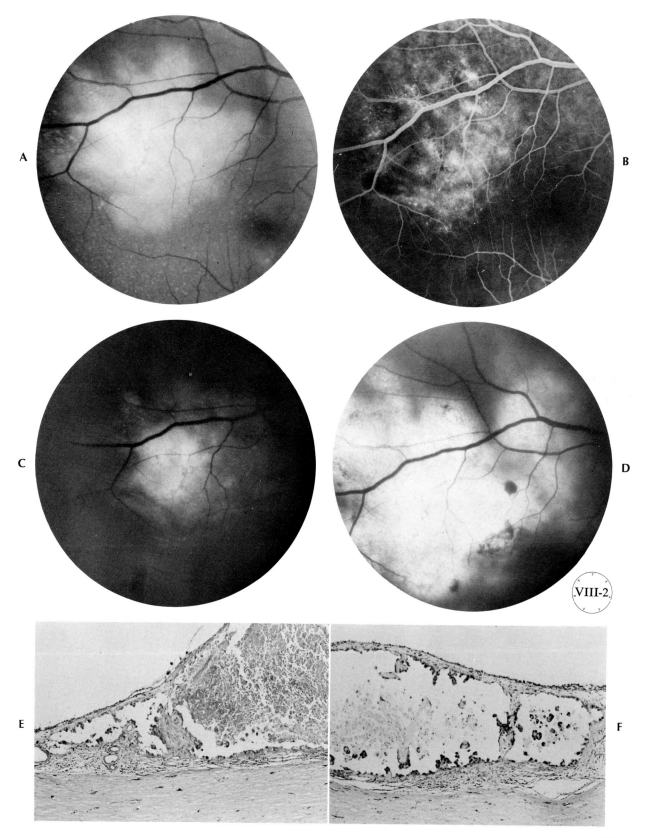

Fig. 5-6. Bilateral hemorrhagic detachment of the macula secondary to metastatic breast carcinoma to the choroid. A 40-year-old black woman with known metastatic breast carcinoma developed bilateral loss of central vision.

A, A large, highly elevated tumor largely covered by subretinal blood and exudate was present inferotemporally to the optic disc in the right eye.

B and **C,** Early angiograms revealed no evidence of fluorescence of the lesion because of the overlying subretinal blood.

D, The 1-hour angiogram revealed some staining of the serosanguinous subretinal exudate.

E, A similar lesion was present in the superotemporal area of the macula of the left eye.

F, Angiography revealed obscuration of the choroidal and tumor fluorescence by the subretinal blood. This lesion might be mistaken for a hemorrhagic and disciform detachment overlying a degenerative or inflammatory lesion.

G, The clinical appearance of the eye illustrated below probably appeared similar to the two eyes above. It was enucleated with the mistaken diagnosis of malignant melanoma. Histopathologic examination revealed a large hemorrhagic detachment of the pigment epithelium and retina (*arrows*) overlying a metastatic carcinoma.

(**E** to **G** from Gass.[2])

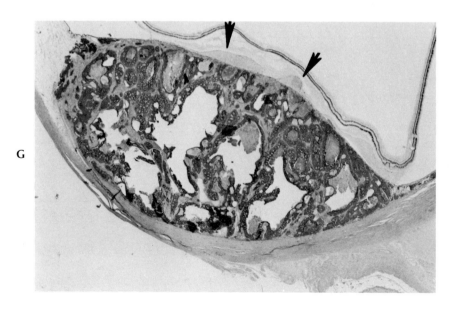

G

152

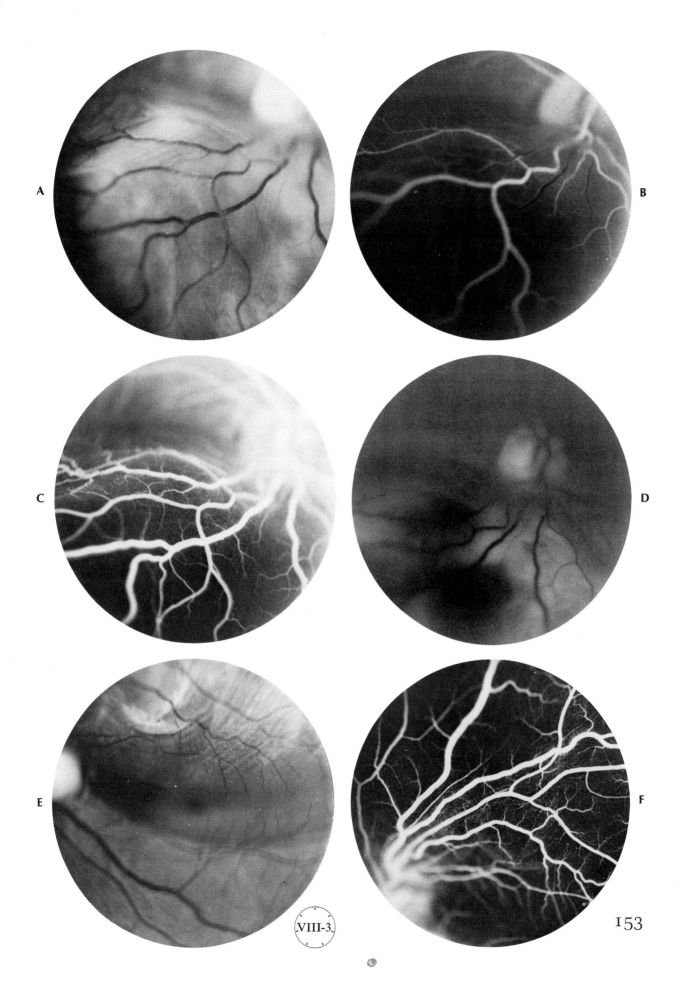

153

Fig. 5-7. Metastatic lung carcinoma to the optic nerve and choroid. A 42-year-old black man with carcinoma of the lung developed complete loss of vision in the left eye.

A, The optic nerve head and surrounding choroid were infiltrated with a white tumor. The large blood vessels on the optic nerve head were obscured by the tumor. There was an exudative detachment of the retina.

B and **D,** Angiography revealed dilatation of some of the capillaries on the optic nerve head and progressive staining of the swollen nerve head. The photograph shows extensive staining of the subretinal exudate.

E, The patient died soon after the above photographic study. A low-power view showed that the nerve fibers of the optic nerve had been completely replaced by the metastatic tumor, which had also invaded the peripapillary choroid. The retina was totally detached.

F, A high-power view of a cross section of the optic nerve revealed complete replacement of the nerve tissue by tumor.

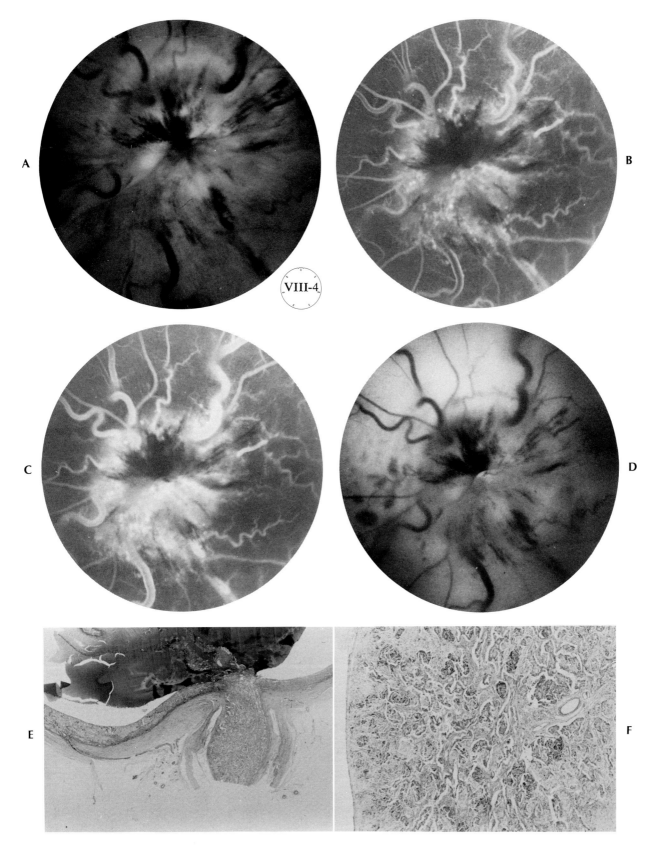

Fig. 5-8. Metastatic skin melanoma to the choroid and ciliary body. A 49-year-old man developed headache, nausea, vomiting, uncinate fits, and severe photophobia. His visual acuity was 20/15 in each eye. Several years previously a pigmented tumor was removed from his back.

A, He had bilateral papilledema and in the left eye had a small white choroidal nodule (*arrows*).

B and **C,** Angiography revealed dilated optic nerve head capillaries and leakage of dye into the subretinal exudate overlying the choroidal tumor.

D, One month later the papilledema was less. The choroidal nodule was larger.

E, At craniotomy there was diffuse infiltration of the meninges and the left temporal lobe by malignant melanoma cells. The patient died soon thereafter.

F, There was a localized nonpigmented tumor composed of amelanotic melanoma cells involving the ciliary processes of the left eye.

G, The choroidal nodule in the left macula area was composed of amelanotic melanoma cells. Note the degenerative changes in the overlying pigment epithelium, the small amount of subretinal exudate adherent to the artifactitiously detached retina, and the three focal areas (*arrows*) where globules of eosinophilic exudate extend through the pigment epithelium.

(**A** to **D** and **G** from Gass.[2])

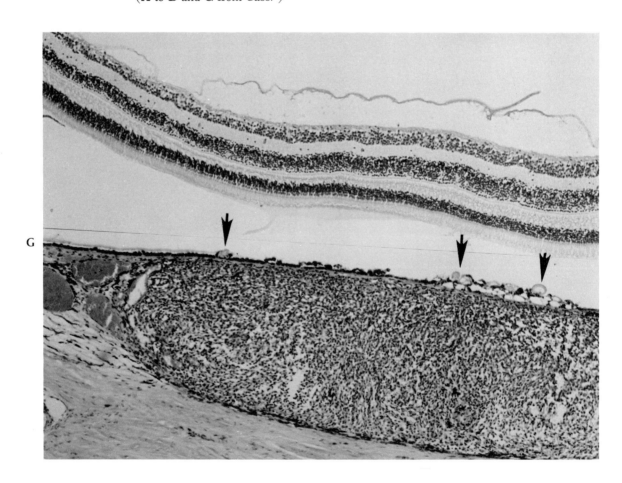

A
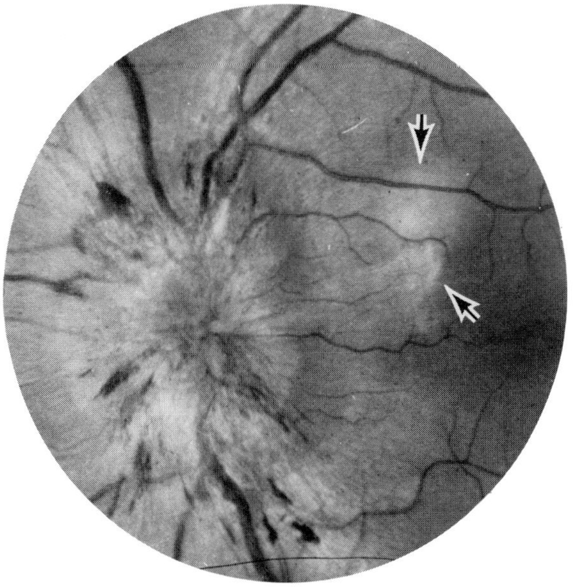
B
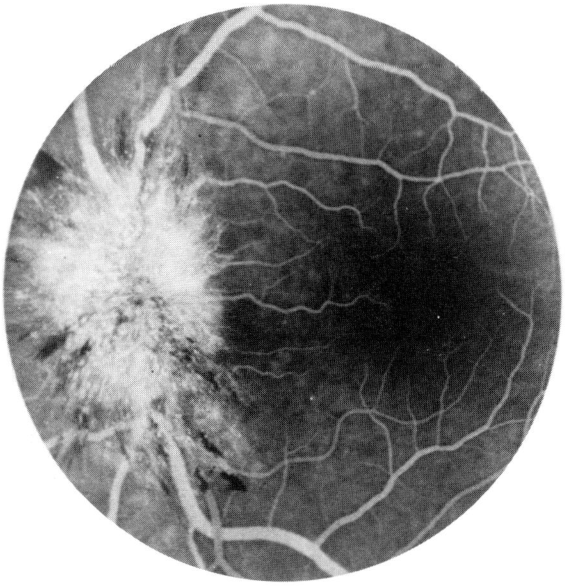
C
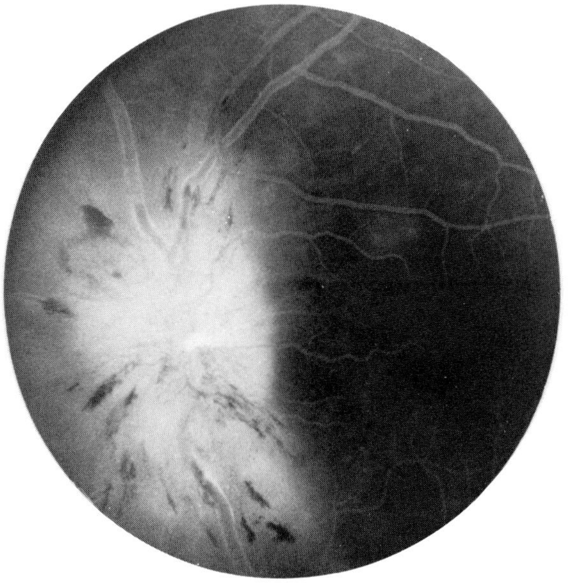
D
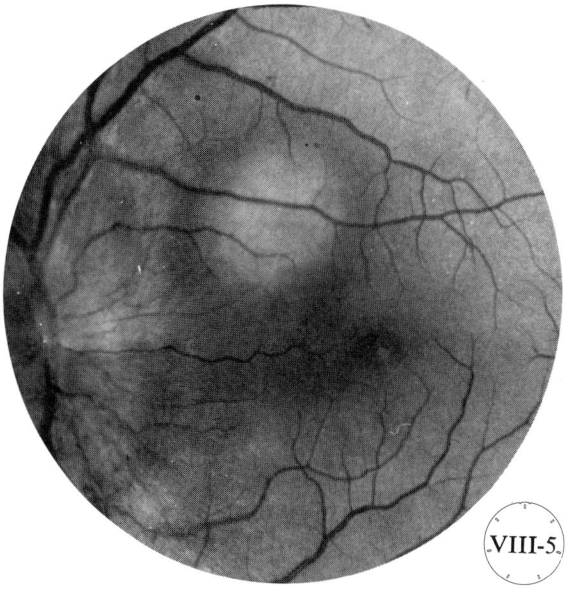

VIII-5

E
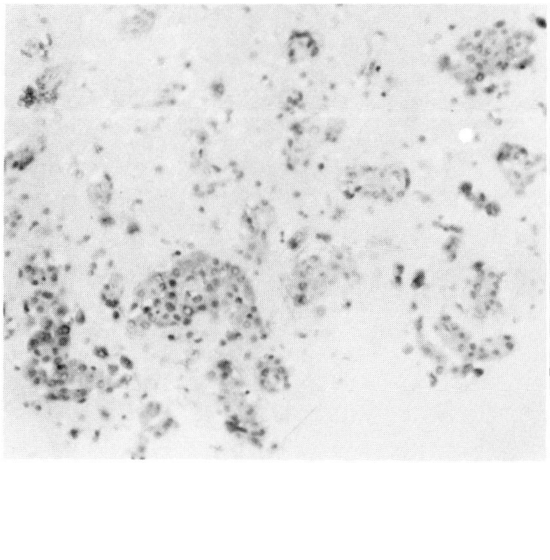
F
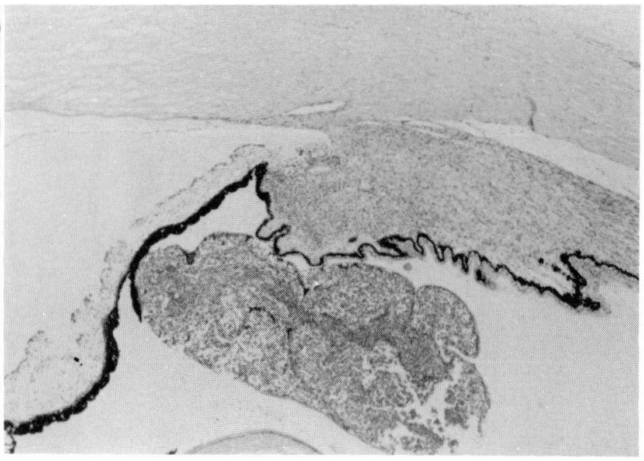

REFERENCES

1. Gass, J. D. M.: Fluorescein angiography: An aid in the differential diagnosis of intraocular tumors, Int. Ophthalmol. Clin. **12**(1): 85-120, Spring 1972.
2. Gass, J. D. M.: Pathogenesis of disciform detachment of the neuroepithelium. VI. Disciform detachment secondary to heredodegenerative, neoplastic, and traumatic lesions of the choroid, Am. J. Ophthalmol. **63:**689-711, 1967.

SUGGESTED READINGS

Bloch, R. S., and Gartner, S.: The incidence of ocular metastatic carcinoma, Arch. Ophthalmol. **85:**673-675, 1971.

Davis, D. L., and Robertson, D. M.: Fluorescein angiography of metastatic choroidal tumors, Arch. Ophthalmol. **89:**97-99, 1973.

Duke, J. R., and Walsh, F. B.: Metastatic carcinoma to the retina, Am. J. Ophthalmol. **47:**44-48, 1959.

Duke-Elder, S.: Textbook of ophthalmology, St. Louis, 1952, The C. V. Mosby Co., vol. 5, p. 5614.

Duke-Elder, S.: System of ophthalmology, St. Louis, 1960, The C. V. Mosby Co., vol. 9, pp. 917-931.

Ferry, A. P.: The biological behavior and pathological features of carcinoma metastatic to the eye and orbit, Trans. Am. Ophthalmol. Soc. **71:**373-425, 1973.

Gass, J. D. M.: Acute posterior multifocal placoid pigment epitheliopathy, Arch. Ophthalmol. **80:**117-185, 1968.

Godtfredsen, E.: On the frequency of secondary carcinomas in the choroid, Acta Ophthalmol. **22:** 394-400, 1944.

Greear, J. N., Jr.: Metastatic carcinoma of the eye, Am. J. Ophthalmol. **33:**1015-1025, 1950.

Jaegar, E. A., Frayer, W. C., Southard, M. E., and Kramer, S.: Effect of radiation therapy on metastatic choroidal tumors, Trans. Am. Acad. Ophthalmol. Otolaryngol. **75:**94-101, 1971.

Levy, R. M., and de Venecia, G.: Trypsin digest study of retinal metastasis and tumor cell emboli, Am. J. Ophthalmol. **70:**778-782, 1970.

Nevins, R. C., Frey, W. W., and Elliott, J. H.: Primary solitary, intraocular reticulum cell sarcoma (microgliomatosis), Trans. Am. Acad. Ophthalmol. Otolaryngol. **72:**867-876, 1968.

Reese, A. B.: Tumors of the eye, New York, 1963, Paul B. Hoeber, Inc., Harper & Row, Publishers, chapter 16, pp. 514-528.

CHAPTER SIX

Leukemia and lymphoma

The retina and uveal tract are frequently involved in patients with leukemia but are rarely affected in patients with malignant lymphomas. Although the fundus may be affected in both the acute and chronic forms of leukemia, the most striking ophthalmoscopic changes occur in acute leukemia. Either or both the retina and choroid may be involved. Occasionally the ocular symptoms may herald the onset of the disease.

LEUKEMIC INFILTRATION OF THE UVEAL TRACT

Although the uveal tract is commonly infiltrated histopathologically, ophthalmoscopic changes are not visible in many patients. If, however, the infiltrate becomes sufficient to cause damage to the overlying pigment epithelium, serous retinal detachment may occur. Such patients may present with a clinical picture resembling either central serous retinopathy (Fig. 6-1), or in the case of more widespread retinal detachment, Harada's disease (Fig. 6-2). Fluorescein angiography is useful in detecting the areas of pigment epithelial damage underlying the serous detachment (Figs. 6-1 and 6-2). The sites of leakage of dye from the underlying choroid are usually multiple. There is nothing, however, peculiar about the angiographic pattern. The choroidal infiltrate may become sufficient to produce a localized (Fig. 6-1) or diffuse choroidal tumor. Leukemic tumefactions of the choroid occur more frequently in the acute lymphatic leukemias.

Occasionally striking changes may occur in the pigment epithelium in patients with extensive choroidal involvement with leukemia (Figs. 6-3 and 6-6, B). It is unclear as to whether the extensive pigment epithelial necrosis and clumping of pigment that occurs in these cases is caused by the leukemic infiltration of the choriocapillaris, chemotherapy, or a combination of both.

Leukemic tumor formation in the ciliary body is rare. Leukemic infiltration of the iris may be diffuse or nodular and may be associated with hyperemia, heterochromia, translucent keratic precipitates, hypopyon, or hyphema.

LEUKEMIC INFILTRATION OF THE RETINA AND OPTIC NERVE HEAD

A variety of changes may be seen in the retina and optic nerve head in acute leukemia. Fullness of the retinal veins and scattered superficial hemorrhages primarily in the posterior fundus are the most frequent retinal abnormalities. White centers within these hemorrhages are common. These white centers have been attributed to cellular debris, capillary emboli, and accumulation of leukemic cells. In some instances these retinal changes may be related directly to the severe anemia rather than leukemic infiltration. Cotton-wool patches, some of which may be caused by ischemia and some of which by localized collections of leukemic cells, may occur. Other retinal changes that may develop include large superficial retinal masses of tumor cells and blood, extensive perivascular leukemic sheathing of the retinal vessels, and ischemic cloudiness of the retina (Figs. 6-4 and 6-5).

Leukemic infiltration may produce a characteristic pale cloudy swelling of the optic nerve head (Figs. 6-3, 6-5, and 6-6). The cloudy swelling typically extends into the surrounding retina. The optic nerve head vessels are often partly obscured by the infiltrate. Visual acuity is usually decreased. Swelling of the nerve head may be associated with widespread evidence of retinal involvement (Fig. 6-5). In one patient with multiple myeloma infiltration of the nerve head there were multiple hemorrhages on the nerve head and peripapillary retina (Fig. 6-6, C).

Treatment for this fatal disease is symptomatic and includes the use of chemotherapeutic agents, corticosteroids, and x-ray irradiation. The fundus changes and visual function may improve during the periods of clinical remission (Figs. 6-5 and 6-6).

INTRAOCULAR INVOLVEMENT OF MALIGNANT LYMPHOMAS

There are very few well-documented cases of either primary or secondary retinal and uveal tract involvement by malignant lymphoma. Reticulum cell sarcoma, lymphosarcoma, and microgliomatosis (a form of lymphoma peculiar to the central nervous system) have been reported.

In microgliomatosis one or more ragged white retinal lesions and cellular infiltration into the vitreous are the characteristic findings, which may simulate those in patients with acute retinitis secondary to toxoplasmosis or cytomegalic inclusion disease. Cellular infiltration of the vitreous may occasionally occur in the absence of a visible retinal lesion and the patient may be misdiagnosed as having a nonspecific uveitis. Tumor infiltration of the choroid occurs less frequently in microgliomatosis, and when it occurs, there is a predilection for tumor cells to extend through Bruch's membrane and to grow beneath the pigment epithelium (Fig. 6-7). Ocular involvement may antedate the onset of central nervous system symptoms. The disease may run a protracted course over a period of months or years. Fig. 6-7 illustrates the clinical and histopathologic findings in an unusual patient in whom proliferation of the reticulum cells was confined to the area between Bruch's membrane and the pigment epithelium. This patient represents the only example of an intraocular lymphoma in the photographic files of the Bascom Palmer Eye Institute.

Some of the patients previously reported as having lymphomatous involvement of the uveal tract probably had instead reactive inflammatory lymphoid hyperplasia (see Fig. 7-13).

Fig. 6-1. Choroidal tumor and serous detachment of the macula secondary to leukemia. A 59-year-old white woman developed blurred vision and metamorphopsis in the left eye.

A, Near the temporal margin of the left optic disc there was a moundlike elevation of the choroid and a shallow serous retinal detachment that extended into the macular region (*black and white arrows*). A small amount of subretinal blood (*black arrow*) was present.

B to **D,** Angiography revealed multiple small pinpoint areas of diffusion of dye from the surface of the tumor as well as evidence of leakage of dye from the optic nerve capillaries into the subretinal exudate. The patient was admitted to the hospital and bone marrow examination revealed acute myelomonocytic leukemia. The patient died soon afterward.

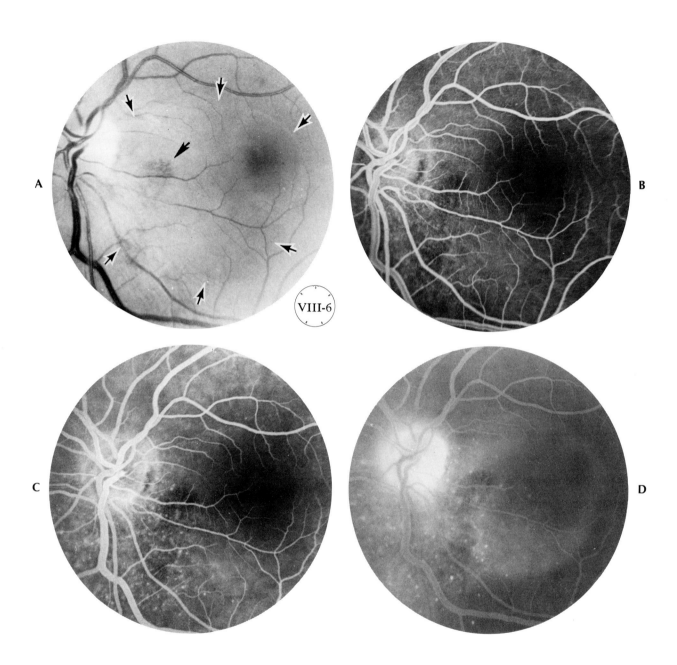

VIII-6

Fig. 6-2. Bilateral bullous retinal detachment simulating Harada's disease in a patient with acute leukemia. A 25-year-old white man developed a central scotoma in his left eye in November 1969. This cleared within 2 weeks. In January 1970, he developed malaise, chills, fever, sweats, weight loss, and blurred vision in both eyes. Visual acuity was 20/70 in the right eye and 20/60 in the left eye. A few cells were present in the anterior chamber and vitreous of both eyes.

A and **B,** There was a bullous detachment of the retina inferiorly in both eyes. The detachment extended into the macular area and there was shifting of subretinal fluid with positioning of the patient. There were no retinal holes and no subretinal masses.

C, Angiography revealed multiple focal as well as diffuse areas of dye leakage from the choroid.

D, One hour after dye injection there were multiple placoid areas of staining at the level of the pigment epithelium. There was some staining of the subretinal fluid.

E and **F,** Similar findings were present in the left eye. Although the ocular findings were suggestive of Harada's disease, the systemic symptoms were more severe than is typically the case. He was hospitalized and a lumbar puncture revealed a spinal fluid protein in 152 milligrams percent and 15 red cells per cubic millimeter. His white blood count was 2,800 and showed atypical lymphocytes present. The bone marrow studies were interpreted as normal. A chest x-ray film showed interstitial pneumonitis. He received 80 milligrams of prednisone and 300 milligrams of isoniazid daily. Most of the subretinal exudate cleared within 1 week. Fine mottling of the pigment epithelium was evident after clearing of the subretinal exudate. His diagnosis at the time of discharge from the hospital was retinal detachment and interstitial pneumonitis probably caused by collagen vascular disease. By April 1970, all subretinal exudate had cleared. In May 1970, he was hospitalized because of urticaria and pneumonia. He died soon after admission and an autopsy revealed acute myelogenous leukemia involving the kidneys, spleen, liver, lymph nodes, and bone marrow. Although the cause of the peculiar placoid pattern of late fluorescein staining is unknown, its appearance suggests that there were multiple relatively flat areas of detachment of the pigment epithelium, which in this patient may have been caused by leukemic infiltration from the choroid into the subpigment epithelial space.

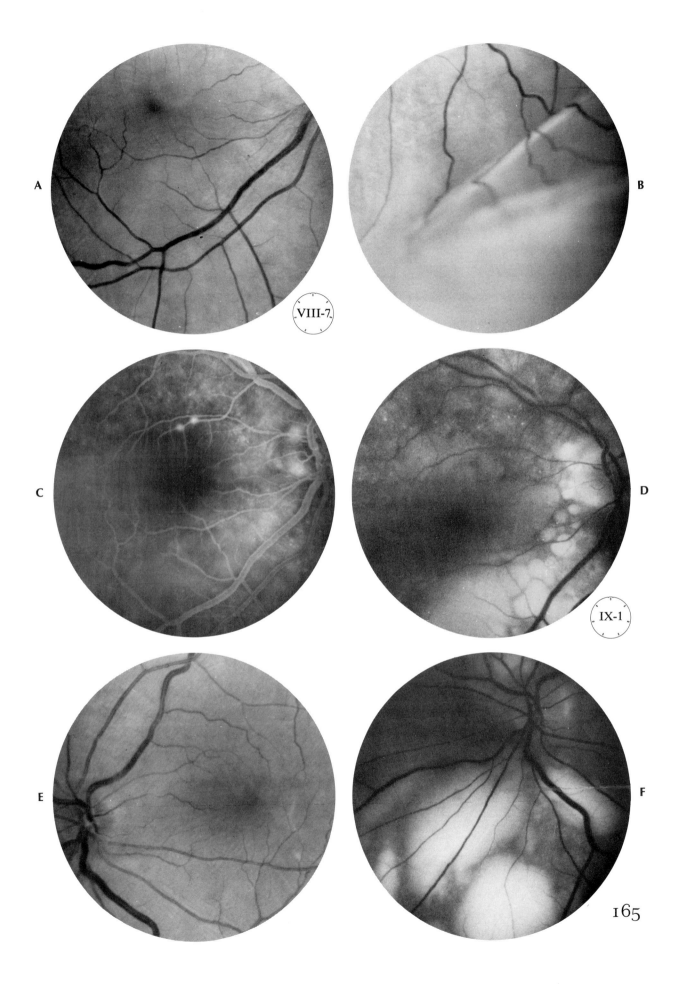

Fig. 6-3. Peculiar clumping of the pigment epithelium in a patient treated for acute leukemia. A 6-year-old white male was diagnosed as having acute lymphocytic leukemia in August 1969. He was treated with vincristine, prednisone, and methotrexate. He remained in remission until April 1970. A relapse at that time responded to cyclophosphamide, vincristine, and prednisone. He developed alopecia and severe visual loss. The visual loss was more noticeable at night than during the day. In May 1970, he developed headaches and papilledema. Spinal fluid pleocytosis was found. He received intrathecal methotrexate. Cytologic examination of the cerebral spinal fluid showed that a remission was achieved. In September 1970, he was seen for the first time at the Bascom Palmer Eye Institute. His visual acuity was 10/40 in the right eye and finger counting in the left eye. There were numerous cells in the vitreous. He presented a striking funduscopic picture in both eyes. He remained essentially unchanged until his death in February 1971. He was last examined on January 15, 1971.

A to **C,** There was massive disturbance of his retinal pigment epithelium with clumping pigment in a pattern suggestive of leopard spots. There was mild papilledema.

D, Fluorescein angiography demonstrated evidence of hypopigmentation of the retinal pigment epithelium and clumping of pigment epithelial cells. The patient died and his eyes were obtained at postmortem examination. **E,** The optic nerve head of the right eye showed evidence of mild papilledema, perivascular infiltration with leukemic cells (*arrow*), and infiltration of the choroid.

F, Clumps of large cells loaded with pigment epithelial pigment granules (*arrow*) corresponded with the leopard spots noted clinically. Note the widespread degenerative changes and necrosis of the pigment epithelial cells. There were patchy areas of destruction of the receptor elements of the retina. There was leukemic infiltration of the retina. There was paucity of the ganglion cells and many areas of gliosis of the inner retinal layers. It is unknown as to whether the changes in the pigment epithelium are primarily attributable to anoxia secondary to the anemia or leukemic infiltration of the choriocapillaris, or to the toxic effects of drugs used in therapy.

(**A** to **C** and **F** from Clayman.[1])

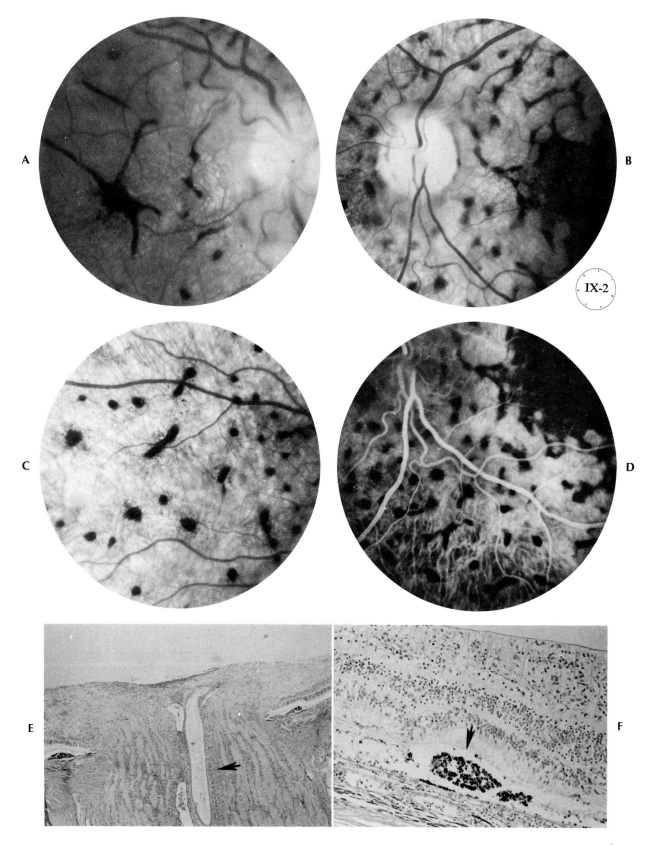

Fig. 6-4. Leukemic infiltration of the retina. An 8-year-old white girl with acute leukemia developed loss of central vision in the left eye.

A, The optic nerve head was blurred and there were scattered retinal hemorrhages in the macula and elsewhere in the fundus.

B, In the periphery there was pronounced perivascular sheathing presumed to be secondary to leukemic infiltration.

C and **D,** Fluorescein angiography revealed dilatation and microaneurysmal formation in the retinal capillary bed and widespread leakage of dye from the capillaries and veins.

E and **F,** A patient with chronic granulocytic leukemia had extensive perivascular infiltration and nodular white and hemorrhagic masses in the retina. Histopathologic examination of the eyes revealed massive perivascular leukemic infiltration and hemorrhagic nodular leukemic tumefactions lying beneath the internal limiting membrane *(arrow)*. (From Kuwabara et al.[2])

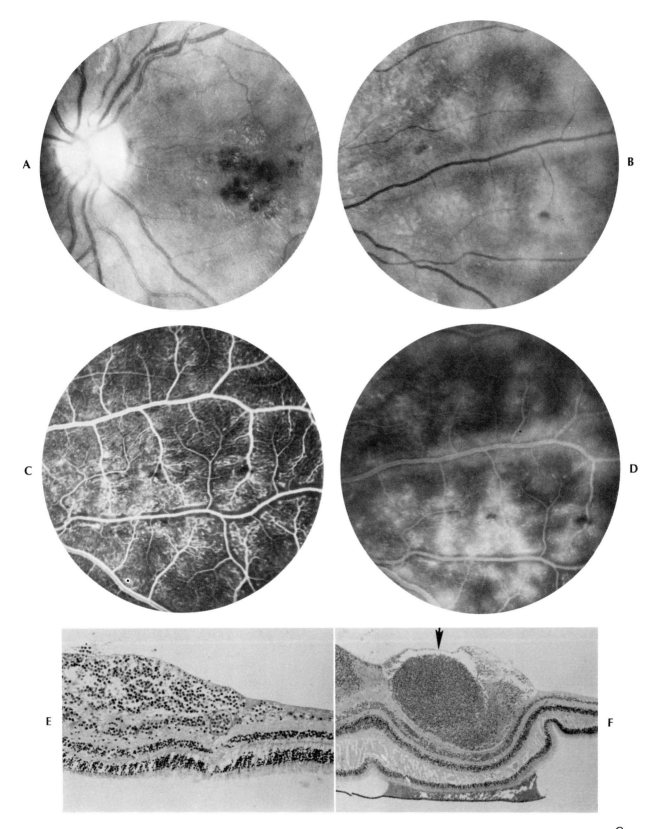

169

Fig. 6-5. Leukemic infiltration of the retina and optic nerve. A 6-year-old girl developed lymphocytic leukemia in December 1966. She was treated with vincristine, prednisone, and methotrexate. Because of visual loss she was seen at the Bascom Palmer Eye Institute on November 8, 1967. Visual acuity in the right eye was finger counting and in the left eye was hand movements.

A and **B,** The optic nerve head in both eyes was obscured by a massive cellular infiltration that extended into the retina in the peripapillary region. There was pronounced perivenous infiltration.

C, By December 13, 1967, the degree of infiltration in the right eye had improved.

D, There was further improvement by March 13, 1968. On June 11, 1968, her visual acuity had returned to 20/20 in this eye.

E, By November 14, 1968, the patient was quite well and was attending school. Her vision in the right eye was 20/20. Most of the perivascular infiltration had disappeared. The optic nerve head was pale and its margins were blurred.

F, The left fundus on November 14, 1968. The patient's visual acuity was 20/200.

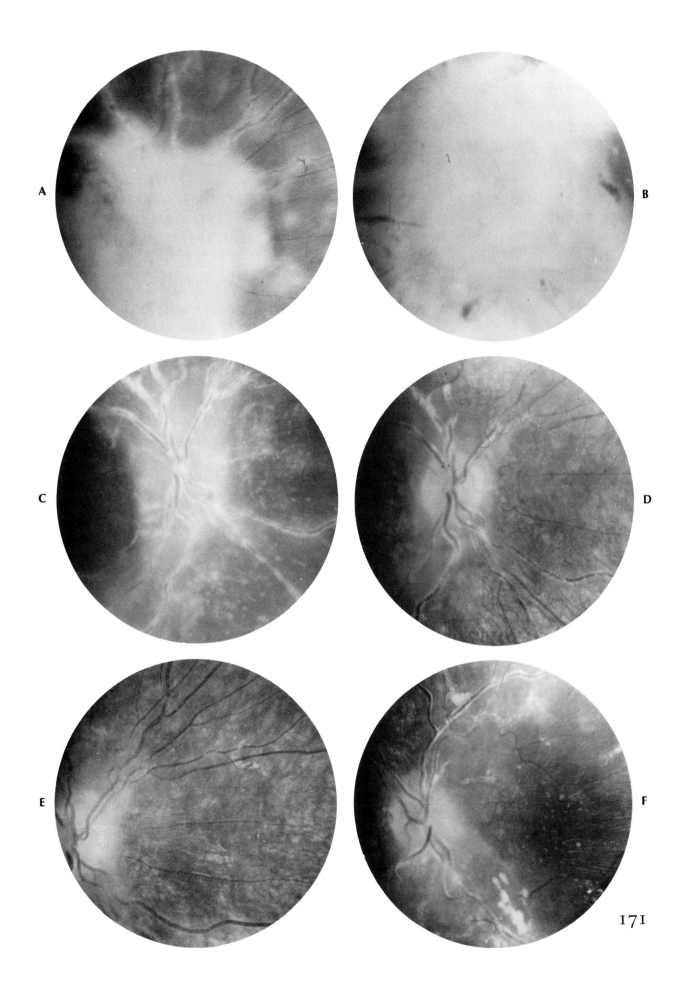

Fig. 6-6. Leukemic infiltration of the optic nerve head. A 6-year-old white girl developed leukemic transformation of a lymphosarcoma of the mediastinum. In June 1970, she was treated with a regimen of vincristine, methotrexate, and prednisone. Remission was achieved, but by September the child developed signs and symptoms of central nervous system involvement. Intrathecal methotrexate was given on September 1, 1970. On September 10, 1970, her vision in the right eye was light perception with projection and the left eye was 20/20.

A, The right optic nerve head and peripapillary retina were swollen and milk-white in color. This is presumed to be related to leukemic infiltration. The optic disc in the left eye was normal. A subconjunctival injection of triamcinolone was given. Two weeks later the vision in the left eye had dropped to 3/200. A course of oral prednisone, 20 milligrams, three times a day was begun.

B, On October 15, 1970, visual acuity was 20/20 in each eye. The swelling of the right optic disc had largely disappeared. There was loss of pigment from the pigment epithelium associated with multiple black clumps of pigment surrounding the optic disc. Her general condition deteriorated. She expired on December 27, 1970. Histopathologic examination of the eyes revealed findings similar to those noted in Fig. 6-3.

C to **E,** Optic nerve infiltration with multiple myeloma.

C, A 67-year-old white woman developed blurred vision on November 23, 1970. She gave a past history of anemia and cobalt therapy for a cyst to the right femur in 1969. The diagnosis was multiple myeloma. She was seen on November 30, 1970. Visual acuity in the right eye was 20/30 and in the left eye was finger counting at 8 feet. The fundus of the right eye was normal. The left optic disc was highly elevated and was largely covered by flame-shaped hemorrhages. The retinal veins were distended. A few cotton-wool patches were present. There were some cells in the vitreous. Note the opacification of the optic nerve head beneath the retinal hemorrhages (*arrows*).

D and **E,** Fluorescein angiography revealed minimal evidence of dilatation of the capillaries of the optic nerve head. There was some staining of the nerve head during the later phases of angiography. The clinical impression was multiple myeloma infiltration of the optic nerve. She had a total dose of 2,000 R of cobalt 60 given to the posterior pole of the left eye over a 2-week period in December 1970. Vision in the left eye improved soon thereafter to 20/70. **F,** March 1971, the visual acuity was 20/70. All of the swelling of the optic nerve head had disappeared. The optic nerve head was slightly pale. The retinal vessels were no longer engorged.

(**B** from Clayman et al.[1])

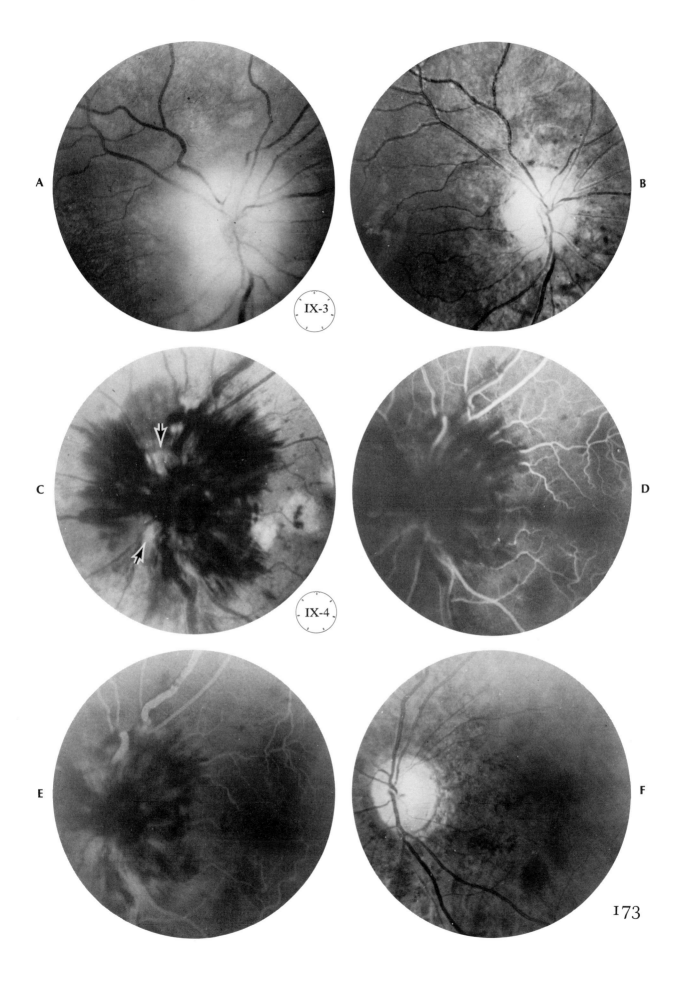

173

Fig. 6-7. Multifocal areas of pigment epithelial detachment secondary to reticulum cell sarcoma (microgliomatosis) occurring over a 4-year period in an apparently healthy woman. In December 1968, a 50-year-old white woman developed blurred vision in the left eye. The initial diagnosis was metastatic carcinoma of the choroid. Soon afterward she was examined by a second physician who diagnosed choroiditis and prescribed corticosteroids orally. Her visual acuity improved. Her general health was good. She was referred to the Bascom Palmer Eye Institute in April 1969. Her visual acuity was 20/20 in each eye. The right eye was normal.

A to **C,** In the left fundus there were multiple discrete, yellowish white, moundlike elevations of the retinal pigment epithelium scattered throughout the midperiphery of the fundus. In the area of the detachments there was a mottled pattern of pigment remaining in the otherwise depigmented pigment epithelium. The disc, retinal vessels, and macula were normal. There was a small area of serous detachment of the retina surrounding some of the pigment epithelial detachments. The vitreous was clear.

D, The early phases of fluorescein angiography revealed the pigment epithelial detachments to be irregularly hypofluorescent. They showed some evidence of staining during the course of angiography. These findings were compatible with a solid rather than a serous exudative detachment of the pigment epithelium. The patient was observed, and after many months the fundus lesions disappeared, leaving a pattern of geographic disturbance of the pigment epithelium. She remained in good health and was without visual symptoms for over 4 years when in July 1973 she returned for follow-up examination. The visual acuity was 20/20 in both eyes. Funduscopic examination of the right eye revealed lesions identical in size, shape, appearance, and distribution to those seen previously in the left eye. No new lesions were present in the left fundus. The patient's general health was good and no treatment was recommended. In late October 1973 she developed focal seizures and was hospitalized. Her neurologic examination and general physical examination were normal except for the fundus changes noted previously. A carotid arteriogram revealed evidence of a subcortical mass in the left parietal region. Craniotomy revealed a localized subcortical blood clot. Multiple biopsies of the brain in this area revealed only reactive gliosis. The postoperative course was complicated by thrombophlebitis. She recovered, however, and was well until mid-December 1973, when she developed a pulmonary embolus and died. An autopsy was not performed, but the eyes were obtained for pathologic examination. Gross examination of the right eye revealed subretinal lesions identical to those depicted in **A** to **C**. Geographic chorioretinal scars were present in the midperiphery of the left fundus.

E and **F,** Histopathologic examination of the right eye revealed multiple mounds of largely necrotic undifferentiated neoplastic tissue lying between the pigment epithelium (*arrow 1*) and Bruch's membrane. A few viable hyperchromatic tumor cells (*arrows 2*) were present along the anterior surface of Bruch's membrane. Note the lymphocytic infiltrate in the choroid (*arrows 3*) beneath the smaller pigment epithelial detachment. The tumor was confined to the subpigment epithelial space. In the left eye there were scattered areas of fibrous tissue lying between atrophic pigment epithelium and Bruch's membrane. There was no viable tumor present in the left eye. The histopathologic diagnosis was probable reticulum cell sarcoma. Despite the negative brain biopsy, this patient probably had the central nervous system form of reticulum cell sarcoma, or microgliomatosis.

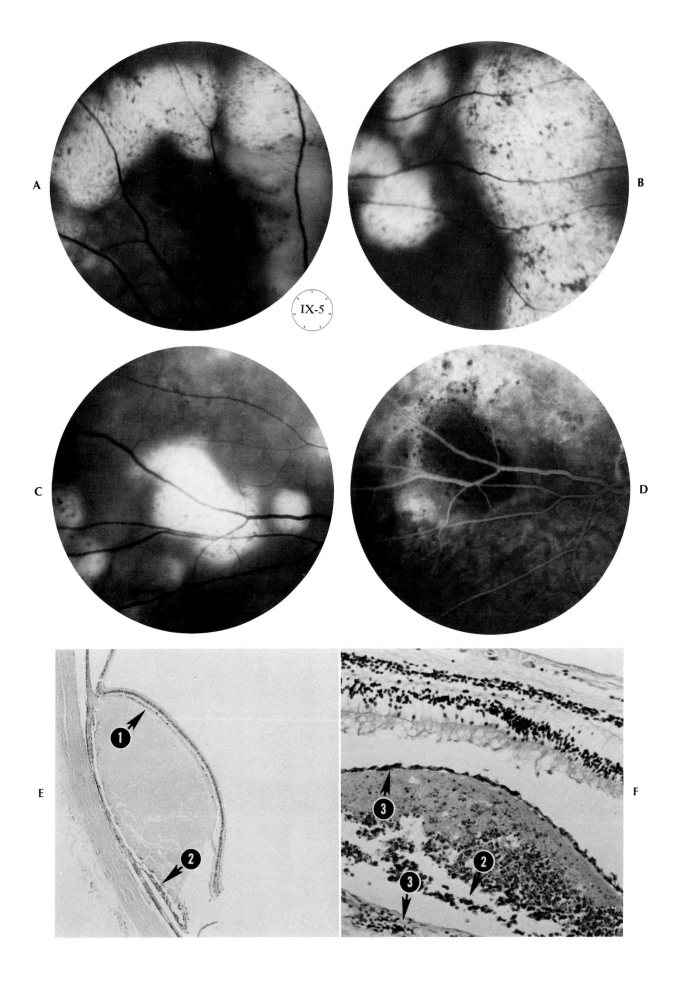

REFERENCES

1. Clayman, H. M., Flynn, J. T., Koch, K., and Isreal, C.: Retinal pigment epithelial abnormalities in leukemic disease, Am. J. Ophthalmol. **74:**416-419, 1972.
2. Kuwabara, T., and Aiello, L.: Leukemia miliary nodules in the retina, Arch. Ophthalmol. **72:**494-497, 1964.

SUGGESTED READINGS

Allen, R. A., and Straatsma, B. R.: Ocular involvement in leukemia and allied disorders, Arch. Ophthalmol. **66:**490-508, 1961.

Ballantyne, A. J., and Michaelson, J. C.: Textbook of fundus of the eye, Baltimore, 1970, The Williams & Wilkins Co., pp. 290-292.

Blodi, F.: The difficult diagnosis of choroidal melanoma, Arch. Ophthalmol. **69:**253-256, 1963.

Clark, E.: Ophthalmological complications of multiple myelomatosis, Brit. J. Ophthalmol. **39:**233-236, 1955.

Duke-Elder, S.: System of ophthalmology, St. Louis, 1966, The C. V. Mosby Co., vol. 9, p. 634.

Duke-Elder, S.: System of ophthalmology, St. Louis, 1967, The C. V. Mosby Co., vol. 10, p. 387.

Ellis, W., and Little, H. L.: Leukemic infiltration of the optic nerve head, Am. J. Ophthalmol. **75:** 867-871, 1973.

Morse, P. H., and McCready, J. L.: Peripheral retinal neovascularization in chronic myelocytic leukemia, Am. J. Ophthalmol. **72:**975-978, 1971.

Zimmerman, L. E.: Lymphoid tumors, in Boniuk, M. (editor): International Symposium on Ocular Tumors, Houston, Texas, 1962. Ocular and adnexal tumors, St. Louis, 1964, The C. V. Mosby Co., pp. 429-446.

Nonneoplastic and nonhamartomatous tumefactions simulating malignant melanoma of the choroid and ciliary body

DISCIFORM SEROUS AND HEMORRHAGIC DETACHMENT OF THE PIGMENT EPITHELIUM AND RETINA

A number of degenerative and inflammatory diseases affecting the choroid may be the underlying cause of localized or disciform serous and/or hemorrhagic detachment of the pigment epithelium and retina. These detachments in some instances may be mistaken for intraocular melanomas (Fig. 7-1).

Serous detachment of the retinal pigment epithelium. Serous detachment of the retinal pigment epithelium presents a characteristic funduscopic picture. It is typically an irregularly round, oval or kidney-shaped, elevated, sharply outlined, smooth, solid-appearing lesion that varies in color from a reddish orange to yellow to white, depending on the pigmentary characteristics of the patient, the duration of the detachment, and the composition of the subpigment epithelial exudate (Figs. 7-1, *A*, and 7-2 to 7-4). A yellowish halo is often present at its margins. These lesions vary in size from barely visible blisters to large elevated lesions occupying most of the posterior pole. They occur most commonly in the macular area, but may occur in the periphery (Fig. 7-3). In patients with senile macular choroidal degeneration small yellowish drusen may be detached along with the pigment epithelium. Usually, however, the drusen fade from view once the pigment epithelium detaches. In long-standing detachments of the pigment epithelium, orange or gray-black pigment may be deposited in the form of an irregular cruciate or Chinese figure on the surface of the pigment epithelial detachment (Fig. 7-2, *A*). Fluorescein angiographic findings in serous detachment of the pigment epithelium are pathognomonic. The early recirculation phases of angiography reveal dye diffusing rapidly from the choriocapillaris across the entire breadth of Bruch's membrane and staining the subpigment epithelium serous exudate. A pigment epithelial detachment is outlined as a sharply defined, hyperfluorescent area that is constant in size and is visible during the entire course of angiography (Figs. 7-2 to 7-4). The intensity of the fluorescence continues to increase during the early stages of angiography and is visible at the end of 1 hour. In many instances where there is a marginal detachment of the overlying retina, the dye may be confined to the subpigment epithelial space, or in some instances, it may spread through small breaks in the pigment epithelium into the subretinal space (Fig. 7-4). In cases where a subpigment epithelial neovascular membrane has extended through a break in the underlying Bruch's membrane, ophthalmoscopic and angiographic evidence of blood pooled in the dependent portion of the pigment epithelial detachment may be present (Fig. 7-2, *D* and *G*). The location of the neovascular membrane may be obscured by the rapid and diffuse staining of the subpigment epithelial exudate. There is a tendency for serous pigment epithelial detachments to enlarge concentrically (Fig. 7-2, *D* and *G*). Serous detachment of the pigment epithelium occurs most commonly in (1) older patients with macular drusen, or so-called senile macular choroidal degeneration, (2) in patients with heredodegenerative diseases associated with angioid streaks, such as pseudoxanthoma elasticum and Paget's disease, and (3) in idiopathic central serous choroidopathy. Large serous detachments of the pigment epithelium are most common in the first two conditions. Rarely do they exceed one disc diameter in size in idiopathic central serous choroidopathy (Fig. 7-4). They rarely occur in the presumed ocular histoplasmosis syndrome. Occasionally in idiopathic central serous choroidopathy the patient may develop a large bullous detachment of the retina and the underlying pigment epithelial detachments may be partly obscured from view (Fig. 7-4). These patients may be mistakenly diagnosed as metastatic carcinoma of the choroid, Harada's disease, or rhegmatogenous detachment. Fluorescein angiography can be invaluable in identifying the pigment epithelial detachments underlying the bullous retinal detachment (Fig. 7-4). Examination of the opposite eye is most important in ruling out the variety of choroidal deseases that may be associated with serous detachment of the pigment epithelium.

Hemorrhagic detachment of the pigment epithelium and retina. There are a variety of causes of breaks in Bruch's membrane and neovascular ingrowth from the choroid into either the subpigment epithelial or subretinal space. Senile macular choroidal degeneration or macular drusen and diseases associated with angioid streaks are the major causes of this complication in the macular area. Hemorrhaging from these neovascular tufts or membranes are responsible for moundlike hemorrhagic detachment or so-called hematomas of the pigment epithelium (Fig. 7-1, *B*). These typically appear as a dark black, smooth subretinal mound (Fig. 7-5). Invariably in 1 to 2 weeks a red halo of subretinal blood develops at the margins of this dark lesion and is evidence that the lesion is a hematoma of the pigment epithelium rather than a choroidal melanoma. If the blood contracts, its surface may be thrown into folds (Fig. 7-5). In senile macular choroidal degeneration drusen are often detached along with the pigment epithelium and can be seen on the surface of the dark black lesion. As the blood beneath the pigment epithelium and retina begins to undergo degradation, it may undergo several color changes. It may change to an irregular splotchy brown color that may closely resemble a pigmented malignant melanoma (Fig. 7-6, *A*) or it may develop a yellowish white color and simulate an amelanotic melanoma or a metastatic carcinoma (Fig. 7-6, *C*). Subsequent organization of the subretinal and subpigment epithelial hematoma may produce a variety of pigmented (Figs. 7-1, *C*, and 7-6, *E*) or nonpigmented disciform lesions that can be confused with a malignant melanoma.

The edge of the optic nerve head is a site where inflammatory and degenerative changes in the peripapillary choroid may stimulate the ingrowth of new capillaries between Bruch's membrane and the pigment epithelium and retina. These neovascular membranes may cause a variety of serous, hemorrhagic, and fibrovascular subretinal peripapillary tumefactions that may be mistaken for neoplastic lesions.

Fluorescein angiography is an invaluable aid in differentiating a localized sub–pigment epithelial hematoma from a malignant melanoma. Angiography reveals the hematoma to be strikingly nonfluorescent throughout the course of angiography (Fig. 7-5). No areas of fluorescence are noted within the tumor except for an occasional small focus of fluorescence somewhere within or often along the superior margins of the detachment in an area where the blood has not completely obscured the underlying choroidal lesion. Even after a change of color has occurred in the various stages of resolution of the hematoma, the degraded blood effectively blocks our background fluorescence and appears as an intensely nonfluorescent area in the fundus (Fig. 7-6). Rarely a layer of serous retinal exudate may overlie the pigment epithelial hematoma and this exudate may stain during the late stages of angiography. The organized hematomas of the pigment epithelium show a variety of angiographic patterns that may simulate closely those seen in a choroidal melanoma (Fig. 7-6, *E* and *F*).

Vascular changes may occur within chorioretinal scars or old organized disciform lesions and produce a funduscopic change that may be mistaken for a malignant choroidal tumor (Figs. 7-1, *D* and *E*, and 7-7). Exudation and further reactive proliferation beneath the retina may cause significant enlargement and elevation of an old cicatricial lesion (Fig. 7-7). Secondary hemorrhage beneath the pigment epithelium near the margin of an old disciform lesion results in the development of a dark black mound at the margins of the lesion and may mislead the clinician into thinking that a previously diagnosed disciform lesion was indeed a malignant melanoma (Fig. 7-1, *D* and *E*). Examination of the opposite eye will usually demonstrate clues to the nature of the tumefaction in the primary eye, such as drusen, angioid streaks, chorioretinal scars, or evidence of choroidal neovascularization in either the macula or peripapillary area.

Bleeding from areas of choroidal neovascularization within or adjacent to small chorioretinal scars secondary to the presumed ocular histoplasmosis syndrome is another less frequent cause of large subretinal hematomas that may resemble a melanoma (Fig. 7-8). Bleeding in these patients occurs beneath the retina rather than beneath the pigment epithelium. It is usually limited to a thin layer of red blood immediately surrounding the choroidal lesion. Only when the bleeding is excessive and blood accumulates in a large mound beneath the retina does it appear as a black mass that may simulate a melanoma.

Although hemorrhagic disciform lesions from whatever cause are typically four to five disc diameters in size, or smaller, and are typically located in the macular area, very large lesions may occur and occasionally may develop in the periphery of the fundus (Fig. 7-8). In patients with large hemorrhagic detachments of the pigment epithelium and retina the blood often spreads through the retina into the vitreous cavity within a month after the hemorrhage occurs. Rarely a severe hemorrhage from a choroidal neovascular membrane will cause massive hemorrhagic detachment of the retina. vitreous hemorrhage, and closed-angle glaucoma (Fig. 7-1, *F*).

Infrequently a neoplastic or hamartomatous choroidal lesion may be the underlying cause of a large serous or hemorrhagic disciform detachment that obscures the tumor from view (Fig. 5-8).

INFLAMMATORY TUMORS SIMULATING MALIGNANT TUMORS OF THE UVEAL TRACT

Posterior rheumatoid scleritis. Rheumatoid scleritis is a peculiar inflammatory disease that may involve the sclera in either a diffuse or circumscribed fashion. The inflammation may result in either an atrophic thinned area of sclera or a massively thickened sclera, so-called brawny scleritis. The inflammation of the sclera is always associated with an underlying uveitis. Most patients have involvement of the sclera anteriorly in the region of the limbus, and the diagnosis of episcleritis, scleritis, or scleral uveitis is easily made. In other patients, however, the focus of scleral uveitis may be confined to the posterior portions of the globe and produce a subretinal tumefaction that may be mistaken for a malignant melanoma (Figs. 7-9 to 7-12). Ocular tenderness, injection of the conjunctiva and episcleral vessels, evidence of intraocular inflammation, and a history of rheumatoid arthritis (present only in 50 percent of patients) are features that should arouse suspicion of an inflammatory lesion. The clinical course varies with the severity of inflammatory reaction. In some patients an acute inflammatory reaction to the focus of necrotic sclera is sufficiently violent that a posterior scleral abscess occurs and produces a rapidly expanding subretinal mass, retinal whitening attributable to necrosis, exudative retinal detachment, and vitritis (Fig. 7-9). This may be accompanied by severe pain and proptosis (Fig. 7-9). In other patients the inflammatory reaction is subacute and fewer inflammatory signs accompany the development of the subretinal mass (Fig. 7-10). In still other patients there may be no clinical history or findings to suggest the presence of an underlying chronic granulomatous mass lesion (Figs. 7-11 and 7-12). In these latter patients the ophthalmoscopic finding of scattered yellow-white nodules (lymphoid follicles in the choroid) on the surface of an orange-colored subretinal tumor may prove to be an important clue to the correct clinical diagnosis (Figs. 7-11 and 7-12). Fluorescein angiography is of little value in differentiating either the acute or chronic lesions from melanomas (Figs. 7-9 to 7-11).

The characteristic histopathologic lesion in rheumatoid scleritis is a zonal type of inflammatory reaction to a focus of necrotic sclera. This reaction varies from an acute purulent destructive process at one end of the spectrum to a chronic, low-grade granulomatous hypertrophic reaction at the other end (Figs. 7-10 and 7-12). The acute and subacute lesions usually respond rapidly to systemic corticosteroids (Figs. 7-9 and 7-10). The large brawny lesions containing much fibrous tissue (Fig. 7-11) do not show a significant response to corticosteroids. The etiology of rheumatoid scleritis is unknown. There may be more than one cause for posterior granulomatous scleritis such as that depicted in Figs. 7-10 and 7-11.

Benign reactive lymphoid hyperplasia of the uveal tract. Diffuse lymphocytic hyperplasia involving the choroid, ciliary body, and iris, usually in one eye of an otherwise healthy individual, is a rare clinical syndrome that is difficult to diagnose and that may resemble in all respects metastatic carcinoma of the choroid, diffuse lymphoma of the uveal tract, or diffuse amelanotic melanoma. These patients may complain initially of recurrent episodes of blurred vision and metamorphopsia secondary to serous detachment of the macula. Initially they may be misdiagnosed as central serous retinopathy. Eventually diffuse thickening of the uveal tract becomes manifest. The fundus develops a gray-yellowish color and there is some mottling of the pigment epithelium (Fig. 7-13). As the ciliary body becomes diffusely involved, the anterior chamber becomes narrowed and the patient may develop acute angle closure glaucoma. Extensive retinal detachment may occur. Early fluorescein angiography reveals irregular mottled areas of hyperfluorescence caused by changes in the pigment epithelium. After development of the retinal detachment, angiography reveals staining of the subretinal fluid not unlike that which might occur overlying diffuse metastatic disease or diffuse melanomas (Fig. 7-13). Histopathologically the entire uveal tract is infiltrated with predominantly lymphocytes (Fig. 7-14). Lymphocytic proliferation is accompanied by varying degrees of plasma cell and reticulum cell proliferation. Lymphoid follicle formation may be present. Infiltration often extends through the emissary canals into the retrobulbar tissue. This tumor histopathologically resembles benign reactive lymphocytic hyperplastic tumors that may arise primarily in the orbit. Since the diagnosis has rarely been made clinically, the value of corticosteroids and low doses of x-ray radiation in the treatment of this disease is unknown. In the past many of these lesions have been misdiagnosed histologically as malignant lymphomas of the uveal tract.

Cysticercosis. Cysticercus cellulosae, the larval form of the pork tapeworm, *Taenia solium,* may invade the eye of patients usually during the first four decades of life. Typically it enters the eye by way of the posterior ciliary arteries and comes to lie in the subretinal space, where over a period of many months it may grow into a large cystic structure. The patient usually presents with a localized retinal detachment with a large yellow-white subretinal cystic mass that may be mistaken for a choroidal melanoma (Fig. 7-15). The head or scolex is often invaginated and appears as a dense white spot within the cystic body of the parasite. Heaving movements of the cyst and undulating movements of the head provide clear-cut evidence of the correct diagnosis. The larva may invade the vitreous cavity and less frequently the anterior chamber. In time the organism incites an inflammatory reaction that will destroy the eye. The treatment consists of surgical removal of the parasite as soon as possible.

Toxocara canis. The larva of the dog ascaris, *Toxocara canis,* may enter the eye, presumably by way of the ciliary arteries, and produce a variety of clinical pictures that may simulate an intraocular neoplasm. Because children are primarily affected, the disease is more likely to be confused with a retinoblastoma than a melanoma. The larva often enters the subretinal space where it may cause a localized eosinophilic granuloma that often extends into the overlying retina and vitreous. The inward extension of the granuloma is often white and may simulate a retinoblastoma (Fig. 7-16, *A*). It may incite a more widespread subretinal inflammatory reaction that may involve the optic nerve head as well (Fig. 7-16, *B*). The larva may migrate into the vitreous cavity and be the cause of a localized granuloma, often in the periphery of the fundus in the vicinity of the ciliary body (Fig. 7-16, *E* and *F*). The white exudative reaction surrounding such a granuloma, particularly when it occurs in the vitreous base inferiorly and is associated with inflammatory cellular infiltrate, may be mistaken for the clinical entity referred to as "pars planitis." This latter disease typically occurs bilaterally and its etiology is unknown. Vitreous bands and a retinal fold may extend from the optic disc to the site of the peripheral granuloma caused by *Toxocara.* Retinal detachment and dense inflammatory vitreous opacities and secondary cataract may occur. The clinical diagnosis of *Toxocara canis* is a presumptive one. Eosinophilia may be present in some patients. Other than corticosteroid therapy to reduce the inflammatory reaction, there is no effective therapy for the intraocular disease.

OTHER LESIONS THAT MAY BE MISDIAGNOSED AS CHOROIDAL MELANOMA

Localized serous retinal detachment. A localized serous retinal detachment unassociated with choroidal disease occasionally has been misdiagnosed as a malignant melanoma. The subretinal exudate is usually sufficiently clear that one may notice that the lesion is not solid. Occasionally, however, the subretinal exudate may be cloudy and the lesion may be misinterpreted as a solid tumor. This mistake should rarely occur if the fundus is examined with indirect ophthalmoscopy. For reasons that are not known, serous detachment of the retina associated with an optic pit may be associated with considerable cloudiness of the subretinal exudate (Fig. 7-17, *A*). On at least one occasion this has led to the misdiagnosis of an amelanotic melanoma (Fig. 7-17, *E*). Fluorescein angiography should clearly differentiate serous retinal detachment attributable either to an optic pit or to a rhegmatogenous detachment from a melanoma (Fig. 7-17). Evidence of diffusion of dye from the choroid does not occur in the last two diseases and is always evident in a choroidal melanoma or other choroidal diseases causing secondary retinal detachment.

Retinoschisis. Retinoschisis is a localized splitting of the retina into an inner and outer layer. Although it may occur anywhere in the fundus, it typically presents as a sharply circumscribed area of cystic elevation of the inner retinal layer extending from the equatorial area out to the ora serrata in the lower temporal quadrant of one or both eyes (Fig. 7-18). The inner retinal layer usually appears quite thin and may have a frosted appearance. Fluid within the cyst may occasionally be cloudy or rarely may contain blood. Visualization of the lesion with indirect ophthalmoscopy and transillumination demonstrates it to be cystic. When the schisis is unassociated with holes in its outer layer, fluorescein angiography reveals no evidence of abnormal fluorescence (Fig. 7-18, *A* and *B*) except for the occasional case where there may be some evidence of abnormal permeability of the retinal vessels in the inner layer. Holes may develop in either the inner or outer layer of the schisis. When a hole develops in the outer layer, the pigment epithelium in the area of the hole becomes depigmented and will appear hyperfluorescent during the early stages of angiography (Fig. 7-18, *C* and *D*).

Choroidal detachment. Choroidal detachment, or more accurately, ciliochoroidal edema, when it presents as a brown, lobular, nonmobile, hemispherical mass in the peripheral fundus, may be misdiagnosed as a pigmented malignant melanoma. It occurs most frequently in patients after surgery for cataracts, retinal detachment, and glaucoma. Occasionally, it develops spontaneously, usually in association with evidence of intraocular inflammation. The ciliochoroidal detachment is often multilobulated and limited to the periphery of the fundus by virtue of the anchoring effect of the vortex veins. Occasionally, however, similar dark mounds of choroidal detachment may spread into the posterior pole. Unlike pigmented uveal melanomas, these detachments transilluminate readily. The dark ciliary band seen normally on transillumination of the pupil disappears in the area of the ciliochoroidal detachment. Hemorrhagic detachment of the ciliary body and choroid produces a funduscopic appearance similar to serous detachment of the ciliary body and choroid. The former lesions, however, do not transilluminate.

Acute posterior multifocal placoid pigment epitheliopathy. This disease typically causes rapid loss of vision in one or both eyes of young adult patients. Though most patients are healthy, a few may give a history of a recent upper respiratory infection. Erythema nodosum and episcleritis have occurred in a few patients. The characteristic ophthalmoscopic picture in those patients, seen within a few days after the onset of the disease, consists of multiple flat, round, oval or geographic, white or yellow-white lesions at the level of the pigment epithelium. Serous retinal detachment does not occur. Vitreous cells may occasionally be present. These lesions undergo rapid and spontaneous resolution over a period of a few days or weeks, and they result in a coarse mottling of the pigment epithelium. Recovery of central vision occurs over a period of several months. The acute placoid lesions that probably are caused by a color change in the pigment epithelium may be mistaken for multiple choroidal metastatic tumors. Fluorescein angiography presents a characteristic picture that clearly differentiates these acute pigment epithelial lesions from choroidal tumors. The acute pigment epithelial lesions are discretely nonfluorescent during the early phases of angiography, and they stain during the later phases. This is in contrast to the irregular pattern of early and late fluorescence seen in metastatic tumors.

Fig. 7-1. Histopathologic condition of disciform detachment of the macula simulating choroidal neoplastic lesions. The eyes with each of the following six lesions were enucleated with the incorrect clinical diagnosis of malignant melanoma of the choroid.

A, A large serous detachment of the pigment epithelium and retina in the macular area.

B, A large hemorrhagic detachment of the pigment epithelium in the macular area.

C, A pigmented disciform scar secondary to organization of subpigment epithelial and subretinal blood.

D and **E,** A large hemorrhagic detachment of the retinal pigment epithelium developing at the temporal margin of an old subretinal disciform scar in the macular area.

F, Massive hemorrhagic detachment of the retina and vitreous hemorrhage secondary to bleeding from a neovascular membrane located in the macular area in a patient with chronic lymphatic leukemia.

(**A** from Zscheile[1]; **B** and **D** to **F** from Gass.[2])

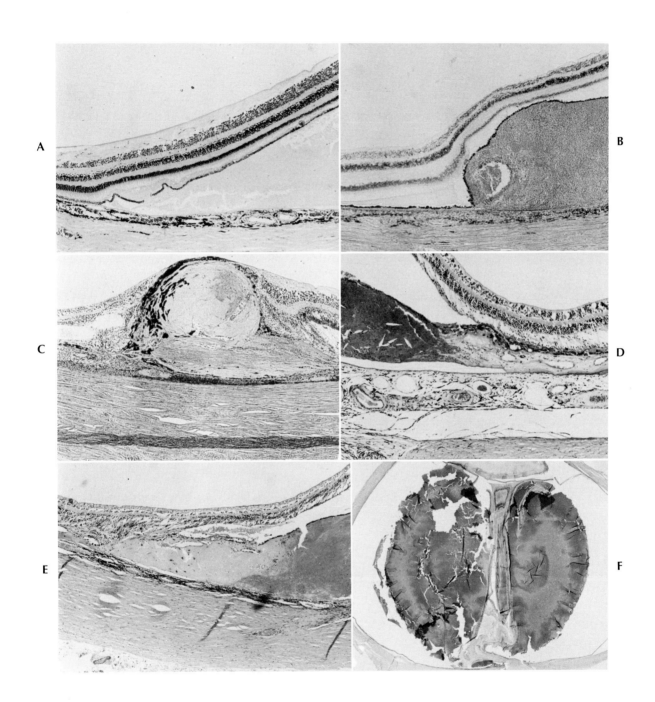

Fig. 7-2. Serous detachment of the retinal pigment epithelium simulating a solid choroidal tumor.

A, This 51-year-old woman presented with blurred vision in her right eye. The visual acuity in the right eye was 20/40. Note the dark pigment figure on the surface of the discretely outlined serous detachment of the retinal pigment epithelium, which has a solid appearance. The dark area inferiorly *(arrow)* is caused by blood present in the subpigment epithelial space. Note the presence of the light-colored halo at the margin of the detachment.

B and **C,** Fluorescein angiography revealed diffuse staining of the subpigment epithelial exudate. The nonfluorescent area inferiorly *(arrow)* and the irregular hypofluorescent area superiorly are secondary to blood present within the subpigment epithelial exudate. The pigment figure is also nonfluorescent.

D, This 52-year-old white man noted blurred vision in his right eye. The visual acuity in that eye was 20/30. Ophthalmoscopic examination revealed a large serous detachment of the pigment epithelium. Note the solid appearance of the lesion and the halo surrounding its margin. There is a small amount of blood in the subpigment epithelial space inferiorly *(arrow)*.

E and **F,** Fluorescein angiography revealed diffuse leakage of dye from the choriocapillaris through the entire width of Bruch's membrane beneath the pigment epithelial detachment. The blood in the subpigment epithelial space is outlined inferiorly *(arrows)*.

G, The same eye depicted in **D** 6 months later. Note the concentric enlargement of the serous detachment of the pigment epithelium and the presence of fine dustlike deposits of orange pigment on its surface inferiorly *(arrow)*. Subpigment epithelial blood was still present inferiorly.

H, Fluorescein angiography revealed hypofluorescence in the region of the blood and the orange pigment.

I, This 70-year-old patient developed loss of central vision in his right eye and was referred to the Bascom Palmer Eye Institute with the diagnosis of metastatic carcinoma of the choroid. Ophthalmoscopic examination revealed a large area of serous detachment of the pigment epithelium in the macula. There was a smaller detachment of the pigment epithelium temporally *(arrow)*.

J and **K,** Angiography confirmed that these lesions were caused by serous detachment of the pigment epithelium.

(**I** to **K** from Gass.[3])

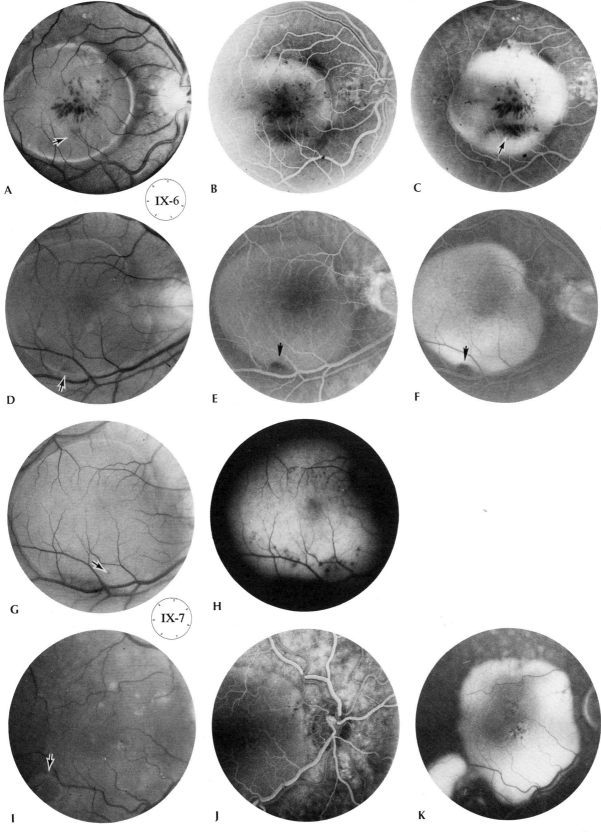

A

B

C

IX-6

D

E

F

G

H

IX-7

I

J

K

187

Fig. 7-3. Peripheral serous detachment of the retinal pigment epithelium simulating malignant melanoma of the choroid. A 61-year-old white woman was seen on August 20, 1963, for routine eye examination. Her past medical history was unremarkable.

A, Funduscopic examination of the left eye revealed a three-disc-diameter-size, well-circumscribed, elevated, orange tumor in the subretinal space. There was mottling of the pigment epithelium over the surface of the lesion. There was an area of loss of pigment from the pigment epithelium posterior to, as well as peripheral to, the lesion. She was examined by numerous ophthalmologists, all of whom believed the lesion was either a malignant melanoma or a metastatic tumor. Because of the absence of retinal detachment and the small size of the tumor, the patient was followed. The lesion transilluminated easily.

B, She was seen at frequent intervals until January 1968. There was no change in the appearance of the lesion except for slight enlargement of several depigmented areas on its surface *(arrows)*. Visual acuity remained 20/20 in both eyes throughout the period of follow-up.

C, Early phase of angiography revealed rapid and diffuse staining of the elevated lesion as well as hyperfluorescence in the areas of depigmentation of the pigment epithelium peripheral to the lesion.

D, The late angiogram revealed staining of the subpigment epithelial exudate. The fluorescence caused by changes in the pigment epithelium surrounding the detachment faded from view. The nature of this lesion was not recognized until 1966. Rapid diffuse staining of the entire mass early in the course of angiography was incompatible with a solid tumor but was characteristic of an exudative detachment of the pigment epithelium.

E, An almost identical but smaller lesion was noted in this 74-year-old white man who came in for a routine eye examination. His visual acuity was 20/20 in both eyes. In the superior temporal quadrant of the right eye, there was a localized, highly elevated, serous detachment of the retinal pigment epithelium *(arrows)* associated with a larger area of depigmentation and mottling of the pigment epithelium. There were multiple drusen on the edges of the pigmented area.

F, Fluorescein angiography confirmed that this elevated lesion was a serous detachment of the pigment epithelium. There was early rapid diffusion of fluorescein dye from the choroid into the subpigment epithelial exudate *(arrows)*. Background choroidal fluorescence was visible in the areas where the pigment epithelium was depigmented peripheral to the tumor. The changes in the pigment epithelium overlying and peripheral to the areas of serous detachment of the pigment epithelium in the two patients illustrated above probably are secondary to previous episodes of recurrent or long-standing retinal detachment surrounding these lesions.

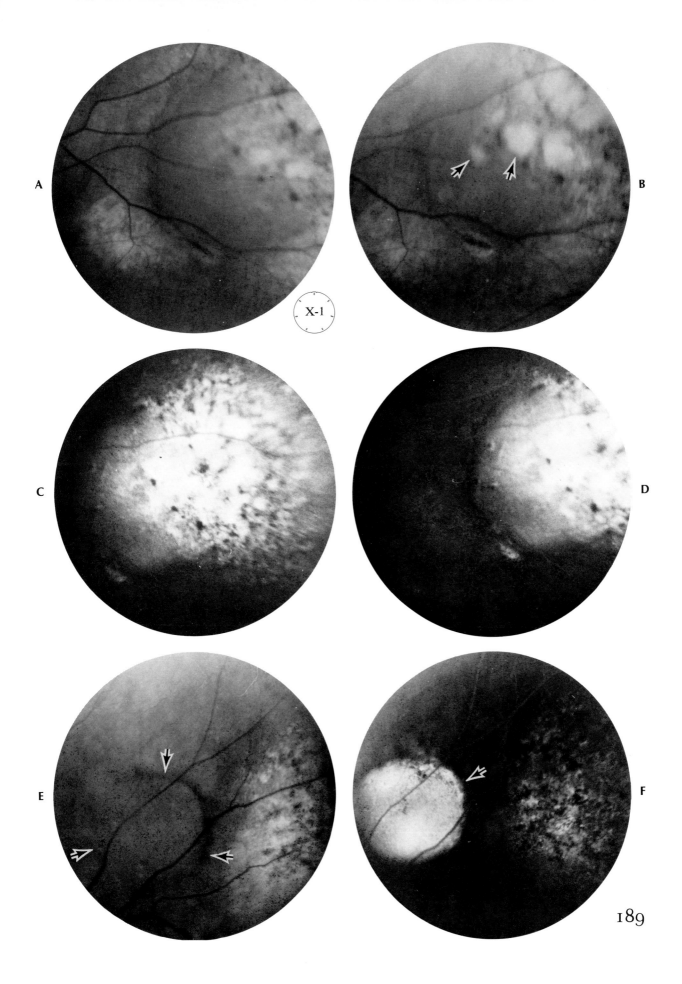

A

B

C

D

E

F

X-1

189

Fig. 7-4. Bilateral bullous retinal detachment with multiple focal serous detachments of the pigment epithelium simulating metastatic carcinoma to the choroid. A tense, 45-year-old white man developed blurred vision first in his left eye and then in his right eye. Soon thereafter he developed loss of his superior field of vision in both eyes. His past medical history was unremarkable. An extensive medical evaluation was within normal limits.

A, Funduscopic examination in the right eye revealed two localized serous detachments of the pigment epithelium *(arrows)* in the macular area and a bullous retinal detachment inferiorly. There was shifting of the subretinal fluid. Note the cloudy subretinal exudate surrounding the pigment epithelial detachments.

B and **C,** Fluorescein angiography showed the typical picture of localized serous detachment of the pigment epithelium *(black and white arrows)* with extravasation of dye through focal defects *(black arrows)* in the overlying pigment epithelium into the subretinal space.

D, In the left eye there was bullous detachment of the retina associated with multiple localized serous pigment epithelial detachments that were obscured by cloudy subretinal exudate.

E, Angiography outlines two large areas of serous detachment of the pigment epithelium *(arrows)* in the left macular area.

F, Macular area of the right eye 9 months later after photocoagulation of the areas of pigment epithelial detachment. The retinal fluid had resolved. The left eye was also treated successfully with photocoagulation. The patient is believed to represent an exaggerated form of idiopathic central serous choroidopathy. When presenting with bilateral bullous retinal detachments, these patients may be misdiagnosed as having Harada's disease, or retinal detachment secondary to metastatic carcinoma or focal choroiditis. (From Gass.[4])

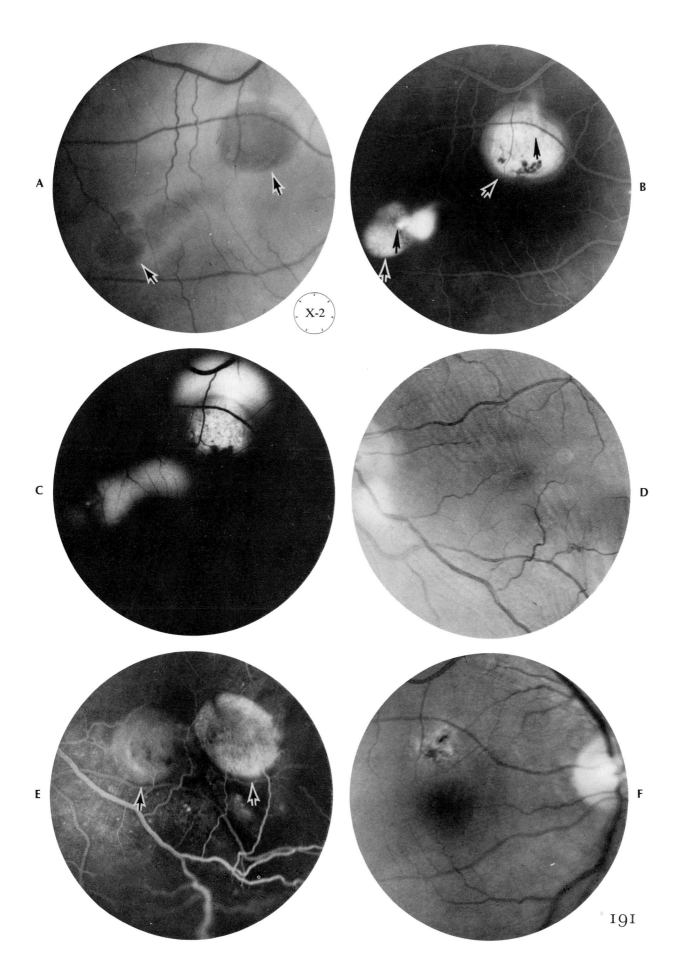

X-2

191

Fig. 7-5. Hemorrhagic detachment of the pigment epithelium and retina simulating malignant melanoma of the choroid. A 63-year-old white woman gave a 6-week history of a large "spot" over her right eye. Visual acuity in the right eye was finger counting. Visual acuity in the left eye was 20/20. Drusen were present in the left macula.

A and **B,** Ophthalmoscopic examination in the right eye revealed a large round elevated black mass secondary to hemorrhagic detachment of the pigment epithelium and retina involving the posterior pole. Note the reddish color of the margins of the lesion.

C and **D,** Fluorescein angiography revealed complete obscuration of the background choroidal fluorescence. There was no evidence in the later photographs of staining in the region of the lesion.

E, A 71-year-old woman noted the sudden onset of loss of central vision in her left eye. Ophthalmoscopic examination revealed a large hemorrhagic detachment of the pigment epithelium and retina. The surface of the subretinal lesion was wrinkled.

F, Fluorescein angiography revealed no evidence of fluorescence of this lesion.

(**A** to **D** from Gass.[5])

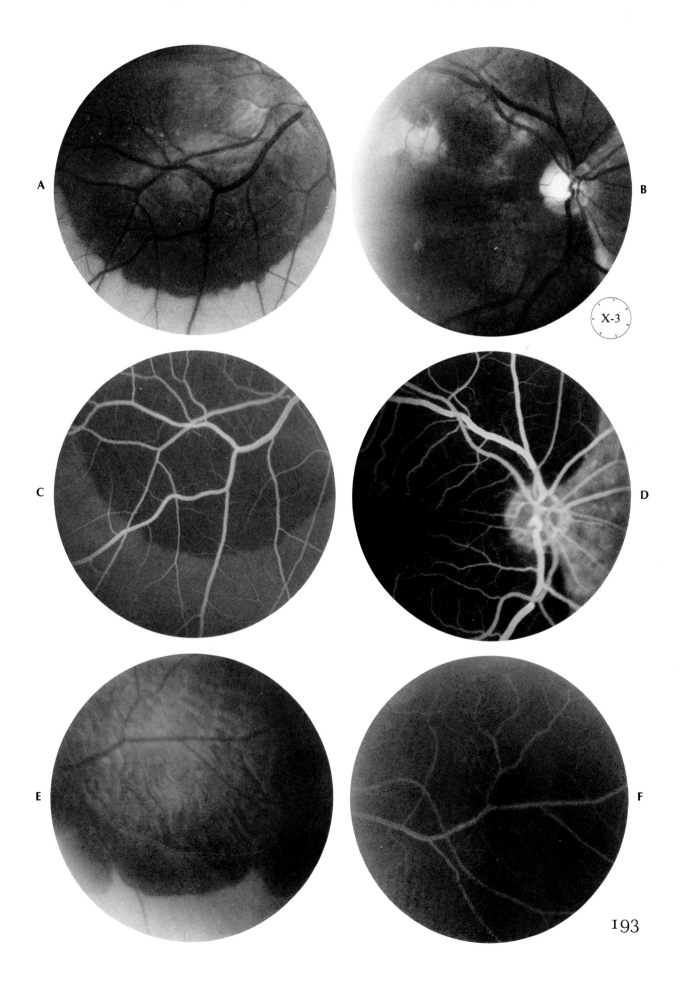

Fig. 7-6. Partly organized hematomas of the pigment epithelium and retina simulating malignant melanoma of the choroid in three patients.

A and **B,** A 76-year-old white woman noted some visual loss in her right eye in November 1970. When she was seen on February 12, 1971, visual acuity in the right eye was less than 20/200. Past medical history was unremarkable.

A, Funduscopic examination revealed a raised, pigmented retinal mass involving the macular area of the right eye. There was some surrounding subretinal blood. The mottled brownish color of this mass of partly decomposed blood closely simulates that which may occur in a malignant melanoma.

B, Angiography revealed complete obscuration of the choroidal fluorescence throughout the angiographic study. This finding was indicative of subretinal and subpigment epithelial blood.

C and **D,** A 59-year-old white woman gave a 6-week history of blurred vision in her right eye.

C, Funduscopic examination revealed a yellowish white subretinal mass inferior to the right macula. It was surrounded by a halo of subretinal blood.

D, Fluorescein angiography revealed obscuration of the choroidal fluorescence by the mound of partly decomposed blood lying in the subretinal and subpigment epithelial space. There was no evidence of fluorescence in the region of this mass throughout the course of the angiographic study.

E and **F,** An 80-year-old white man was seen by his local ophthalmologist because of blurred vision in the right eye. He gave a history of poor vision in his left eye for at least a 1-year duration. His local physician noted a serous detachment of the right macula and an elevated pigmented lesion in the left macula, which was suspected of being a melanoma. When he was seen at the Bascom Palmer Eye Institute, the patient had a serous detachment of the right macula associated with drusen and a small subretinal neovascular membrane.

E, In the left eye he had an elevated nodular brown mass *(arrows)* surrounded by subretinal fluid in the macular area. There were some drusen and considerable depigmentation of the surrounding pigment epithelium.

F, Early fluorescein angiography revealed minimal fluorescence on the surface of the lesion. There was some staining of the subretinal fluid in the 1-hour angiogram. This patient was followed for a number of years and the pigmented disciform scar did not increase in size.

(**E** and **F** from Gass.[2])

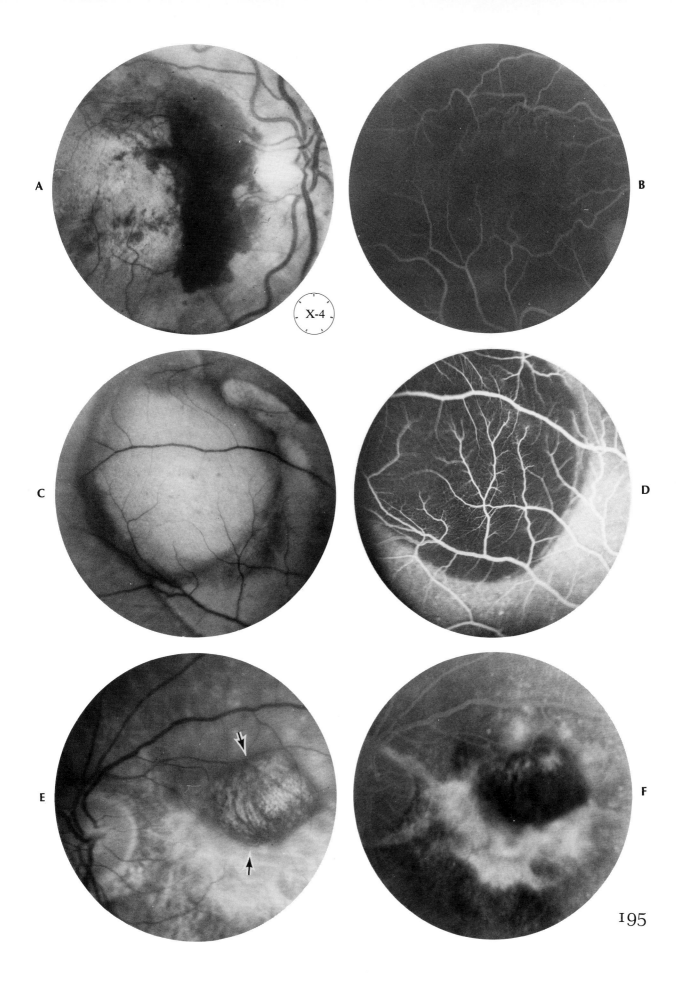

A

B

C

D

E

F

X-4

195

Fig. 7-7. Exudative detachment of the retina overlying a chorioretinal scar simulating an amelanotic choroidal tumor. A 26-year-old white woman was examined on December 3, 1970, complaining of flashing lights in her left eye. At 15 years of age she developed loss of central vision in her right eye. Examination at that time revealed a hemorrhagic detachment of the right macula and evidence of the presumed ocular histoplasmosis syndrome in both eyes. She was hospitalized at that time and a chest x-ray examination revealed a small active infiltrate in her right lower lobe. A tuberculin test was negative. A histoplasmin skin test was strongly positive. Multiple sputum and gastric washes were negative for fungi and acid-fast bacilli. The macular lesion resolved, leaving her with a macular scar and 20/400 vision. She had no further trouble until December 1970, when she complained of photopsia and headaches.

A, On December 3, 1970, ophthalmoscopic examination revealed an atrophic chorioretinal scar in the right macular area and multiple peripheral atrophic chorioretinal lesions in both eyes. Her clinical diagnosis at that time was migraine headache associated with photopsia in the left eye.

B, She returned on February 17, 1971, to report decrease in acuity in the right eye. Examination at that time revealed an elevated nonpigmented lesion that largely obscured the underlying chorioretinal scar from view. There was a small amount of subretinal blood. She was treated with subconjunctival injections of cortisone.

C, She returned 1-month later with further decrease in vision. At this time there was a very large nonpigmented lesion in the right macula. The pigmented edge of the scar was still barely visible *(arrows)*. Because of the pronounced enlargement and opacification of the lesion, there was some concern that the patient might have a neoplastic lesion of the choroid.

D, By July 1971, however, much of the exudate had resolved. The outlines of the previous pigmentary changes surrounding the atrophic scar were again visible *(arrows)*. This patient illustrates an unusual degree of exudative reaction occurring at the site of a chorioretinal scar. (Courtesy Dr. D. Jones, Houston, Texas, and Dr. J. Elliott, Nashville, Tenn.)

196

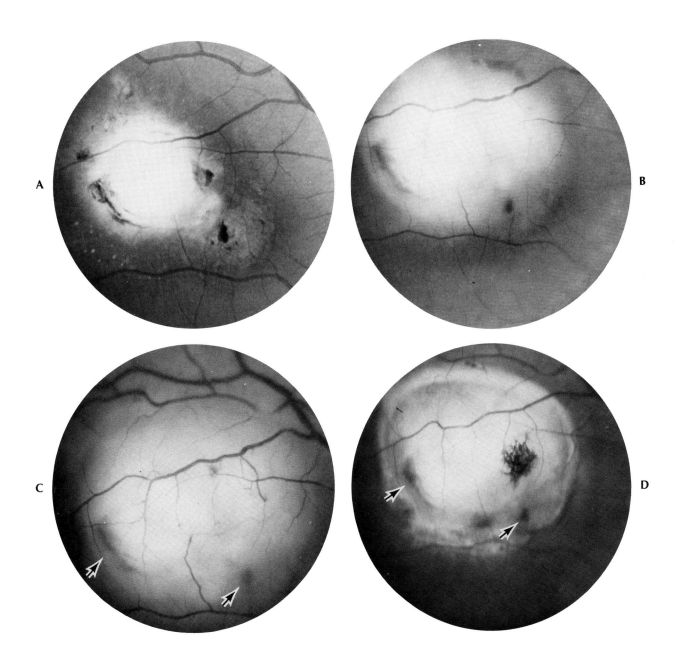

197

Fig. 7-8. Pseudomelanoma secondary to a large subretinal hemorrhage from a peripheral chorioretinal scar in a patient with the presumed ocular histoplasmosis syndrome. A 66-year-old white man gave a 3-week history of a nasal field defect in his right eye. His local physician diagnosed a malignant melanoma. He was examined at the Bascom Palmer Eye Institute in May 1966. His past medical history and family history were unremarkable. Visual acuity in his right eye was 20/20 and in his left eye was 20/20.

A, Ophthalmoscopic examination of the right eye revealed a large, elevated, brown and black subretinal mass in the superior temporal quadrant. A number of focal, atrophic chorioretinal scars associated with varying degrees of pigmentation were scattered throughout the fundi. There was a halo of peripapillary atrophy of the pigment epithelium in the right eye.

B and **C,** Fluorescein angiography revealed no evidence of fluorescence in the region of the pigmented mass, indicating that it was blood. There was hyperfluorescence surrounding a small atrophic chorioretinal scar *(arrow)*.

D, The patient was last seen in December 1970. Ophthalmoscopic examination at that time revealed extensive pigmentary change in the superotemporal quadrant. In addition to the atrophic chorioretinal scar noted previously in **C,** there was a gray fibrovascular membrane lying beneath the retina *(arrows)*. This patient is believed to have the presumed ocular histoplasmosis syndrome. The large subretinal hemorrhage apparently occurred at the site of a small subretinal neovascular membrane, which was associated with one of the chorioretinal scars.

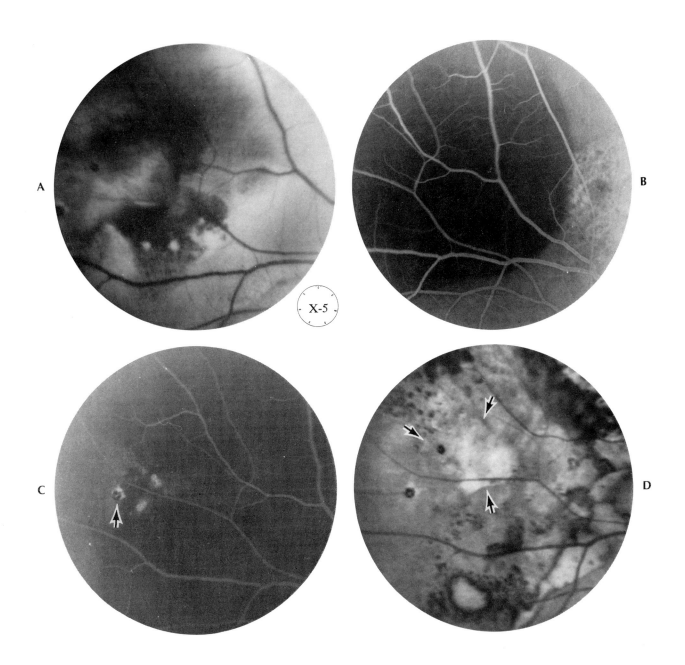

X-5

A

B

C

D

199

Fig. 7-9. Acute posterior rheumatoid scleral abscess simulating a choroidal tumor. A 19-year-old white woman had a splenectomy for idiopathic thrombocytopenic purpura at age 13 years. She was well thereafter until March 1972, when she developed polyarthritis, bilateral episcleritis, and pneumonia. She was treated with antibiotics and developed erythema multiforme. The clinical diagnosis was rheumatoid arthritis. She showed a good response to corticosteroid therapy but was subject to intermittent episodes of episcleritis particularly in the left eye. By January 1973, she had developed a marginal corneal ulcer inferiorly associated with nodular episcleritis in the left eye. There was a serous detachment of the retina inferiorly. By February 1973, she had developed intractable pain and redness in the left eye. On slit-lamp examination she had minimal reaction in the anterior chamber. There was pronounced episcleritis.

A and **B,** Funduscopic examination of the left eye revealed a large highly elevated white subretinal mass with an irregular surface and scattered overlying retinal hemorrhages temporal to the macular area. There was a moderate inflammatory cell infiltration of the vitreous.

C and **D,** Fluorescein angiography showed minimal evidence of fluorescence during the early phases of the study, but there was extensive staining of the subretinal exudate and the mass during the later stages. She continued to have intractable pain despite corticosteroid and azathioprine therapy. She developed proptosis in the left eye, and surgical drainage of a posterior scleral abscess was done. After this the inflammatory reaction and pain subsided. She developed progressive perilimbal scleral thinning, which required treatment with a scleral patch by July 1973. In September 1973, her visual acuity was 20/300.

E, Funduscopic examination of the left eye revealed an atrophic staphylomatous chorioretinal scar temporally in the region of the previous scleral abscess.

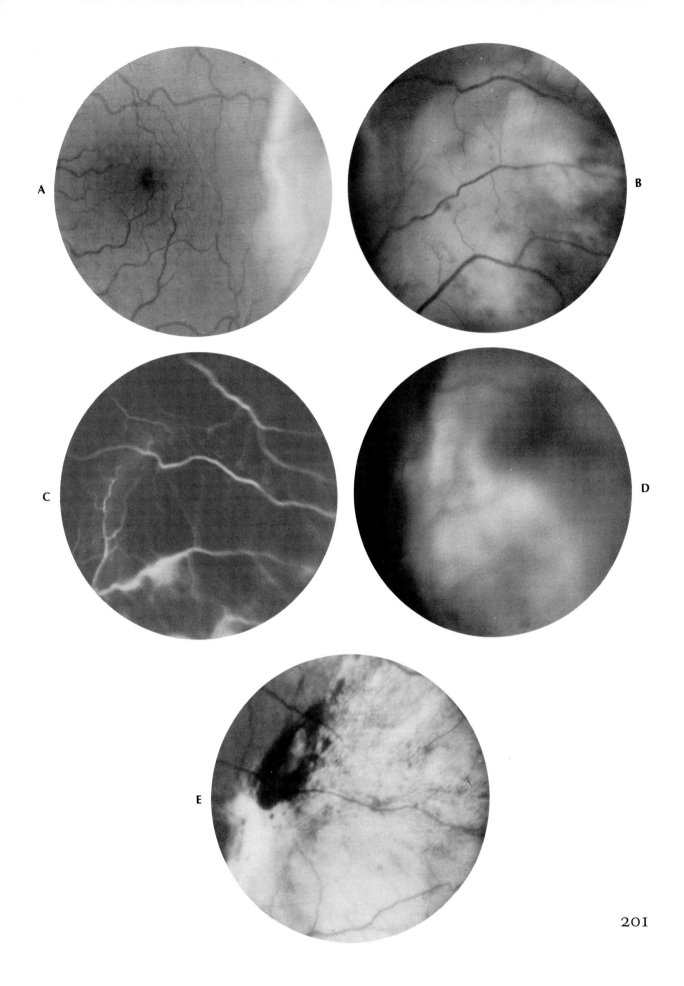

Fig. 7-10. Exudative detachment of the retina and choroid associated with scleritis. A 31-year-old white man developed redness and decreased vision in his right eye. Within 2-weeks he had developed angle-closure glaucoma in the right eye and was admitted to the hospital. At this time he had evidence of scleritis extending from the limbus posterior to the equator in the superior temporal quadrant of the right eye. His visual acuity in the right eye was 20/30 and in the left eye was 20/20. Ocular tension in the right eye was 38 mm Hg and in the left eye it was 15 mm Hg.

A, In the inferotemporal quadrant there was a large subretinal mass protruding into the vitreous cavity. There was a thin layer of subretinal fluid overlying the mass. The mass had a slightly irregular surface and appeared orange in color.

B to **D,** Fluorescein angiography showed staining on the surface of the mass and eventual staining of the subretinal fluid. His past medical history was unremarkable. His general physical examination revealed that his blood pressure was 270/130. He had electrocardiographic and radiographic evidence of left ventricular hypertrophy. Laboratory examination revealed a white blood count of 15,400 with a shift to the left. He had proteinuria. His BUN was 26 milligrams percent. The sedimentation rate was 7 millimeters per hour. A protein electrophoresis was normal. He was treated with subconjunctival and systemic corticosteroid. The choroidal mass rapidly decreased in size. The anterior chamber angle opened spontaneously within 5 days after admission to the hospital. No cause was found for the hypertension.

E and **F,** A 78-year-old white woman gave a 7-month history of decreased vision in her left eye. Her vision in the right eye was 20/70 and in the left eye was hand movements. She had received corticosteroid treatment for 7 months because of ocular inflammation. Because of failure of the lesion to respond to treatment her physician became suspicious of a malignant melanoma and enucleated the eye. At the time of enucleation, a transillumination defect was present and a radioactive phosphorus uptake test was negative.

E, Histopathologic examination of the eye revealed diffuse thickening of the sclera and choroid posteriorly, secondary to a granulomatous scleral uveitis. There were several dome-shaped areas of exudative detachment of the retina (*arrows*).

F, High-power view showing the typical picture of rheumatoid scleral uveitis. Note the zonal type of granulomatous reaction surrounding the necrotic sclera (*arrows*). (AFIP Accession No. 1067300; courtesy Dr. J. Shields, Philadelphia, and Dr. L. E. Zimmerman, Washington, D. C.)

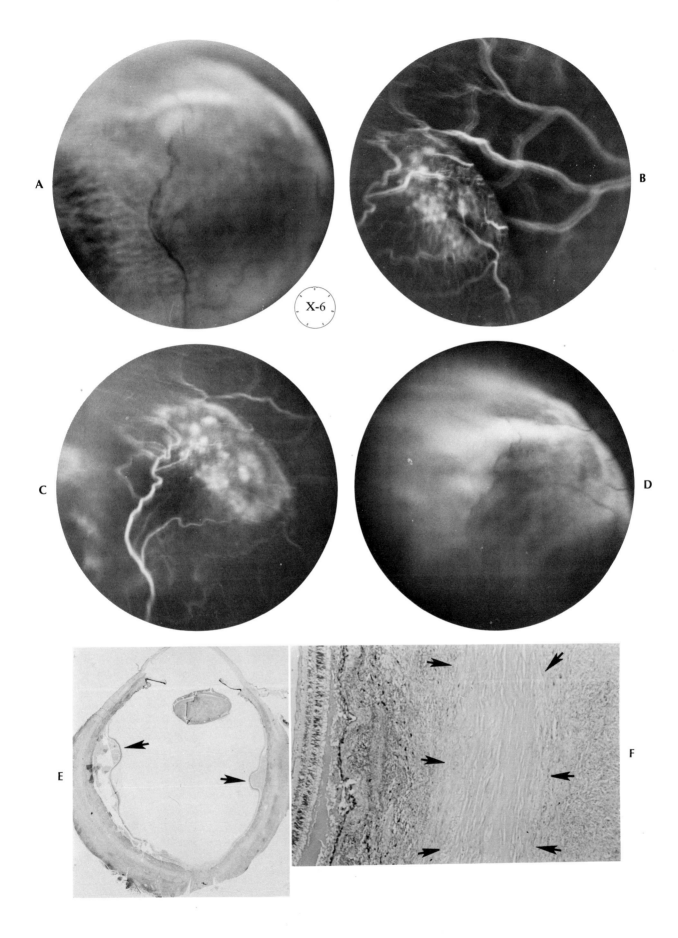

A

B

C

D

E

F

X-6

Fig. 7-11. Hypertrophic posterior granulomatous scleritis simulating malignant melanoma of the choroid. A healthy 54-year-old Cuban woman was examined on January 13, 1973, because of decreased vision in the right eye of uncertain duration. Her acuity in the right eye was 20/50 and in the left eye was 20/20. She was wearing a hyperopic correction of 4.5 diopters in the right eye and 2.5 diopters in the left eye.

A to C, There was a large, nonpigmented, orange subretinal mass in the superior temporal quadrant. The mass extended posterior to the macular area. Oblique chorioretinal folds extended through the macular area *(black and white arrows).* A number of fine, very lightly pigmented lines *(black arrows)* and scattered small gray nodules were present on the surface of the lesion.

D and **E,** The early phases of fluorescein angiography revealed hyperfluorescence in the area of the mass and evidence of chorioretinal folding *(arrows).*

F, Late phases of angiography, however, showed minimal evidence of fluorescein staining. The left fundus was normal except for an old peripheral chorioretinal scar. The initial clinical diagnosis was amelanotic melanoma or metastatic carcinoma. She was admitted to the hospital and no evidence of a primary lesion was found. She did have evidence of Hashimoto's thyroiditis and cystolithiasis. Because of the absence of retinal detachment and the peculiar appearance of the lesion, she was followed until June 1973. There was no chance in the appearance of the lesion.

G, She was reevaluated elsewhere and an ultrasonogram was interpreted as showing a posterior mass *(arrows)* with possible extraocular extension. Malignant melanoma could not be ruled out. On July 15, 1973, right eye was enucleated. Histopathologic diagnosis was hypertrophic posterior scleritis (Fig. 7-12). (Courtesy D. J. Coleman, New York.)

H, Vertical sagittal section of the formalin-fixed right eye revealed an orange subretinal tumor *(small black and white arrows)* with multiple yellow-white nodules *(black arrow)* on the surface. On cut section the tumor was white and was caused by massive thickening of the sclera. The nodules on the anterior surface of the tumor were lying within the choroid, which was displaced anteriorly by the scleral tumor. Similar nodules *(large black and white arrow)* were present in the thickened episcleral tissue overlying the tumor. The histopathologic findings are presented in Fig. 7-12. The histopathologic diagnosis was hypertrophic posterior scleritis.

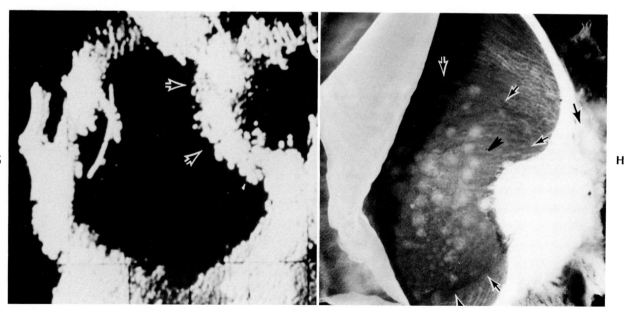

G   H

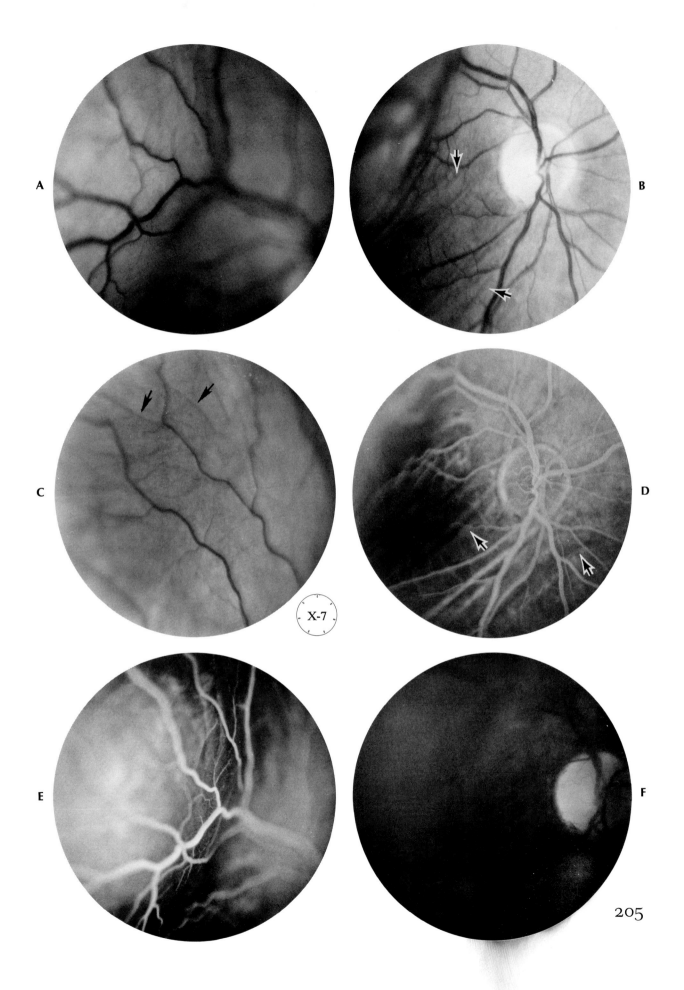

A

B

C

X-7

D

E

F

205

Fig. 7-12. Histopathologic findings in a patient with hypertrophic posterior scleritis, which was mistakenly diagnosed as malignant melanoma (same patient as in Fig. 7-11).

A, Low-power view showing extensive thickening of the posterior sclera. There were scattered lymphoid follicles in the choroid and episcleral region (*arrows*). These large follicles in the choroid were responsible for the nodules noted on the tumor surface ophthalmoscopically and grossly in Fig. 7-11, *H*. The retina was artifactitiously detached in sectioning.

B, High-power view of the choroid overlying the scleral mass showing a focal collection of lymphocytes and a ridgelike elevation of the pigment epithelium, which is believed to correspond with the fine pigmented lines noted in Fig. 7-11, *C*.

C, There were a few scattered areas of granulomatous inflammation within the center of the mass. Note the round cell infiltration and giant cells (*arrow*) surrounding the organized scleral tissue.

D, Cross section of the optic nerve and meninges. Note the thickening of the dural sheath and the presence of multiple lymphoid follicles within the dura and optic nerve head (*arrows*).

E, Well-defined lymphoid nodules (*arrows*) located adjacent to a posterior ciliary artery near the margins of the tumor. The ophthalmoscopic finding of multiple small yellow-white nodules on the surface of an orange subretinal tumor is probably an important sign in differentiating hypertrophic posterior scleritis from other subretinal tumors.

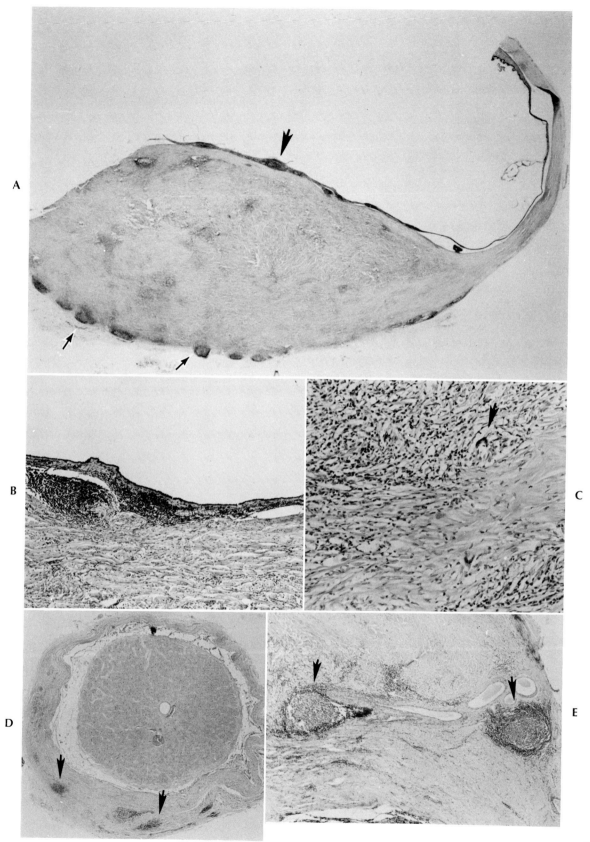

Fig. 7-13. Reactive lymphoid hyperplasia of the uveal tract simulating diffuse malignant melanoma or metastatic carcinoma. A 55-year-old woman gave a 2½-year history of recurrent episodes of unexplained metamorphopsia and blurred vision in the right eye. In March 1962, she developed retinal detachment and closed-angle glaucoma in the right eye. Ten years previously she had had bilateral mastectomy for multiple intracanulicular fibromas. Twenty-eight years previously a subtotal thyroidectomy had been performed for exophthalmic goiter. Her general physical examination was within normal limits. Multiple laboratory studies were normal. These included complete blood counts, blood chemical determinations, and a metastatic bone series. Her vision in the right eye was 20/40 and in the left eye was 20/20. Her exophthalmometric readings were right eye 20, left eye 19. The extraocular movements were full. The eyes were not inflamed. Gonioscopy revealed a totally occluded angle on the right. The ciliary processes and pars plana were readily visible through an undilated pupil. The intraocular pressure was 35 mm Hg in the right eye and 17 mm Hg in the left eye prior to and after pupillary dilatation.

A and **B,** There was a diffuse yellow discoloration of the fundus attributable to choroidal thickening and alteration of the normal choroidal pigmentary pattern. These changes were most conspicuous at the posterior pole. There was a serous macular detachment. The fundus of the left eye was normal.

C and **D,** Fluorescein angiography revealed early and widespread areas of hyper-fluorescence and evidence of staining along the surface of the choroidal lesion. Note the mottled pattern of pigment similar to that seen in metastatic carcinoma. By June 1962, visual acuity in the right eye was reduced to 20/200. By December 1962, the choroid appeared to be of three or four times normal thickness. The pars plana and pars plicata were greatly thickened. The tension in the right eye was 42 mm Hg. By March 1964, the retina was completely detached and the eye was enucleated. (See Fig. 7-14 for the histopathologic condition.)

(From Gass.[6])

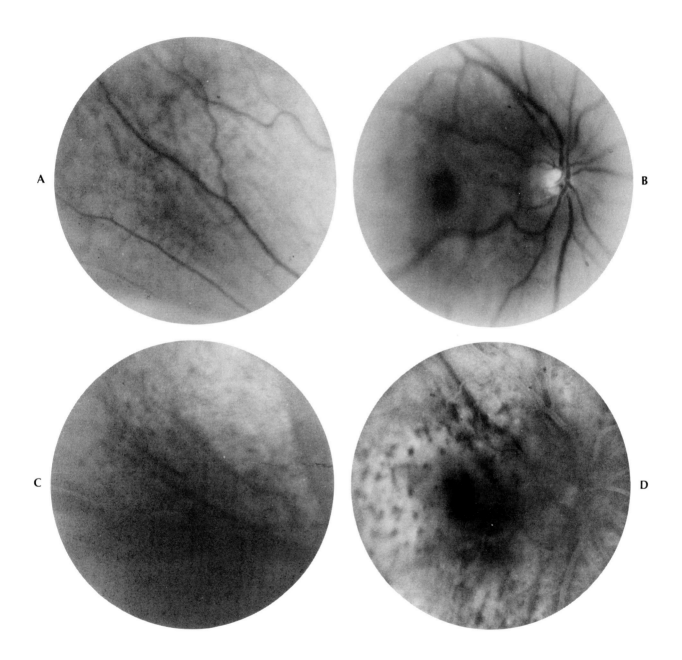

Fig. 7-14. Histopathologic condition of reactive lymphoid hyperplasia of the uveal tract in the same patient shown in Fig. 7-13.

A, Gross specimen of the right eye sectioned horizontally revealed a totally detached retina and diffuse thickening of the uveal tract.

B, Horizontal histologic section of the eye. Note the diffuse thickening and cellular infiltration of the uveal tract, the exudative retinal detachment, and infiltration of the retrobulbar tissues.

C, There was dense cellular infiltration of the ciliary body and iris. There was a well-developed lymphoid follicle in the pars plicata.

D, The choroid was thickened by a small round cell infiltration and deeply eosinophilic exudate.

E, High-power viewing showing cellular detail of the uveal tract infiltration that was composed primarily of lymphocytes. Plasma cells, plasmacytoid cells, Russell's bodies, and reticulum cells were scattered throughout the uveal infiltration. This cellular pleomorphism and the presence of lymphoid follicles are important findings in differentiating this inflammatory lesion from a lymphosarcoma. This patient was alive and well without evidence of recurrence 9½ years later. Eyes with identical findings have been previously reported in the literature as a malignant lymphoma arising in the eye.

(From Gass.[6])

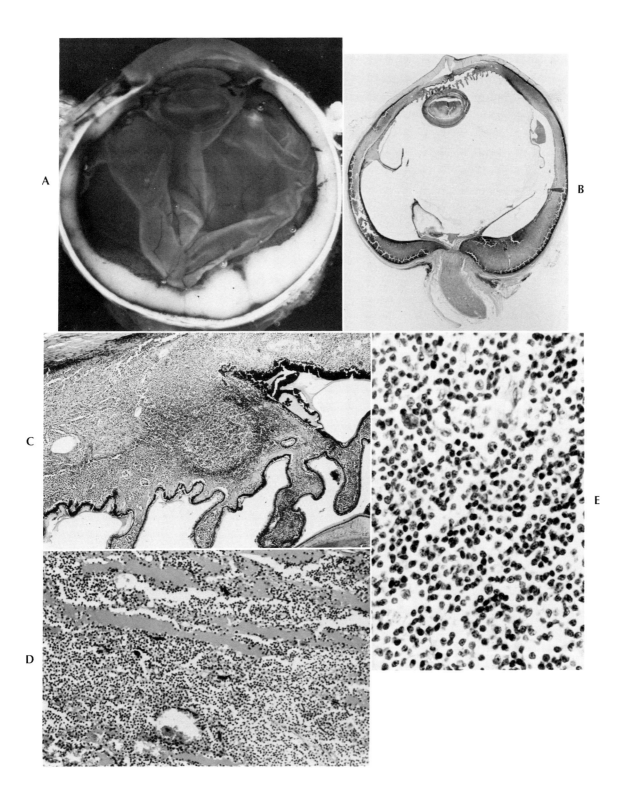

Fig. 7-15. Subretinal cysticercosis simulating a nonpigmented tumor of the choroid. A 38-year-old white male was examined on June 18, 1969, with a 15-day history of a shadow in his left eye. His past history was normal. Vision in the right eye was 20/15 and in the left eye was 20/25. Laboratory studies revealed a 2-percent eosinophilia.

A, There was a serous detachment of the retina superiorly in the left eye. Beneath the retina there was a large, round, whitish cystic mass. It was only after recognizing movement of an invaginated scolex *(arrows)* that the examiner realized that this mass was caused by the cysticercosis organism.

B to **D,** Fluorescein angiography revealed no abnormality in the region of the organism but did show evidence of fluorescence caused by changes in the pigment epithelium and staining of the subretinal fluid inferior to the cysticercus larva. On June 24, 1969, the parasite was removed through a combined scleral and choroidal incision. The retina reattached spontaneously and by February 24, 1971, the visual acuity was 20/25 and the retina was flat.

E, Histopathologic condition of an eye enucleated in another patient whose clinical diagnosis was malignant melanoma of the choroid. Histopathologic examination revealed a viable cysticercus in the subretinal space. The scolex *(large arrows)* was invaginated inside the cystic body of the parasite *(small arrows).* (From Kirk and Petty.[7])

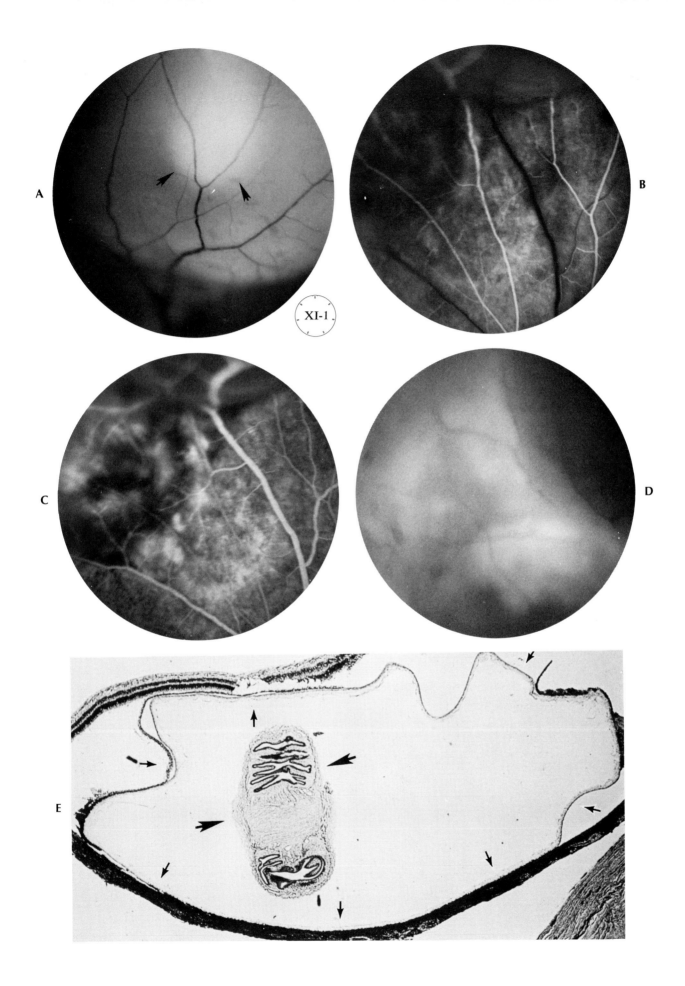

Fig. 7-16. Eosinophilic granuloma secondary to *Toxocara canis* simulating retinoblastoma. A 4-year-old white boy was in excellent health when his parents noted a white reflex in the pupil of the right eye. The child was the product of a full-term normal pregnancy and delivery and his growth and development were normal. His local physician noted a white mass in the right eye and made a diagnosis of probable retinoblastoma.

A, Funduscopic examination under general anesthesia revealed a circumscribed three-disc-diameter-size, gray, subretinal mass in the macular region of the right eye. The central one third of the lesion was white where it had extended into the retina and overlying vitreous. Vitreoretinal folds extended from the dome of the lesion to the optic nerve head, which was displaced in a temporal direction. The vitreous was grossly clear. The left eye was normal. Routine blood counts revealed a white blood count of 13,000 with 38 percent eosinophilia. The presumptive diagnosis was probably intraocular *Toxocara canis*. A pediatric evaluation revealed no evidence of systemic disease.

B and **C,** A 4-year-old white girl was examined in August 1968, because of blindness in her left eye of a 5-month duration. Swelling of the left optic disc had been noted in March 1968. Her general health and physical examination were normal. A blood count and differential count were normal. In August 1968, visual acuity in the right eye was 20/20 and the left eye was blind. The vitreous in the left eye contained many inflammatory cells.

B, A yellowish mass involving and surrounding the optic disc was seen in the left fundus. The initial clinical impression was neuroretinitis. The patient was given oral prednisone, 50 milligrams, on alternate days for 2 weeks. The vitreous inflammatory reaction improved, but the fundus lesion was unchanged. Because of the possibility of retinoblastoma, enucleation was performed.

C, Histopathologic examination revealed a subretinal eosinophilic granulomatous mass that involved the optic nerve head. A nematode larva identical to that depicted in **F** was found (*arrow*).

D to **F,** A 3½-year-old black girl presented with iris seclusion and occlusion, cataract, a flat anterior chamber, and a slightly enlarged left eye. The right eye was normal. Because of the possibility of retinoblastoma, the eye was enucleated.

D, Gross examination of the left eye revealed a white mass overlying the pars plana and pars plicata. The mass extended on the back surface of the cataractous lens (*arrow*).

E, Histopathologic examination revealed a granulomatous mass involving the ciliary processes and the posterior surface of the iris. Several small eosinophilic granulomas were present within this mass (*arrow*).

F, High-power view of the granuloma, indicated by arrow in **E,** revealed a larva compatible with *Toxocara canis* (*arrow*). Note the massive eosinophic infiltration.

(**A** from Gass[8]; **C** from Bird et al.[9])

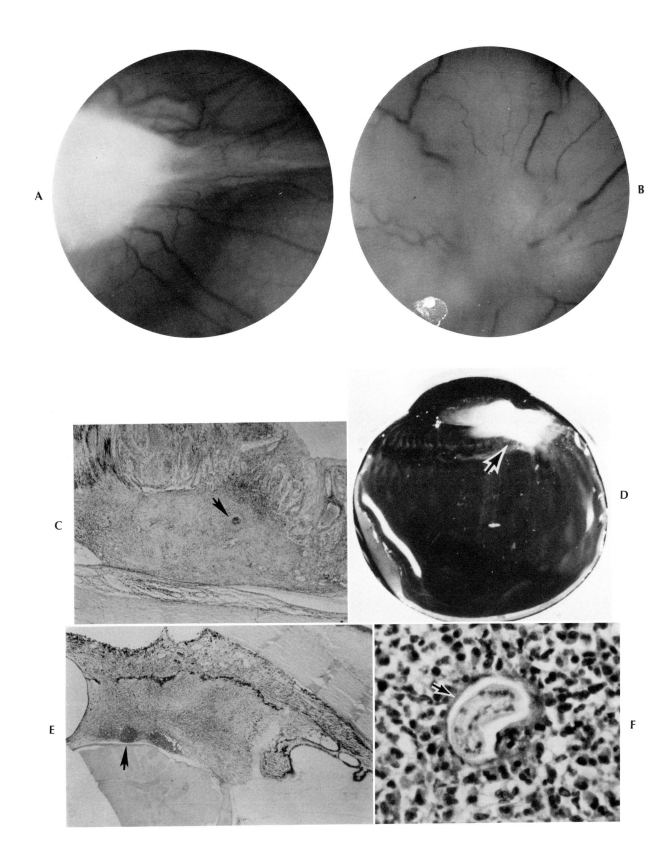

Fig. 7-17. Serous detachment of the retina associated with congenital pit of the optic nerve head: a possible cause for misdiagnosis of a choroidal tumor. A 29-year-old white man was seen on October 15, 1973, with a 6-month history of metamorphopsia and blurred vision in the right eye. His general health was excellent. His past medical history was unremarkable. Visual acuity in the right eye was 20/200 and in the left eye was 20/20.

A, There was a localized serous detachment of the retina in the macular region. The detachment extended nasally to the edge of the optic disc. There were yellow lines deep to the retinal vessels indicative of wrinkling of the outer retinal layers, and cloudiness of the subretinal fluid, which gave the lesion a solid appearance. The optic disc was slightly enlarged and was oval in configuration. There was a small optic pit present at the 9:30 margin of the optic disc *(arrow)*.

B, The left optic nerve and fundus were normal.

C and **D,** Fluorescein angiography revealed absence of capillaries in the region of the optic pit, gradual staining of the optic nerve head and pit, but no evidence of any pigment epithelial abnormality in the area of the detachment. The solid appearance of the retinal detachment may be primarily secondary to heavy precipitation of proteinaceous exudate on the posterior surface of the retina. This solid appearance may cause a misdiagnosis as occurred in the following patient.

E, A 39-year-old white woman was seen because of loss of vision in her eye. An elevated lesion of the macula was noted, and because a malignant melanoma was suspected, the eye was enucleated. Histopathologic examination revealed an optic pit *(arrow)*, and a retinal detachment extending from the optic pit into the temporal portion of the fundus. Retinal detachment in these patients is believed to be secondary to fluid entering the subretinal space at the site of the pit. The origin of the subretinal fluid is unknown, but it may be cerebrospinal fluid, fluid vitreous, or serous exudate from the blood vessels in the area of the pit. (From Ferry[10]; AFIP Neg. No. 62-2328.)

216

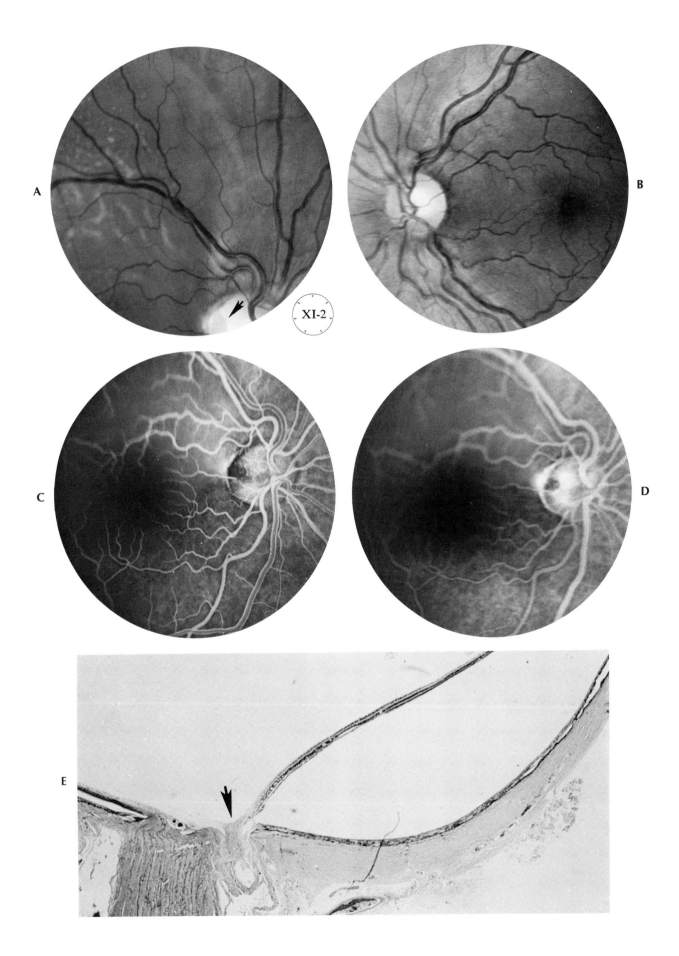

XI-2

Fig. 7-18. Retinoschisis simulating a choroidal tumor. A 62-year-old man was seen for routine eye examination.

A, In the inferotemporal quadrant of the left eye there was a highly elevated cystic lesion that extended out to the ora serrata. The retinal vessels coursed over the surface of the lesion. There was a slight haziness of the fluid within this lesion. The choroidal pattern could be discerned, however, in the area of the lesion. With scleral depression there was evidence of an outer retinal layer. There were no retinal holes. If viewed monocularly this lesion might be mistaken for a solid choroidal tumor.

B, Fluorescein angiography revealed no alteration in the background choroidal fluorescence in the region of the lesion and in this particular patient there was no evidence of leakage of dye from the retinal vessels in the inner wall of the schisis. Use of the binocular indirect ophthalmoscope and fundus stereophotography should always enable the clinician to differentiate a retinoschisis from a solid choroidal tumor. Angiography is useful in differentiating a localized area of retinoschisis unassociated with a retinal tear from a long-standing peripheral rhegmatogenous retinal detachment. In the former the pigment epithelium is normal. In the latter the underlying pigment epithelium becomes depigmented and angiography reveals hyperfluorescence in the area of long-standing detachment. (See Fig. 1-1.)

C and **D,** A 52-year-old white woman was seen because of a large area of retinoschisis in the periphery of the right eye. (From Gass.[11])

C, Ophthalmoscopic examination revealed retinoschisis with a large round hole with rolled edges in the outer retinal layer (*large arrows*). There was a smaller hole in the inner retinal layer (*small arrows*). There was a serous detachment of the retina, not only in the area of the schisis, but beyond.

D, Fluorescein angiography showed hyperfluorescence in the area of the hole in the outer retinal layer. The fluorescence gradually faded from view during the course of angiography. This hyperfluorescence was caused by loss of pigment from the pigment epithelium in the area of the long-standing large hole in the outer retinal layer. The absence of evidence of hyperfluorescence beyond the area of the hole indicates that the serous detachment of the retina is of relatively short duration. In this patient, the localized area of hyperfluorescence lying beneath the retinal detachment and schisis might be confused with fluorescence caused by an underlying choroidal tumor.

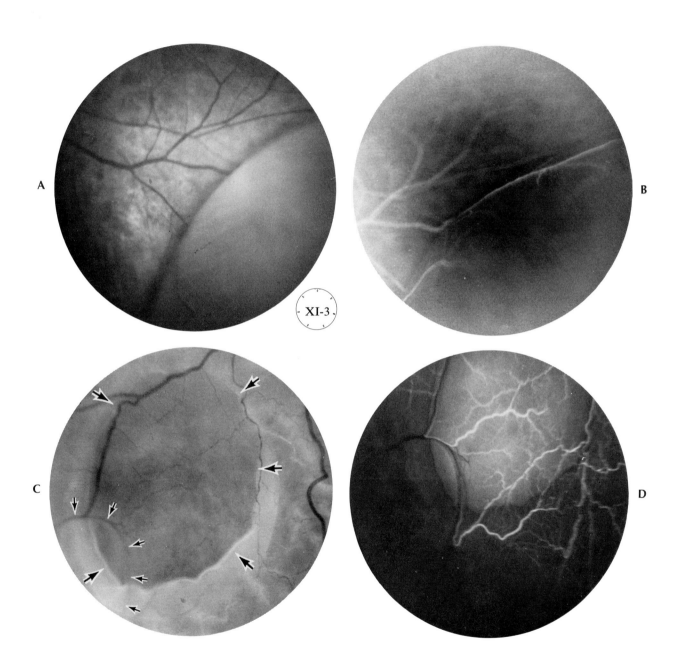

A

B

C

D

XI-3

REFERENCES

1. Zscheile, F. T.: Disciform lesion of the macula simulating a melanoma, Arch. Ophthalmol. **71:**505-507, 1964.
2. Gass, J. D. M.: Pathogenesis of disciform detachment of the neuroepithelium. III. Senile disciform macular degeneration. Am. J. Ophthalmol. **63:**617-644, 1967.
3. Gass, J. D. M.: Pathogenesis of disciform detachment of the neuroepithelium. IV. Fluorescein angiographic study of senile disciform macular degeneration, Am. J. Ophthalmol. **63:**645-673, 1967.
4. Gass, J. D. M.: Bullous retinal detachment. An unusual manifestation of idiopathic central serous choroidopathy, Am. J. Ophthalmol. **75:**810-821, 1973.
5. Gass, J. D. M.: Stereoscopic atlas of macular diseases, St. Louis, 1970, The C. V. Mosby Co., p. 43.
6. Gass, J. D. M.: Retinal detachment and narrow-angle glaucoma, Am. J. Ophthalmol. **64:**612-621, 1967.
7. Kirk, H. Q., and Petty, R. W.: Malignant melanomas of the choroid; a correlation of clinical and histological findings, Arch. Ophthalmol. **56:**843-860, 1956.
8. Gass, J. D. M.: Pathogenesis of disciform detachment of the neuroepithelium. V. Disciform macular degeneration secondary to focal choroiditis, Am. J. Ophthalmol. **63:**661-689, 1967.
9. Bird, A., Smith, J. L. S., Curtin, V. T.: Nematode optic neuritis, Am. J. Ophthalmol. **69:**72-77, 1970.
10. Ferry, A. P.: Macular detachment associated with congenital pit of the optic nervehead, Arch. Ophthalmol. **70:**346-357, 1963.
11. Gass, J. D. M.: Fluorescein angiography: An aid to the retinal surgeon, Proceedings of the 25th anniversary congress of the Retina Service. (In press.)

SUGGESTED READINGS

Andersen, S. R.: Medulloepithelioma of the retina, Int. Ophthalmol. Clin. **2:**483-505, 1962.

Ashton, N.: Larval granulomatosis of the retina due to *Toxocara*, Brit. J. Ophthalmol. **44:**129-148, 1960.

Berkow, J. W., Font, R. L.: Disciform macular degeneration with subpigment epithelial hematoma, Arch. Ophthalmol. **82:**51-56, 1969.

Bettman, J. W., and Fellows, V.: The differential diagnosis of dark lesions of the posterior fundus, Am. J. Ophthalmol. **41:**975-980, 1956.

Boniuk, M., and Zimmerman, L. E.: Problems in differentiating idiopathic serous detachments from solid retinal detachments, Int. Ophthalmol. Clin. **2:**411-430, 1962.

Duguid, I. M.: Features of ocular infestation by *Toxocara*, Brit. J. Ophthalmol. **45:**789-796, 1961.

Ferry, A. P.: Macular detachment associated with congenital pit of the optic nerve head: Pathologic findings in two cases simulating malignant melanoma of the choroid, Arch. Ophthalmol. **70:**346-357, 1963.

Ferry, A. P.: Lesions mistaken for malignant melanoma of the posterior uvea: A clinicopathologic analysis of 100 cases with ophthalmoscopically visible lesions, Arch. Ophthalmol. **72:**463-469, 1964.

Gass, J. D. M.: Hemorrhage into the vitreous, a presenting manifestation of malignant melanoma of the choroid, Arch. Ophthalmol. **69:**778-779, 1963.

Gass, J. D. M., Norton, E. W. D., and Justice, J., Jr.: Serous detachment of the retinal pigment epithelium, Trans. Am. Acad. Ophthalmol. Otolaryngol. **70:**990-1015, 1966.

Harper, J. Y.: Recurrent scleritis with elevation of the retina, Arch. Ophthalmol. **63:**663-667, 1960.

Reese, A. B.: Spontaneous cysts of the ciliary body simulating neoplasms, Am. J. Ophthalmol. **33:**1738-1746, 1950.

Reese, A. B., and Jones, I. S.: The differential diagnosis of malignant melanoma of the choroid, Arch. Ophthalmol. **58:**477-482, 1957.

Reese, A. B., and Jones, I. S.: Hematomas under the retinal pigment epithelium, Trans. Am. Ophthalmol. Soc. **59:**43-79, 1961.

Ryan, S. J., Jr., Frank, R. N., and Green, W. R.: Bilateral inflammatory pseudotumors of the ciliary body, Am. J. Ophthalmol. **72:**586:591, 1971.

Ryan, S. J., Jr., Zimmerman, L. E., and King, F. M.: Reactive lymphoid hyperplasia: An unusual form of intraocular pseudotumor, Trans. Am. Acad. Ophthalmol. Otolaryngol. **76:**652-671, 1972.

Sanders, T. E.: Intraocular juvenile xantho-granuloma (neoxanthoendothelioma), Am. J. Ophthalmol. **53:**455-462, 1962.

Scheie, H. G.: Gonioscopy in the diagnosis of tumor of the iris and ciliary body with emphasis on intra-epithelial cysts, Trans. Am. Ophthalmol. Soc. **51:**313-331, 1953.

Shields, J. A., and Zimmerman, L. E.: Lesions simulating malignant melanoma of the posterior uvea, Arch. Ophthalmol. **89:**465-471, 1973.

Tredici, T. J., and Fenton, R. H.: Hematoma beneath the retinal pigment epithelium: Report of a case mistaken clinically for a malignant melanoma of the choroid, Arch. Ophthalmol. **72:**796-799, 1964.

Wadsworth, J. A. C.: Epithelial tumors of the ciliary body, Am. J. Ophthalmol. **32:**1487-1501, 1949.

Wilder, H. E.: Nematode endophthalmitis, Trans. Am. Acad. Ophthalmol. Otolaryngol. **54:**99-109, 1950.

Wilkinson, C. P., and Welch, R. B.: Intraocular *Toxocara*, Am. J. Ophthalmol. **71:**921-930, 1971.

Zimmerman, L. E.: Problems in the diagnosis of malignant melanoma of the choroid and ciliary body, Am. J. Ophthalmol. **75:**917-929, 1973.

Zimmerman, L. E., and Spencer, W. H.: The pathologic anatomy of retinoschisis: With a report of two cases diagnosed clinically as malignant melanoma, Arch. Ophthalmol. **63:**10-19, 1960.

CHAPTER EIGHT

Tumors of the retinal pigment epithelium

A variety of primary and reactive tumors of the pigment epithelium may simulate malignant melanoma of the choroid.

HYPERTROPHY OF THE PIGMENT EPITHELIUM

These hypertrophic lesions, which have been described also as congenital hyperplasia and benign melanoma of the pigment epithelium, are typically round or oval, sharply outlined, flat, black lesions that may be located anywhere in the fundus (Figs. 8-1 to 8-3). Although they are usually one to three disc diameters in size, very large lesions may occur (Fig. 8-3). Viewed monocularly they may be misinterpreted as being elevated. They usually occur as solitary lesions in one eye, but multiple lesions may be present. These may be grouped in a cluster and have been likened to animal tracts (Fig. 8-1, *F*). The overlying retinal vasculature is typically normal, although occasionally pigment may surround vessels and obscure them from view. Some lesions show an irregularly hypopigmented ring just inside of the periphery of the lesion (Figs. 8-1, *B* to *D*, and 8-2, *A* and *C*). Others may show more generalized hypopigmentation (Figs. 8-1, *E*, and 8-2, *E*). In the latter case, there is a peripheral zone of hyperpigmentation and the thin zone of hypopigmentation may not be present. It is uncertain as to whether the hypopigmented ring and the generalized areas of hypopigmentation are congenital or are acquired. The areas of fenestration, however, progressively enlarge (Figs. 8-1, *B*, and 8-2, *A*). Dense visual field defects corresponding with these lesions may be present. There is some clinical and histopathologic evidence to suggest that slowly progressive degenerative changes occur in the retina overlying these lesions. The lesions have no potential for growth.

Areas of hypertrophy of the pigment epithelium obscure the choroidal fluorescence from view except in the fenestrated areas and in the hypopigmented ring area (Figs. 8-2 and 8-3).

Histopathologically these lesions are caused by a focal area of hypertrophy rather than hyperplasia of the pigment epithelium (Fig. 8-4). The enlarged pigment epithelial cells are filled with large, round, black pigment granules of various sizes (Fig. 8-4, *B*, *C*, and *F*). There is a sharp zone of transition between these cells and normal pigment epithelium, which contains uniform football-shaped pigment granules (Fig. 8-4, *D* and *F*). A marginal zone of depigmentation may be present (Fig. 8-4, *B*). Atrophy and degeneration of the outer layers of the overlying retina may (Fig. 8-4, *B*) or may not be present (Fig. 8-4, *E*). The basement membrane of the hypertrophied pigment epithelial cells may be thickened. The fenestrated areas of depigmentation (Fig. 8-4, *G*) correspond histopathologically with focal areas of loss of the pigment epithelium and adherence of the atrophic retina to the underlying Bruch's membrane by means of proliferating glial cells (Fig. 8-4, *H*).

The changes seen clinically and histopathologically suggest that hypertrophy of the pigment epithelium is a congenital defect in the structure of the pigment epithelium. During life, degenerative changes occur in both the hypertrophied pigment epithelium and overlying retina. Since the lesion is slightly elevated histopathologically, one may consider it technically as a hamartoma of the pigment epithelium.

CONGENITAL HYPOPLASIA (AMELANOTIC FRECKLE) OF THE RETINAL PIGMENT EPITHELIUM

A peculiar flat, sharply circumscribed, usually round or oval, white lesion caused by focal hypopigmentation and hypoplasia of the pigment epithelium (Fig. 8-5) may be confused with nonpigmented choroidal nevi, metastatic carcinoma, or other nodular lesions of the choroid.

Histopathologically these lesions are the result of a sharply circumscribed area of absence or near absence of the pigment granules in a slightly flattened but otherwise viable pigment epithelium (Fig. 8-5). The overlying retina and underlying choroid appear normal. These lesions are presumed to be congenital malformations of the pigment epithelium.

COMBINED PIGMENT EPITHELIAL AND RETINAL HAMARTOMAS

A group of peculiar sessile tumors involving the pigment epithelium, retina, and overlying vitreous may occur anywhere in the fundus, although most have been reported in the region of the optic nerve head (Figs. 8-6 and 8-7). Although the etiology of these tumors is unknown, they probably are developmental tumors (hamartomas) involving the pigment epithelium and retina.

Juxtapapillary pigment epithelial and retinal hamartomas. Patients with these lesions are typically asymptomatic until late childhood or early adulthood when they present because of blurring and distortion of central vision in one eye. The visual acuity in the eye is decreased and an enlarged blind spot is demonstrable. Ophthalmoscopic examination reveals an ill-defined, slightly elevated, finely mottled pigmented tumor of the optic nerve head and adjacent retina (Figs. 8-6 and 8-7). The pattern of pigmentation gives the lesions a mossy or filigree appearance. Many fine dilated capillaries are evident within the tumor and the tumor surface is partly covered by a thin gray membrane. Prominent retinal striae radiate away from the edges of this membrane into the macula, which is displaced toward the lesion. The pigment epithelium surrounding the tumor may be irregularly depigmented. Small superficial hemorrhages may be present if the patient is examined soon after the onset of blurred vision. Fluorescein angiography demonstrates many small dilated capillaries within the tumor (Fig. 8-6). Some leakage of dye from these capillaries occurs.

Histopathologic examination reveals considerable disorganization of the normal architecture of the optic nerve and retina corresponding to the tumor (Fig. 8-7). The tumor is composed of an admixture of glial, blood vessel, and pigment epithelial proliferation. Cords and sheets of pigment epithelial proliferation are intertwined throughout the tumor and they show a predilection for surrounding the blood vessels and extending along the plane of nerve fibers (Fig. 8-7, *B*). The layer of pigment epithelium underlying the tumor may be doubled (Fig. 8-7, *C*). Fibrocellular tissue presumed to be glial proliferation is present along the inner surface of the tumor. The tumor underlying this tissue is thrown into folds.

Spontaneous contraction of the glial tissue lying within and on the surface of these tumors is probably responsible for the surrounding traction lines in the retina and distortion of the macula. This distortion may increase gradually over a period of months and years (Fig. 8-6). These lesions are most likely to be mistaken for juxtapapillary choroidal melanomas (Fig. 3-18) and melanocytomas (Figs. 2-19 and 2-20). In some cases the tumor is nonpigmented clinically, and histopathologically the hyperplastic pigment epithelium contains little or no pigment. I have seen one patient who had a large nonpigmented mass of the optic nerve head as well as a partly pigmented tumor in the periphery of the fundus (Fig. 8-8). These tumors have not changed in appearance over a period of several years and they are presumed to be hamartomas of the pigment epithelium and retina.

Peripheral pigment epithelial and retinal hamartomas. Tumors believed to be related to the juxtapapillary lesions described above may occur in the macula or elsewhere in the fundus. These lesions are typically discovered in one eye of otherwise healthy young children presenting with monocular strabismus and amblyopia. There is usually no history of permaturity or exposure to high levels of oxygen. These children typically have lesions that share the following features (Figs. 8-9 to 8-11): (1) They are slightly elevated, black or charcoal gray masses involving the pigment epithelium, retina, and overlying vitreous; (2) they extend in a fanlike projection from either the optic disc or from the direction of the optic disc into the periphery; (3) the outer portion or base of the lesion is composed of a relatively flat sheet of highly pigmented tissue that blends imperceptively into the surrounding pigment epithelium; (4) the outer pigmented portion of the tumor is obscured centrally by varying amounts of thickened gray-white retinal and preretinal tissue; and (5) the surface of the inner portion of the lesion is contracted and is associated with distortion and displacement of the neighboring retina, retinal vessels, and optic nerve head toward the center of the lesion. Retinal detachment, exudation, hemorrhage, and vitreous inflammatory cells are absent. Unlike the juxtapapillary lesions, migration of pigment into the inner portions of the tumor does not occur. Fluorescein angiography typically depicts dilation, tortuosity, central displacement, and in some cases permeability alterations of the retinal blood vessels within the tumor (Fig. 8-10). The peripheral retina of these patients, unlike that seen in retinopathy of prematurity appears to be normally vascularized. These lesions may be misdiagnosed as retinoblastoma, choroidal melanoma, or reactive proliferation of the pigment epithelium secondary to trauma, inflammation (such as from *Toxocara canis*), or retrolental fibroplasia. These lesions have no growth potential. The early onset of ocular signs and symptoms; the absence of evidence of inflammation, injury, prematurity, or exposure to neonatal oxygen; unilaterality of the lesion; the similarity of their appearance; and their failure to grow suggest that these lesions are present at birth and that they are hamartomas composed of malformed retina and pigment epithelium. The histologic feature of these peripheral lesions are unknown, but they are probably similar to those arising in the juxtapapillary area. While their pathogenesis is uncertain, their clinical features are sufficiently characteristic that they should not be mistaken for either a melanoma or a retinoblastoma.

Fig. 8-1. Variations in the clinical appearance of congenital hypertrophy of the retinal pigment epithelium.

A, A jet-black, well-circumscribed area of hypertrophy of the pigment epithelium associated with an absolute scotoma was present in the paramacular region of this young white woman. Note the small nonpigmented fenestrations *(arrow)*.

B, Hypertrophy of the pigment epithelium showing a peripheral nonpigmented ring and several fenestrations *(arrows)*.

C, Multiple fenestrations *(arrows)* and a peripheral nonpigmented ring in hypertrophy of the pigment epithelium.

D, Hypertrophy of the pigment epithelium showing generalized hypopigmentation and a nonpigmented peripheral ring.

E, Hypertrophy of pigment epithelium showing widespread hypopigmentation in an elderly patient.

F, Multiple areas of hypertrophy of the pigment epithelium.

(**A** courtesy Dr. L. Yanuzzi, New York, N. Y., and Dr. B. Esterman, Far Rockaway, N. Y.; **F** from Buettner.[1])

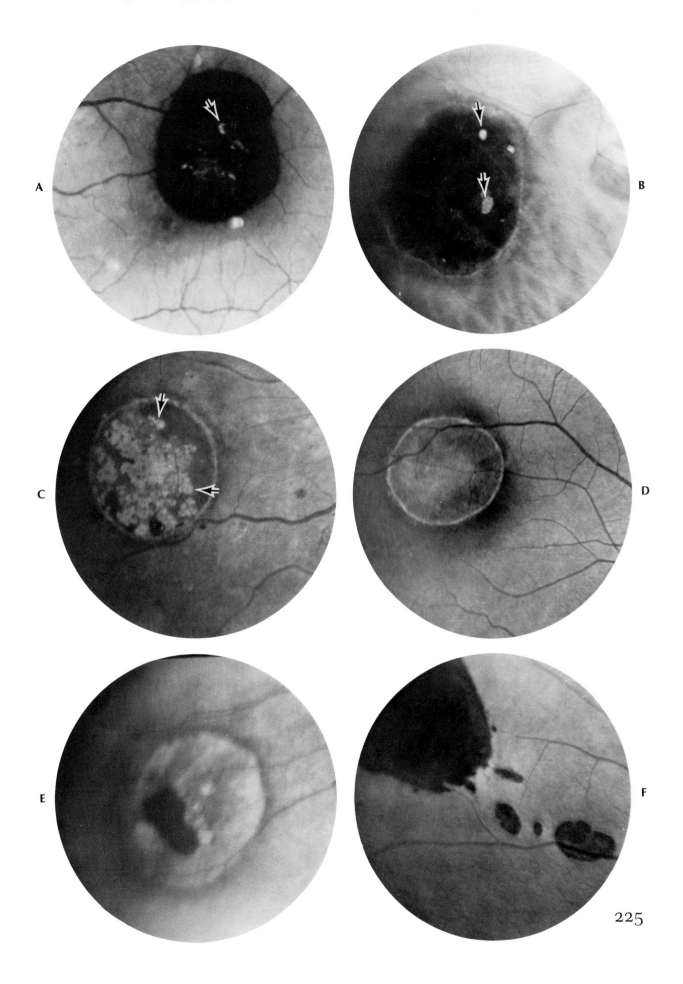

225

Fig. 8-2. Hypertrophy of the retinal pigment epithelium.

A, This is the same lesion depicted in Fig. 8-1, *B,* as it appeared 4 years later. The three nonpigmented fenestrations *(arrows)* have enlarged slightly.

B, Angiography revealed that the lesion obscured the background choroidal fluorescence except in the areas of the nonpigmented halo and fenestrations.

C, This peripapillary hypertrophy of the retinal pigment epithelium was associated with a very faint nonpigmented halo and large nonpigmented fenestrations. This patient had an enlarged blind spot on field examination in this eye.

D, Angiography of patient depicted in **C.**

E, Hypertrophy of the pigment epithelium showing generalized hypopigmentation that extended out to and includes the area where one would normally expect to see a nonpigmented halo.

F, Angiography reveals evidence of hypopigmentation centrally. Note the peripheral ring of hypofluorescence that is greater than might be expected from the clinical appearance of the lesion.

(**C** and **D** from Buettner.[1])

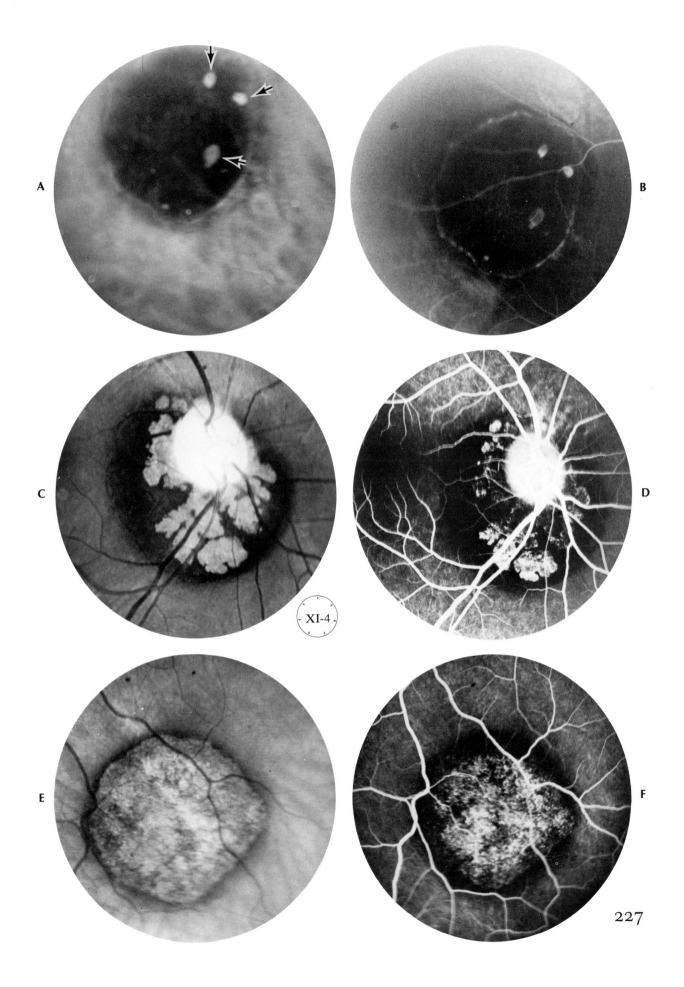

Fig. 8-3. Large area of hypertrophy of the pigment epithelium mistaken for a malignant melanoma. A 59-year-old woman had a routine eye examination. A large pigmented tumor was observed in the right eye and the patient was referred with the possible diagnosis of malignant melanoma. Her visual acuity was normal in both eyes.

A, In the superotemporal quadrant of the right eye there was an eight-disc-diameter-size, flat, black area of hypertrophy of the retinal pigment epithelium. There were several areas of thinning of the pigment within the central portion of the lesion *(arrows)*. There was no evidence of serous detachment. There was an absolute field defect corresponding with the lesion.

B to **D,** Fluorescein angiography revealed that the lesion completely obscured the background choroidal fluorescence except in those few areas where there was thinning of the pigment epithelium *(arrows)*.

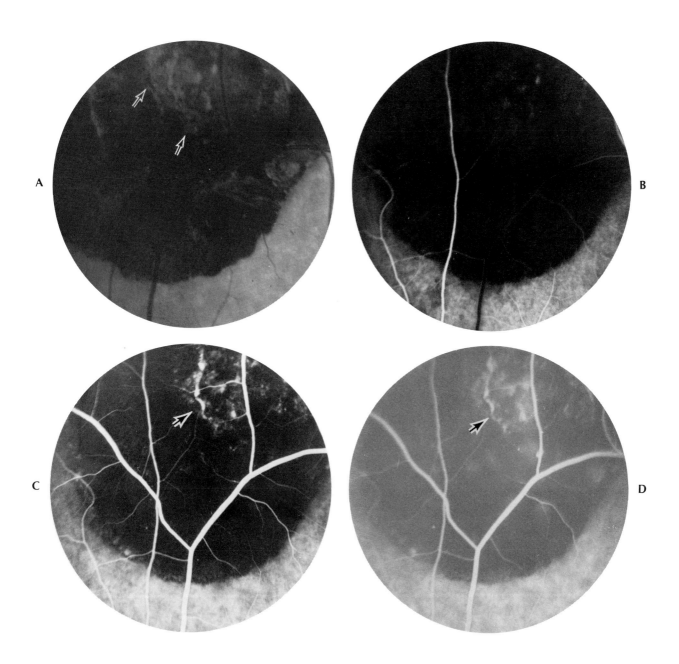

Fig. 8-4. Histopathologic condition of hypertrophy of the retinal pigment epithelium.

A, A coin-shaped, flat pigmented lesion was an incidental finding on gross examination of an autopsy eye. Note the nonpigmented halo just inside the margins of the pigmented lesion.

B, Histopathologic examination revealed the pigmented tumor illustrated in **A,** to be composed of a single layer of large retinal pigment epithelial cells filled with enlarged, round pigment granules (right half of photomicrograph). The main body of the lesion was separated from the normal surrounding pigment epithelium by a halo of partly depigmented pigment epithelium *(arrows)*. There was extensive degeneration of the outer layers of the retina overlying the entire lesion. There were scattered large cells filled with pigment granules lying on the surface of the pigmented lesion and in some areas they were present in the inner retinal layers.

C, High-power view of the lesion showing the large pigment epithelial cells packed with large round melanin granules. Note the loss of the outer layers of the overlying retina.

D, High-power view (same magnification as in **C**) of the retina and normal pigment epithelium adjacent to the pigment epithelial lesion shown in **A** and **C.**

E, Histopathologic condition of another patient with hypertrophy of the pigment epithelium. In this case there is a sharp line of junction *(arrow)* separating the normal pigment epithelium on the left side of the photomicrograph and the hypertrophy of the pigment epithelium on the right side. Probably the clinical appearance of this lesion was more like those without depigmented halos depicted in Figs. 8-1, *A* and *F,* and 8-3, *A.* Note also in this case the retina overlying the hypertrophy of the pigment epithelium appears normal. In this case, Bruch's membrane appears thickened and there is some atrophy of the underlying choriocapillaris.

F, Electron microscopic view of the normal pigment epithelium *(left side)* and the hypertrophied pigment epithelium *(right side)* (same case as in **A**). Note the thickening of the basement membrane *(bm)* of the pigment epithelium.

G, Hypertrophy of the retinal pigment epithelium associated with a large central fenestrated area noted in gross examination of an autopsy eye.

H, Electron microscopy of the margin *(arrow)* of the hypertrophied pigment epithelium *(to left of arrow)* and the central fenestrated areas showing loss of the pigment epithelium in the fenestrated area and proliferation of glial cells along the inner surface of Bruch's membrane.

(**A** to **C** and **F** to **H** from Buettner.[1])

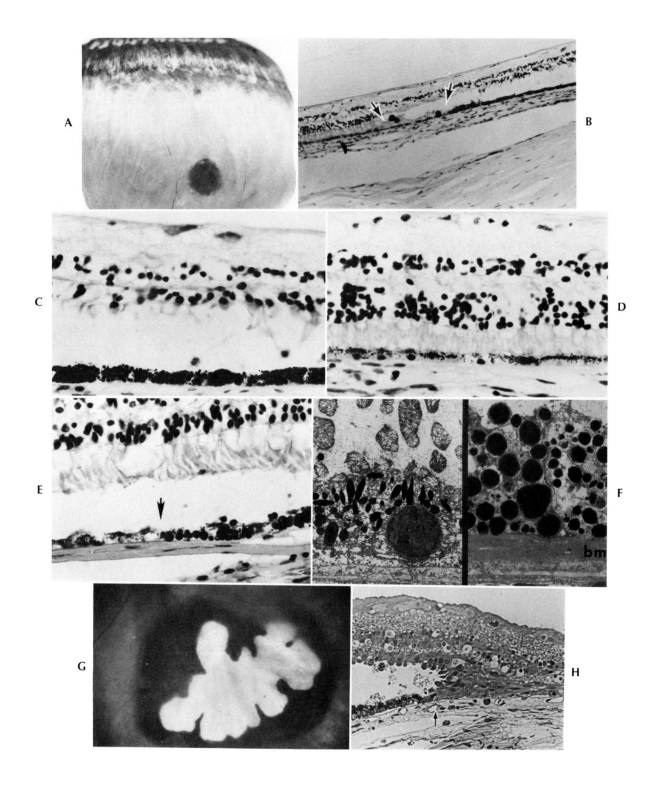

Fig. 8-5. Amelanotic freckle of the pigment epithelium.

A, Note the sharply circumscribed nonelevated white subretinal lesion noted in gross examination of a fresh eye removed at autopsy. (Same eye as in Fig. 2-17, *E.*)

B, Histopathologic condition showing a focal area of depigmentation of the artifactitiously detached retinal pigment epithelium corresponding with the lesion shown in **A** *(arrows).*

C and **D,** High-power views showing the sharp transition *(arrows)* between the nonpigmented flattened pigment epithelial cells and the relatively normal surrounding pigment epithelial cells.

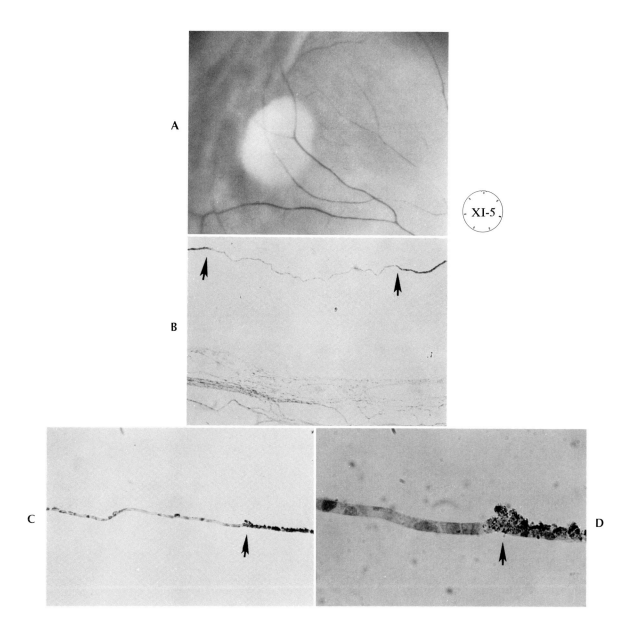

XI-5

Fig. 8-6. Juxtapapillary retinal and pigment epithelial hamartoma simulating a malignant melanoma. A 21-year-old white man noted progressive distortion of vision and a negative paracentral scotoma in his left eye for approximately 1 year. His unaided vision had been 20/20 in each eye 2 years previously. There was no history of previous injury of inflammation. There was no history of strabismus. He was the product of a full-term, normal pregnancy and delivery. His birth weight was 8 pounds. He had had a number of flat, darkly pigmented spots on his buttocks and arms since early childhood. His general health was excellent. His family history was normal. Uncorrected visual acuity in his right eye was 20/20+2 and in the left eye was 20/50. The vision could not be improved with lenses. Amsler grid examination demonstrated a negative scotoma nasal to fixation and metamorphopsia centrally. The right fundus was normal.

A, In the left eye there was a circumscribed, slightly elevated, finely mottled, pigmented lesion involving the retina and margins of the optic disc between 6 and 3 o'clock. Flecks of pigmented tissue extended anteriorly into the thickened retina and optic nerve tissue and partly covered the major retinal vessels as they entered the optic nervehead. The preretinal membrane covered the surface of the lesion. Prominent retinal traction folds extended from the area of the preretinal membrane into the macula. There were many fine dilated tortuous capillaries within the tumor. No cells were present in the vitreous. The pigment epithelium surrounding the nasal and superior margin of the lesion was irregularly hypopigmented. There was no evidence of serous detachment.

B to **D,** Fluorescein angiography showed dilated capillaries within the tumor and minimal evidence of leakage of dye from these vessels.

E and **F,** Seven years later the patient's visual acuity in the left eye was 20/70. The lesion appeared slightly shrunkened. The gray membrane covering the surface of the lesion was more prominent. The superior half of the optic nerve head was pale. Note evidence of further displacement of some of the retinal vessels *(arrows)* toward the lesion (compare with **A**).

(**A** to **D** from Vogel et al.[2])

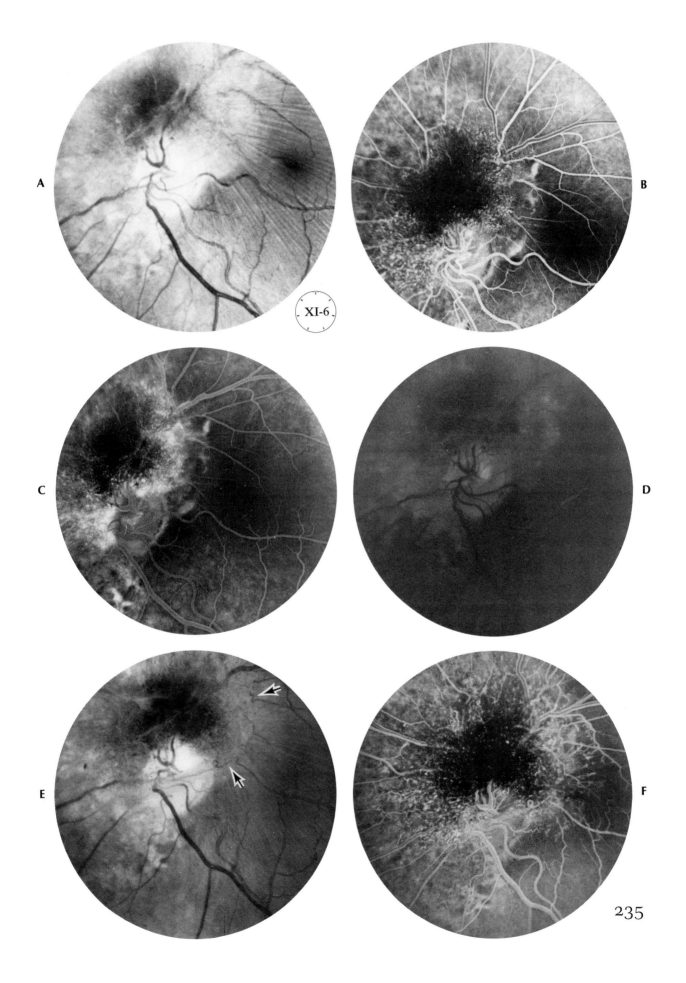

235

Fig. 8-7. Hamartoma of the pigment epithelium and retina simulating a malignant melanoma. A 29-year-old man gave an 8-week history of blurred vision in his left eye.

A, There was a dirty gray, brownish, slightly elevated, well-defined lesion involving the nasal half of the optic disc and surrounding retina. There were retinal folds extending into the macular area. Dilated capillaries were present within the tumor. There were salt-and-pepper changes in the surrounding pigment epithelium. Melanoma was suspected and the eye was enucleated.

B, Histopathologic examination revealed disorganization of the normal architecture of the optic nerve head and retina associated with hyperplasia of the retinal blood vessels, retinal pigment epithelium, and glial tissue. Cords and sheets of pigment epithelial proliferation extended throughout the tumor and surounded blood vessels. Note the proliferation of fibrous tissue near the surface of the retina.

C, A 49-year-old man had an ophthalmoscopic picture similar to that depicted in **A.** Note the similarity of the histopathologic findings. In addition, there is duplication of the underlying pigment epithelium *(arrows)*. Note the multiple folds in the inner retinal layers secondary to the fibrocellular membrane along the inner retinal surface.

(**A** from Machemer[3]; **B** from Machemer[3]; and **C** from Vogel et al.[2])

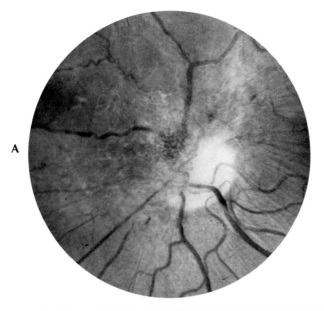

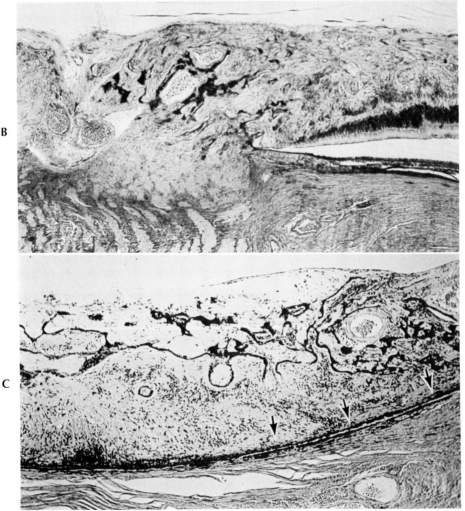

237

Fig. 8-8. Optic nerve head tumor presumed to be hamartoma of the pigment epithelium and retina. A 70-year-old white woman gave a history of poor vision in her left eye for at least 10 years. There was no previous history of injury. Visual acuity in the right eye was 20/40 and in the left eye was finger counting. She had a Marcus Gunn pupillary reaction on the left. There were drusen present in the right macula.

A, In the left eye she had a slightly gray, elevated, fibrovascular mass that involved the upper half of the optic disc and surrounding retina. There were patchy areas of hyperpigmentation at the base of the lesion. There was a zone of atrophy of the pigment epithelium surrounding the lesion. The retinal vessels superiorly were buried within the substance of the lesion. In the macula there was a pigmented disciform scar.

B, In the temporal periphery of the left eye there was an elevated irregularly pigmented lesion involving the pigment epithelium and retina.

C and **D,** Fluorescein angiography revealed many blood vessels within the optic nerve head tumor.

E, There was minimal staining of the tumor 1 hour after injection of the dye. This was evidence that the tumor was probably composed of rather densely packed tumor cells rather than collagen, which would have been stained intensely with dye. Note the choroidal staining surrounding the tumor where the pigment epithelium was depigmented. This patient has been followed for a period of 2 years with no change in either the optic nerve head or peripheral lesions. The diagnosis is that the cause is unknown, but it is presumed that both lesions probably represent hamartomas involving the pigment epithelium and retina. The absence of pigment in the optic nerve head lesion does not exclude the possibility of the hamartoma's being largely the result of hyperplastic pigment epithelium since, in some cases, the abnormal pigment epithelium does not produce melanin. Possibly the peripheral lesion is a pigmented disciform scar secondary to a previous hemorrhage from a peripheral choroidal neovascular membrane similar to that in the patient's left macula.

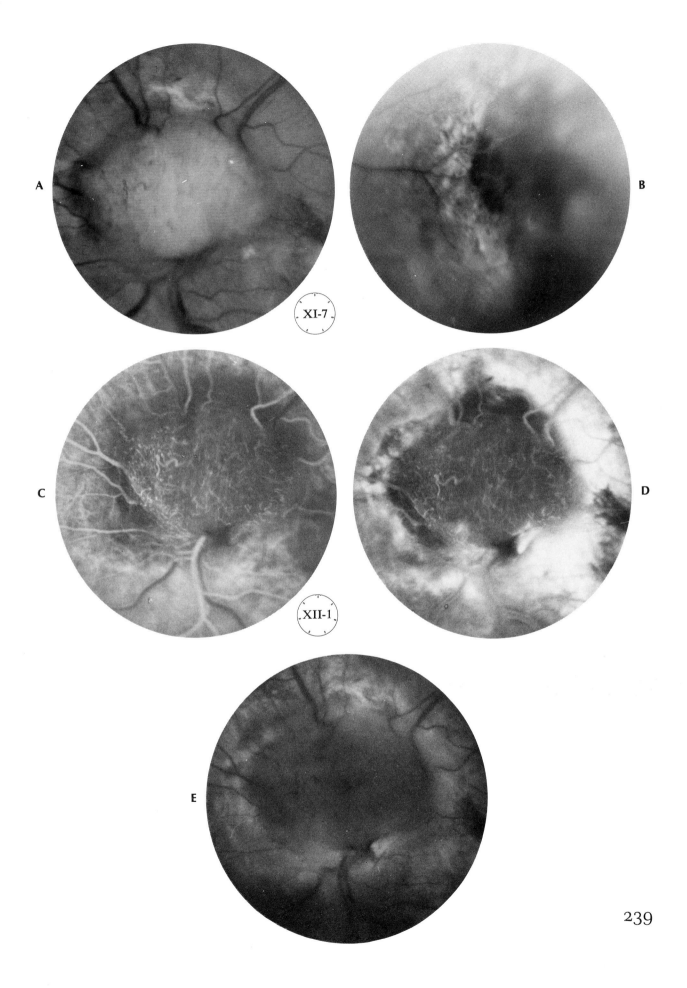

239

Fig. 8-9. Probable hamartoma of the pigment epithelium and retina simulating retinoblastoma and malignant melanoma of the choroid. A 19-month-old white girl was referred to the Bascom Palmer Eye Institute because of the possibility of retinoblastoma. She was the product of an uncomplicated, full-term pregnancy and delivery. Her birth weight was 8 pounds. No supplemental oxygen was used. Her growth and development were normal until age 5 months when intermittent exotropia was noted. Her first cousin was "blinded from pressure on the nerve head." A maternal aunt had visual loss secondary to a brain tumor. The patient's general health was good. Vision in the right eye appeared to be normal. She was unable to fix steadily with the left eye. Cycloplegic retinoscopy of the right eye was −1.25 and in the left eye was −10.00 +2.50 × 90. The left eye was slightly smaller than the right eye. The fundus of the right eye was normal.

A to **C,** The fundus photographs were made with the patient lying on her right side. In the left eye there was pronounced displacement of the major retinal vessels, optic nerve head, and the macula (*arrow in* **A**) in a superotemporal direction toward a partly pigmented tumor that extended from the temporal portion of the macula in a fanlike projection to the equator. Much of the central portion of the pigmented lesion was obscured by a mound of gray-white, semitranslucent, thickened retinal tissue and a preretinal membrane along its inner surface. The retinal vessels within the tumor were slightly dilated and tortuous and appeared to be gathered together beneath the contracted preretinal vitreous membrane. Fine traction folds of the retina radiated outward from the margins of the tumor. There was some straightening of the retinal vessels that coursed beyond the tumor anterior to the equator. The peripheral margins of the tumor presented a feathery appearance where the flat highly pigmented portion of the lesion blended imperceptively into the normal pigment epithelium (*arrows* in **C**). There were no hemorrhages, exudates, or subretinal fluid. The vitreous was clear. By age 40 months the child's visual acuity in the right eye was 20/40 and in the left eye was finger counting. The retinal lesion was unchanged.

D to **F,** A 30-month-old white girl was referred to the Bascom Palmer Eye Institute with the diagnosis of possible retinoblastoma or malignant melanoma. She was the product of a full-term normal pregnancy and delivery. At age 2 months a left exotropia was noted. Her growth and development were otherwise unremarkable. Her past medical history showed one episode of pneumonia and a febrile convulsion. She had one sibling who had an exotropia. The family history was otherwise normal. Visual acuity in the right eye appeared to be normal. Fixation with the left eye was poor. She was unable to locate a penny at 2 feet with the left eye. A left exotropia was present. Funduscopic examination of the right eye was normal. Funduscopic examination of the left eye revealed inferotemporal displacement of the optic nerve head and retinal vessels toward a large, eight-disc-diameter-size, elevated, partly pigmented mass in the macula and paramacular areas. The base of the lesion was black in color and relatively flat and was at the level of the pigment epithelium. The central portion of the pigmented lesion was obscured by thickened semitranslucent retinal tissue and a gray-white preretinal membrane. There was no evidence of retinal detachment, exudation, or hemorrhage. The peripheral margins of the pigmented lesion were feathery and blended imperceptively with the normal pigment epithelium. (From Gass.[4])

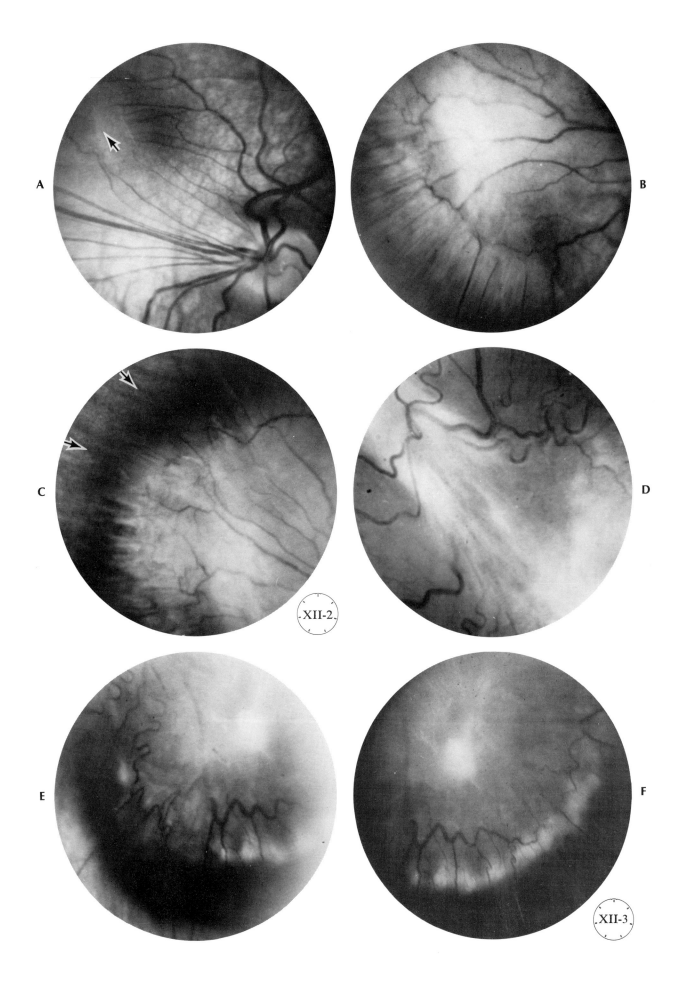

Fig. 8-10. Hamartoma of the pigment epithelium and retina in the macular region. An 8-year-old white boy in good ocular health was referred to the Photographic Laboratory of the Wills Eye Hospital (Philadelphia) in 1967 because of a lesion in the left macula. There was no accompanying history and the patient was lost to follow-up examination. His right fundus was normal.

A, The left fundus showed a lesion almost identical to that depicted in Fig. 8-9.

B to **D,** Fluorescein angiography demonstrated exceptional tortuosity, dilatation, and abnormal permeability of the retinal vessels in the region of the tumor. *Arrows* indicate the temporal border of the flat pigmented portion of the tumor.

(From Gass.[4])

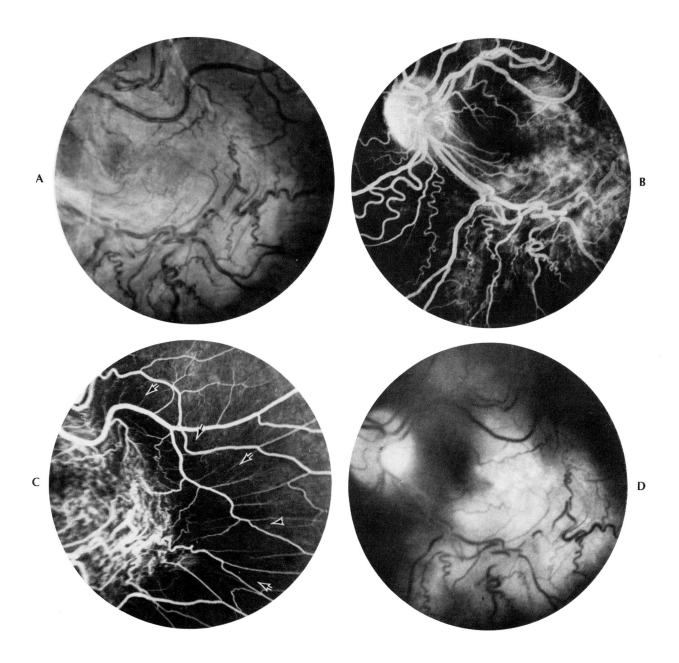

Fig. 8-11. Peripheral hamartoma of the pigment epithelium and retina simulating a malignant melanoma in a child. A 6-year-old white boy was referred to the Bascom Palmer Eye Institute because of a pigmented mass in the periphery of the right eye. He was the product of a 7-month pregnancy and a breach delivery. His birth weight was 5 pounds, 15 ounces. He was maintained in an isolette for several days. A small red lesion, presumed to be a hemangioma, was present on the right temporal area at birth. It increased in size to about 20 millimeters and was excised when he was 9 months of age. The boy's general health was good. His growth and development were normal. One sibling, age 16, had esotropia and amblyopia. Two other siblings were normal. Visual acuity in the right eye was 20/400 and in the left eye was 20/20. He had 10 prism diopters of right esotropia.

A, Ophthalmoscopic examination revealed considerable displacement of the major retinal vessels and macula (*arrow*) in a superotemporal direction.

B and **C,** In the superotemporal quadrant of the right eye there was a slightly elevated, black lesion that extended along the equator between 9 and 12 o'clock. This was associated with slight tortuosity of the retinal vessels overlying the tumor. Some of the vessels were partly obscured by a few areas of gray semitranslucent tissue interpreted as preretinal vitreous condensation. The edges of the tumor blended imperceptively into the normal pigment epithelium. There was no evidence of retinal detachment, hemorrhages, or exudates. The left fundus was normal.

D, Fluorescein angiography revealed scattered areas of focal dilatation of the retinal capillary bed over the peripheral aspect of the lesion. There was no evidence of dye leakage from these vessels. The retinal vessels appear to extend normally into the periphery of the fundus in the area of the tumor. When the boy was reexamined at age 12 years, the lesion was unchanged.

E and **F,** A 3-month-old white boy was referred to the Bascom Palmer Eye Institute because of a pigmented lesion in the right eye. He was the product of an 8-month pregnancy that was otherwise uncomplicated. His birth weight was 5 pounds, 13 ounces. There was no history of supplemental oxygen therapy. His growth and development were normal except for an esotropia that developed at age 6 months. On examination he had central fixation in both eyes. There was no strabismus demonstrable. In the right fundus there was a slightly elevated, poorly circumscribed, dark gray lesion, about two to three disc diameters in size along the inferonasal retinal vessels (*arrows*). The retinal vessels traversing the lesion were slightly tortuous, and they and the underlying pigmented lesion were partly obscured by a light gray membrane. There was no subretinal exudation and hemorrhage. There was a slight inferonasal displacement of the inferior major retinal vessels. The left eye was normal. At age 7 years the visual acuity in the right eye was 20/70 and in the left eye 20/20. A small-angle esotropia was present. The fundus lesion in the right eye was unchanged.

(From Gass.[4])

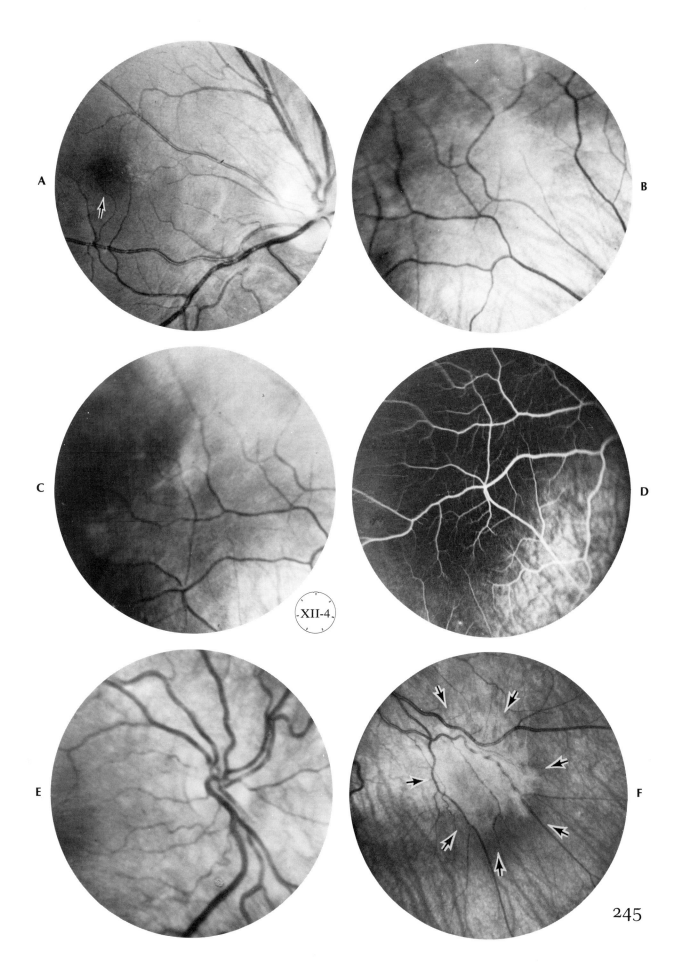

PRIMARY ADENOMAS AND ADENOCARCINOMA OF THE RETINAL PIGMENT EPITHELIUM

Primary hyperplastic and neoplastic tumors involving solely the retinal pigment epithelium are extremely rare.

REACTIVE HYPERPLASIA OF THE PIGMENT EPITHELIUM

The rare primary tumors of the pigment epithelium may be difficult in some cases to distinguish from the more common reactive hyperplasias of the pigment epithelium secondary to trauma, intraocular foreign body, inflammation, underlying choroidal tumors, and degenerative lesions associated with subpigment epithelial and subretinal bleeding (Fig. 7-6, *E*).

REFERENCES

1. Buettner, H.: Congenital hypertrophy of the retinal pigment epithelium, Amer. J. Ophthalmol. (In press.)
2. Vogel, M. H., Zimmerman, L. E., and Gass, J. D. M.: Proliferation of the juxtapapillary retinal pigment epithelium simulating malignant melanoma, Doc. Ophthalmol. **26:**461-481, 1969.
3. Machemer, R., Die primäre retinale Pigmentepithelhyperplasie, Graefe Arch. Ophthalmol. **167:** 284-295, 1964.
4. Gass, J. D. M., An unusual hamartoma of the pigment epithelium and retina simulating choroidal melanoma, Trans. Am. Ophthalmol. Soc. **LXXI:** 171-185, 1973.

SUGGESTED READINGS

Duke, J. R., and Maumenee, A. E.: An unusual tumor of the retinal pigment epithelium, Am. J. Ophthalmol. **47:**311-317, 1959.
Fair, J. R.: Tumors of the retinal pigment epithelium, Am. J. Ophthalmol. **45:**495-505, 1958.
Garner, A.: Tumors of the retinal pigment epithelium, Brit. J. Ophthalmol. **54:**715-723, 1970.
Graham, G. C.: Juxtapapillary retinal pigment epithelial tumor, Arch. Ophthalmol. **85:**299-301, 1971.
Kurz, G. H., and Zimmerman, L. E.: Vagaries of the retinal pigment epithelium, Int. Ophthalmol. Clin. **2:**441-464, 1962.
Reese, A. B.: Hyperplasia and neoplasia of the pigment epithelium. In Boniuk, M. (editor): International symposium on ocular tumors, Houston, Texas, 1962: Ocular and adnexal tumors, St. Louis, 1964, The C. V. Mosby Co., p. 303.
Reese, A. B.: Pigmented tumors; de Schweinitz lecture, Am. J. Ophthalmol. **30:**537-565, 1947.
Reese, A. B., and Jones, I. S.: Benign melanomas of the retinal pigment epithelium, Am. J. Ophthalmol. **42:**207-212, 1948.
Schlernitzauer, D. A., and Green, W. R.: Peripheral retinal albinotic spots, Am. J. Ophthalmol. **72:**729-732, 1971.
Vogel, M. H., and Wessing, A.: Die Proliferation des juxtapapillaren retinalen Pigmentepithels, Klin. Monatsbl. Augenheilkd. **162:**736-743, 1973.

CHAPTER NINE

Retinal telangiectasis

Retinal telangiectasis is a congenital anomaly of the retinal vessels that typically occurs in one eye of an otherwise healthy boy or young man (Figs. 9-1 to 9-5 and 9-7). Less than 20 percent of cases occur in females and less than 20 percent are bilateral. The disease is usually discovered during the first two decades of life, although some patients may remain symptom free until beyond 60 years of age. The disease is rarely familial and has seldom been associated with other diseases. It has been reported in multiple family members who also had muscular dystrophy (Fig. 9-4, A to C). I have seen one patient who also had facial hemiatrophy and multiple other anomalies (Fig. 9-4, D to F). These patients present a great variety of clinical pictures depending on the severity of the retinal vascular involvement. Those with minimal retinal involvement often present in the second decade of life, or later, with cystoid macular edema and exudation (Fig. 9-1), a localized peripheral retinal detachment, or a peripheral subretinal mass, usually in the inferior half of the eye (Fig. 9-6). Those patients with more widespread involvement usually present early during the first decade of life because of strabismus, a white pupillary reflex, or failure to pass an eye examination in school. Retinal telangiectasis always involves the retinal capillary bed and, in addition, may involve the major retinal arteries and veins. In some patients only a small segment of the retinal capillary bed is affected and the patient may be asymptomatic for years before vascular decompensation leads to cystoid macular edema, circinate retinopathy, and localized retinal detachment (Fig. 9-1). The small irregularly dilated retinal capillaries simulate those seen in other retinal angiopathies, such as diabetes, branch vein occlusion, and so forth. Retinal capillary changes in retinal telangiectasis may be widespread and may involve the optic nervehead as well. In some patients large aneurysmal dilation of the major retinal vessels as well as the capillary bed may occur (Figs. 9-2 to 9-4). Patients with prominent aneurysms have been referred to in the past by some authors has having Leber's miliary aneurysms. These areas of aneurysmal involvement may be surrounded by localized retinal exudation, exudative detachment, and circinate retinopathy. As the degree of exudation increases, a mound of dark greenish exudative detachment develops beneath the telangiectatic vessels. Amorphous yellow exudate is deposited beneath and within the retina near the periphery of the detachment. Large quantities of yellow exudate derived from the peripheral telangiectasis may form a disciform macular lesion that eventually organizes (Figs. 9-2 and 9-3). The findings of a yellowish white exudative mound in the macula of one eye in a child should always suggest the possibility of peripheral retinal telangiectasis. Massive yellowish or white exudative detachment of the retina secondary to retinal telangiectasis is the most common cause of so-called Coats' disease or more accurately, Coats' syndrome (Figs. 9-2, 9-4, 9-5, and 9-7). The demonstration of the telangiectatic vessels is important in differentiating this form of telangiectasis from exophytic retinoblastoma. In severe cases subretinal hemorrhage, retinitis proliferans, total retinal detachment, and glaucoma may occur (Fig. 9-7). Visual function may be extremely low or absent. Subretinal exudate in the macular area and in the periphery of the fundus may organize to form gray subretinal mounds that may simulate postinflammatory or neoplastic subretinal tumors (Figs. 9-3 and 9-6).

Fluorescein angiography is helpful in demonstrating the structural and permeability alterations of the retinal vascular abnormality (Figs. 9-1 to 9-4 and 9-6). The permeability of the telangiectatic vessels to fluorescein is variable. Portions of the affected capillary bed may be absent (Figs. 9-2 and 9-3). There may be a slight delay in perfusion of the telangiectatic segment of the retina. The dye stains both the intraretinal and subretinal exudate in the vicinity of the telangiectatic vessels. Retinal exudate remote from the telangiectasis may not stain. The yellowish subretinal and intraretinal exudate does not show angiographic evidence of staining. Organized subretinal exudative masses do stain with fluorescein (Fig. 9-3, F).

The course of retinal telangiectasis is quite variable. Generally it is a slowly progressive disease once exudation commences. Some patients may remain stable for a number of years. In a few patients there may be a spontaneous remission of the exudation (Fig. 9-1, E and F). A zone of noticeable pigmentary disturbance surrounding the margins of an organized subretinal mass can be seen as evidence of spontaneous resolution of exudative retinal detachments in some patients.

Photocoagulation as well as transscleral cryotherapy and diathermy are useful in destroying localized areas of peripheral retinal telangiectasis to reduce the degree of intraretinal and subretinal exudation (Figs. 9-1, 9-2, 9-4, and 9-6). Treatment of peripheral lesions is successful in reducing the heavy deposit of yellowish exudate in the macular area (Fig. 9-2), and good visual acuity may return if treatment is done prior to the development of retinal degeneration and organization of the exudate. Photocoagulation may also be used in the treatment of paramacular telangiectasis outside the papillomacular bundle area to reduce cystoid macular edema and exudation (Fig. 9-1). Photocoagulation of paramacular lesions, however, probably should be delayed if only minor visual loss is present, since in some patients the visual loss may not progress and spontaneous improvement may occur (Fig. 9-1, E and F).

The localized form of retinal telangiectasis affecting only the capillary bed may simulate but usually can be differentiated from similar microvascular changes occurring in diabetes, branch vein occlusion, x-ray irradiation, and hypertension. Cases with large aneurysms involving the major retinal vessels should be differentiated from cavernous hemangioma of the retina (see Chapter 11) and acquired macroarterial aneurysms of the retina. Patients with this latter disease are typically middle aged or older, and they present with a solitary retinal artery aneurysm usually in association with evidence of hypertensive retinal vascular changes. Patients presenting with yellow-white disciform macular lesions secondary to peripheral retinal telangiectasis may be misdiagnosed as having an inflammatory disciform detachment secondary to *Toxocara canis* or to trauma. Infants and children presenting with large areas of white or yellow exudative retinal detachment may be misdiagnosed as exophytic retinoblastoma. The presence of telangiectatic vessels in the detached retina, the absence of vitreous opacities, and the presence of a normal opposite eye are findings against but not entirely excluding retinoblastoma (see Chapter 13). These patients also must be differentiated from other causes of Coats' syndrome, such as retinal angiomatosis (Chapter 10) and senile macular degeneration with extensive yellowish exudative detachment of the retina. A peripheral organized exudative mass secondary to retinal telangiectasis can be misdiagnosed as choroidal melanoma or other subretinal tumors when it is first discovered in an adult (Fig. 9-6). These lesions are usually located in the inferior fundus. Such lesions would be less likely to cause macular detachment and symptoms early in life. Telangiectatic vessels may not be clearly visible in these organized lesions.

The histopathologic findings in the advanced exudative stages of retinal telangiectasis are demonstrated in Figs. 9-5 and 9-7. An outpouring of PAS-positive exudate surrounds the dilated telangiectatic retinal vessels and appears to stream into the outer retinal layers, which appear degenerated and disorganized. The exudate extends into the subretinal space where it contains masses of lipid and pigment-laden macrophages and cholestrol clefts. These lipid-laden macrophages may be found beneath the retina as well as within the outer retinal layers in areas quite remote from the telangiectatic vessels. Presumably, these macrophages are responsible for the yellow exudate seen clinically. Massive endothelial proliferation and obstruction of the telangiectatic vessels may be associated with hemorrhagic infarction of the retina in severe cases (Fig. 9-7). Retinal gliosis, fibrous metaplasia of the pigment epithelium, and organization of the subretinal exudate may eventually occur. In the late organized stages the histopathologic diagnosis of retinal telangiectasis may be difficult or impossible to make. The choroid is not primarily involved in retinal telangiectasis.

Fig. 9-1. Exudation and detachment secondary to localized retinal telangiectasis. A 48-year-old white man was in good ocular health until July 1970, when he noted metamorphopsia in the right eye. His eye examination in March 1966 was said to be normal. His visual acuity was 20/20 in each eye at that time. When he was seen initially at the Bascom Palmer Eye Institute in February 1973, his visual acuity in the right eye was 20/70 and in the left eye was 20/15.

A, Ophthalmoscopic examination revealed circinate retinopathy that was centered just temporal to the right macular area. Within this area of circinate retinopathy there were many telangiectatic retinal capillaries. There was some serous detachment of the underlying retina and cystoid macular edema.

B and **C,** Fluorescein angiography confirmed the presence of the retinal telangiectasis and cystoid macular edema. Argon laser photocoagulation was used to treat many of the telangiectatic vessels outside the central macular area in February 1973. There was gradual resolution of the circinate exudate and intraretinal edema.

D, Despite apparent resolution of the exudate, when the patient was last seen on September 11, 1973, his visual acuity in the right eye was still 20/70.

E and **F,** A 21-year-old white man noted sharp loss of visual acuity in his right eye at age 16.

E, He had a localized area of exudative detachment of the retina involving the temporal half of his right macula. There were dilated vessels in the center of this lesion, which was surrounded by circinate exudate. The cause at that time was unknown. No treatment was prescribed and over a period of several years his central vision gradually returned. He was initially examined at the Bascom Palmer Eye Institute at age 21 years. At that time his visual acuity was 20/20. There was retinal telangiectasis involving the temporal half of the macula that extended almost to the equator. He had only a few small yellowish intraretinal exudates. There was no cystoid macular edema or detachment. He was last seen at age 26 years, and at that time his visual acuity was 20/20.

F, Ophthalmoscopic examination revealed retinal telangiectasis and no evidence of intraretinal exudation or retinal detachment. This patient illustrates that in some cases, at least, spontaneous regression of intraretinal exudation may occur in retinal telangiectasis.

(**E** and **F** from Gass.[1])

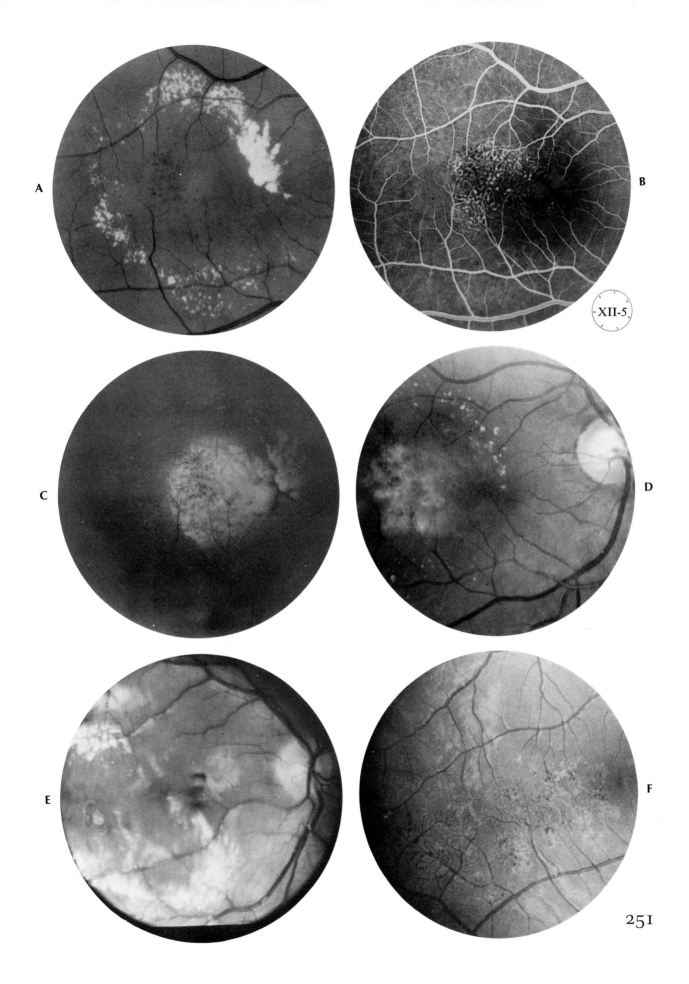

251

Fig. 9-2. Total exudative retinal detachment secondary to retinal telangiectasis. A 2½-year-old white boy developed right exotropia at age 2 years. He was the product of a full-term normal pregnancy and delivery. His general growth and development were normal. Visual acuity was light perception in the right eye. The vision in the left eye was normal.

A, Ophthalmoscopic examination of the right eye revealed a total exudative detachment of the retina. There were large deposits of yellowish exudates within and beneath the retina posteriorly. Note the slight engorgement of the retinal vessels.

B, In the periphery of the fundus, temporally, there was an elevated dark greenish subretinal exudative mass covered with many dilated tortuous and partly sheathed telangiectatic vessels.

C, Angiography outlined the telangiectatic vessels, which leaked dye during the later stages of the study. Note the dark areas where no capillary perfusion was present. The telangiectatic vessels were treated with xenon photocoagulation and the subretinal exudate resolved.

D, When the boy was 10 years of age, a small subretinal disciform scar remained in the macula. Visual acuity in the eye was finger counting at 6 feet.

(From Gass.[2])

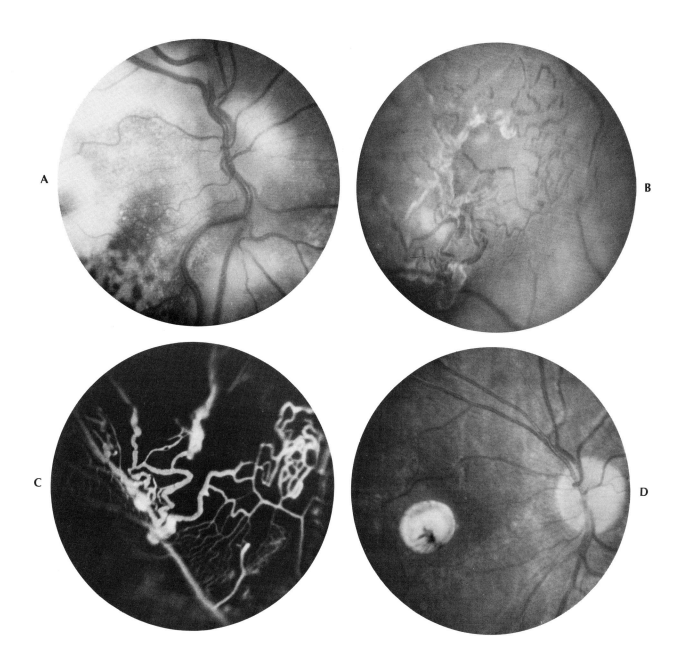

Fig. 9-3. Organized disciform macular scar secondary to retinal telangiectasis. A 12-year-old black boy was examined because of poor vision in his left eye.

A, Ophthalmoscopic examination revealed a large, elevated, partly organized disciform subretinal scar involving the posterior pole of the left eye. There was serous and yellowish subretinal exudate surrounding the superior half of the lesion. The right fundus was normal.

B, In the periphery of the left eye superiorly there were dilated telangiectatic retinal vessels overlying subretinal exudate, which extended into the posterior pole. Note the large aneurysms located on both the arterial and venous side of the circulation.

C to **E,** Angiography demonstrated partial loss of the capillary bed in the area of the telangiectasis and leakage of dye from the telangiectatic vessels.

F, One-hour angiogram showing staining of the disciform macular lesion.

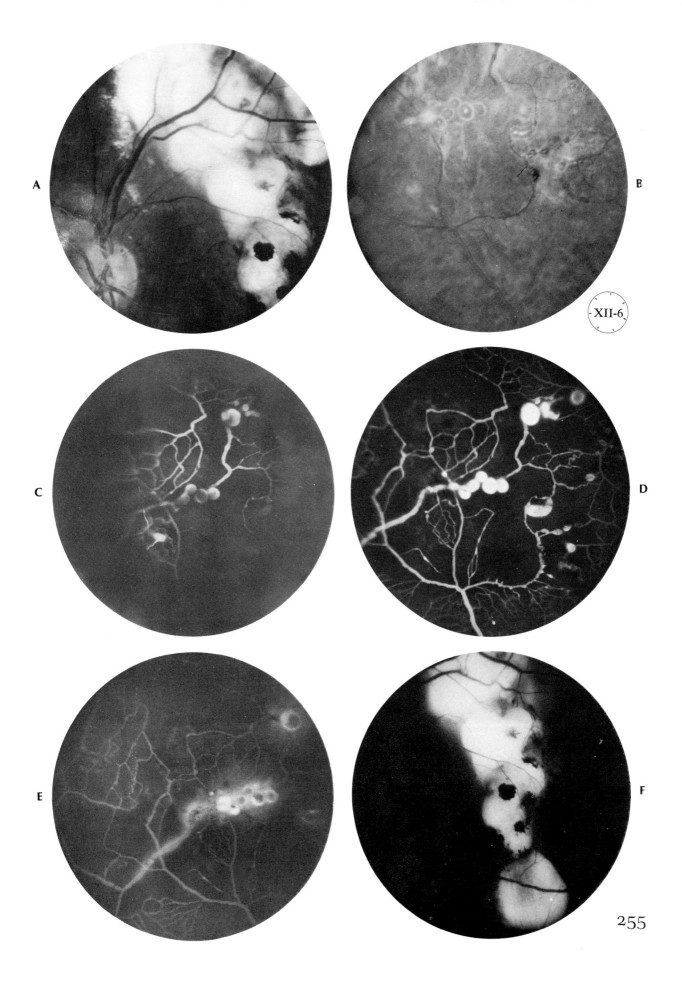

Fig. 9-4. Massive exudative retinal detachment secondary to retinal telangiectasis simulating retinoblastoma. A 6-year-old white boy was examined because of poor vision in his left eye. He and his brother and a maternal uncle had muscular dystrophy. There were several other members of the mother's side of the family with muscular dystrophy. The patient had a cutaneous spider on one cheek. He had numerous cafe-au-lait spots and some elevated pigmented nevi. Visual acuity in the right eye was normal, and in the left eye was light perception only. The right fundus was normal.

A and **B,** Funduscopic examination of the left eye revealed a massive yellowish exudative detachment of the retina. In the superotemporal quadrant there was a yellow-white elevated subretinal mass associated with massive telangiectasis involving the major retinal vessels and capillary bed.

C, Fluorescein angiography outlined the areas of retinal telangiectasis overlying the peripheral mass. The subretinal exudate was drained transsclerally and the telangiectatic vessels were partly destroyed with transscleral cryopexy. Nine months later the retina was reattached. When he was last seen 3 years later, however, he had again developed a small area of localized peripheral retinal detachment. Because of the poor visual function in the eye, no further treatment was recommended.

D to **F,** A 13-year-old white boy was examined because of an exudative detachment and a peripheral subretinal mass in his right eye.

D, There were multiple congenital defects including facial hemiatrophy, left esotropia, left deafness, a congenital bowel defect requiring bowel resection and colostomy, and hypospadias. He had strabismus surgery at age 11 years. He had no visual symptoms until 5 months prior to his examination when he noted blurred vision in the right eye. Visual acuity in the right eye was 20/40 and in the left eye was 20/30.

E and **F,** Funduscopic examination of the right eye revealed an elevated exudative subretinal mass between 5:30 and 8 o'clock. There was yellowish subretinal exudate surrounding the mass and a serous retinal detachment that extended into the posterior pole. He had a similar but smaller lesion in the nasal periphery of his left eye. The lesion in the right eye was treated with transscleral cryotherapy. This was complicated by vitreous hemorrhage. He never regained central vision in his left eye and this eye was treated successfully using argon laser.

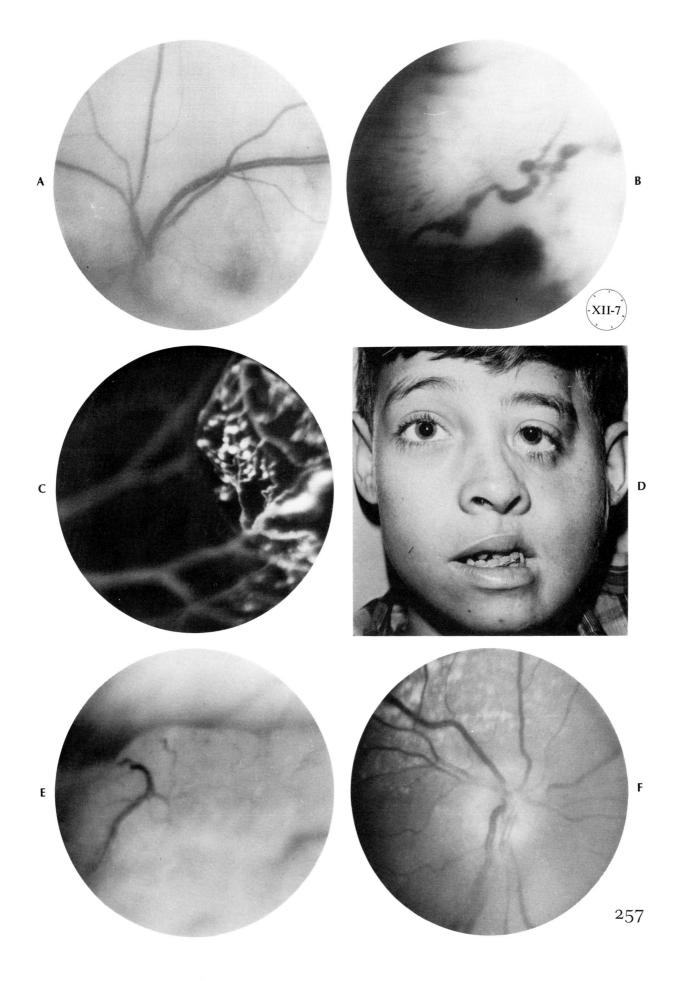

Fig. 9-5. Peripheral exudative subretinal masses secondary to retinal telangiectasis in a child whose eye was enucleated with the mistaken diagnosis of retinoblastoma. A 2½-year-old black boy had a history of exotropia of an 8-month duration. On initial examination, a yellowish exudative retinal detachment was noted and the initial impression was that it was probably Coats' disease. Soon thereafter, however, he developed several masses in the peripheral fundus. The eye was enucleated because of suspected retinoblastoma.

A, Gross examination of the eye revealed a multilobulated yellow-white subretinal mass (*black and white arrows*) located in the periphery of the eye. The surface of this lesion was covered with dilated, telangiectatic retinal vessels (*black arrow*). An exudative detachment extended into the posterior pole of the eye.

B, Histopathologic condition of the mass shown in **A**. Note the retinal thickening and the subretinal exudate in the temporal periphery of the eye. The dilated telangiectatic vessels evident in **A** are located at *arrow 1*. The detachment extended posteriorly as far as *arrow 2*. Lipid-laden macrophages were present within the outer retinal layers posteriorly (*arrow 3*).

C, High-power view of *area 1* in **B**. There were dilated retinal vessels (*arrows*) in the degenerated retina, which was greatly thickened by exudate containing pigment and lipid-laden macrophages and cholesterol slits. A similar exudate was present in the subretinal space.

D, High-power view of a telangiectatic capillary (*arrow*). Note the exudate within the extensively degenerated and disorganized retina.

E, High-power view of *area 3* in **B,** showing lipid-laden macrophages within the outer retinal layers in the macular area.

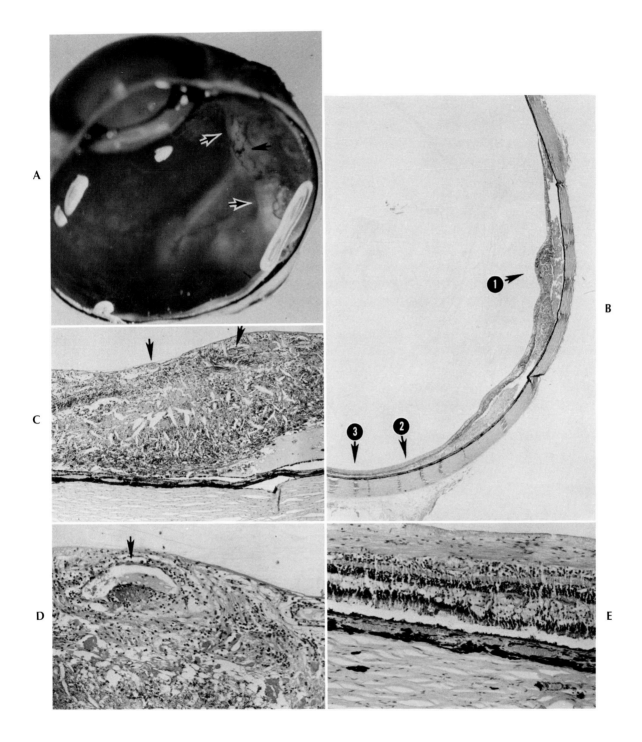

Fig. 9-6. Peripheral organized subretinal exudative mass simulating a malignant melanoma in an adult patient with retinal telangiectasis. A 44-year-old white man gave a 6-day history of a superior shadow in the right eye. His past history and family history were unremarkable. Visual acuity in both eyes was 20/20.

A and **B,** There was a serous detachment of the inferior one third of the retina in the right eye. There was yellowish exudate beneath and within the retina along the superior edge of the detachment. At 6 o'clock in the far periphery there was an elevated, multilobulated, gray, subretinal mass that extended posterior to the equator *(arrows).* There was telangiectatic capillaries overlying the mass.

C and **D,** Angiography showed evidence of retinal capillary telangiectasis and permeability to fluorescein overlying the mass. The peripheral telangiectatic vessels were treated with cryotherapy and resolution of the exudative retinal detachment occurred within several months.

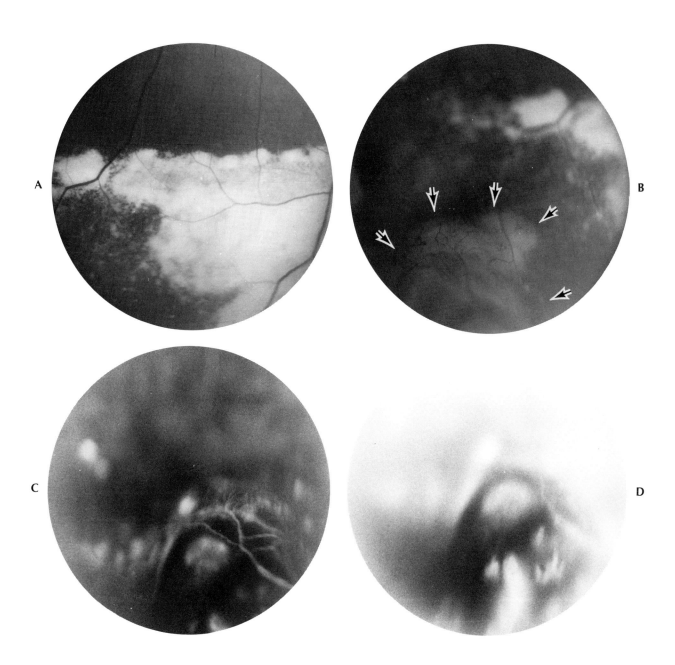

Fig. 9-7. Retinal exudation and hemorrhagic infarction secondary to retinal telangiectasis simulating an exophytic retinoblastoma. A 3-year-old white boy had a 3-week history of a white pupillary reflex in the left eye. His past medical history and family history were unremarkable. Visual acuity in the right eye was 20/15 and in the left eye was no light perception. Funduscopic examination of the right eye was normal.

A and **B,** Ophthalmoscopic examination of the left eye revealed evidence of retinal ischemia and massive intraretinal and subretinal exudation with areas of perivascular hemorrhage throughout the fundus. In areas, the retinal blood vessels were dilated and irregular in caliber. Note the cyanotic appearance of the obstructed arterioles (*arrows*). The initial clinical impression was that it was probable retinal telangiectasis. The patient returned 1 month later with infection of the conjunctiva of the left eye. His pupil was irregularly dilated and there was no light perception. The retina was totally detached and hemorrhagic. Because of the possibility of a retinoblastoma the eye was enucleated.

C, Histopathologic examination of the eye revealed endothelial proliferation of the retinal blood vessels throughout the eye. Note the prominent eosinophilic intraretinal exudation in the outer layers of the retina characteristic of retinal telangiectasis.

D, There was extensive hemorrhagic infarction and necrosis of the retina. Note the conspicuous vascular endothelial proliferation (*arrow*).

E, This figure shows a dilated, partly necrotic retinal vessel (*arrows*) and thickening of the retina secondary to intraretinal hemorrhage and exudation.

F, In several areas there was hemorrhagic detachment of the internal limiting membrane of the retina (*arrows*).

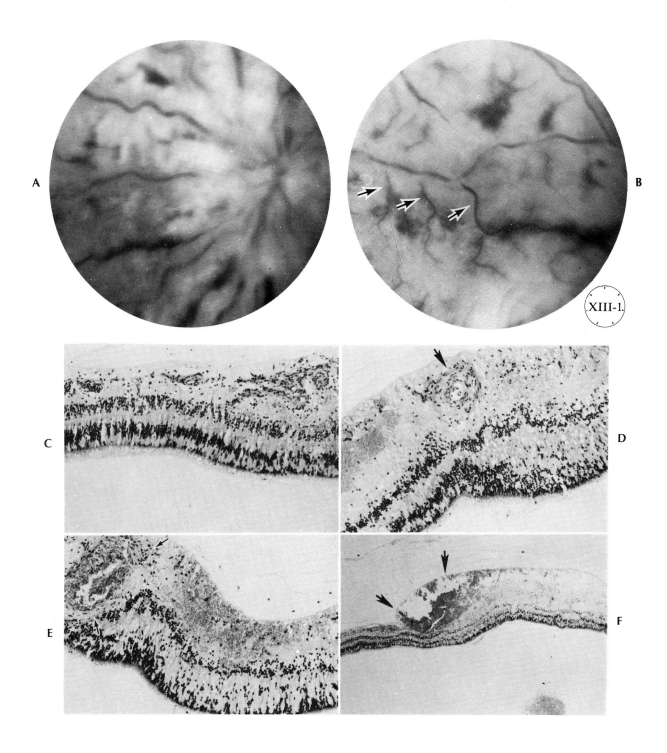

XIII-1.

REFERENCES

1. Gass, J. D. M.: Stereoscopic atlas of macular diseases, St. Louis, 1970, The C. V. Mosby Co., p. 155.
2. Gass, J. D. M.: A fluorescein angiographic study of macular dysfunction secondary to retinal vascular disease. V. Retinal telangiectasis, Arch. Ophthalmol. **80:**592-605, 1968.

SUGGESTED READINGS

Coats, G.: Forms of retinal disease with massive exudation, Royal London Ophthalmol. Hosp. Rep. **17:**440-525, 1907-1908.

Elwyn, H.: Coats' disease. In: Diseases of the retina, Philadelphia, 1946, Blakiston Division, McGraw-Hill Book Co., pp. 148-157.

Farkas, T. G., Potts, A. M., and Boone, B. S.: Some pathologic and biochemical aspects of Coats' disease, Am. J. Ophthalmol. **75:**289-301, 1973.

Frenkel, M., and Russe, H. P.: Retinal telangiectasia associated with hypogammaglobulinemia, Am. J. Ophthalmol. **63:**215-220, 1967.

Gautier-Smith, P. C., Sanders, M. D., and Sanderson, K. V.: Ocular and nervous system involvement in angioma serpiginosum, Brit. J. Ophthalmol. **55:** 433-443, 1971.

Reese, A. B.: Telangiectasia of the retina and Coats' disease, Am. J. Ophthalmol. **42:**1-8, 1956.

Small, R. G.: Coats' disease and muscular dystrophy, Trans. Am. Acad. Ophthalmol. Otolaryngol. **72:** 225-231, 1968.

Tripathi, R., and Ashton, N.: Electron microscopical study of Coats' disease, Brit. J. Ophthalmol. **55:** 289-301, 1971.

CHAPTER TEN

Angiomatosis retinae (von Hippel's disease)

Angiomatosis retinae and von Hippel's disease are terms used synonymously to describe congenital, hereditary, capillary angiomatous hamartomas of the retina and optic nerve. When associated with central nervous system and other organ involvement, this condition is referred to as von Hippel–Lindau disease. Lindau established that cystic capillary angiomas of the cerebellum were the isolated manifestation of a generalized developmental disease characterized by the occurrence of multiple angiomatous tumors of the retina, medulla, pons, and spinal cord, as well as polycystic or angiomatous lesions of the pancreas, lungs, liver, kidneys, adrenal glands, ovaries, and epididymis. Some authors have suggested that these lesions should be classified as neoplastic rather than hamartomatous lesions because of their unusual ability to grow in some cases. Pheochromocytomas and polycythemia are unusual components of this disease. Twenty to 25 percent of patients with retinal angiomas develop clinical evidence of central nervous system involvement. Probably a significantly higher percentage of patients have lesions in the central nervous system. The retinal lesions are reported to be bilateral in 50 percent of the patients. The retinal angiomas usually become manifest prior to 30 years of age. Central nervous system symptoms frequently manifest later than the ocular symptoms. The mode of transmission of the disease is autosomal dominant with incomplete penetrance and variable expressivity. The capillary angiomas may present in the retina, optic nerve head, or retrobulbar portion of the optic nerve. They may arise from the inner (endophytic) or outer (exophytic) retinal layers

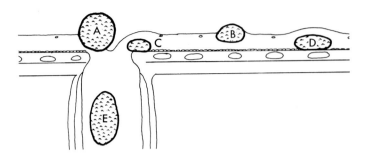

Fig. 10-1. Sites of origin of capillary angiomas in von Hippel's disease. **A,** Endophytic angioma of the optic nerve head. **B,** Endophytic peripheral retinal angioma. **C,** Exophytic juxtapapillary angioma. **D,** Exophytic peripheral retinal angioma. **E,** Intraneural angioma.

(Fig. 10-1). Early, the orange-red retinal tumor may be minute and unassociated with exudate or evidence of dilatation of the major retinal vessels. Later as arteriovenous shunting of blood develops within the tumor, the arteries and veins supplying and draining the angioma become tortuous, dilated, and similar in color (Figs. 10-2 to 10-7). Intraretinal and subretinal exudation and hemorrhage may eventually develop. The exudate is proteinaceous and contains lipid material that precipitates in a yellowish circinate pattern at the outer margins of the area of intraretinal and subretinal exudates surrounding the tumor. As the retinal detachment increases in size, yellowish exudate may accumulate beneath as well as within the retina in the macular area remote from the site of the angioma (Fig. 10-2). Dilatation and tortuosity of the feeder vessels do not occur or are not visible in those angiomas arising within (Fig. 10-8) or immediately adjacent to the optic nerve head (Figs. 10-9 to 10-11). An exophytic tumor in the juxtapapillary area may be relatively flat and inapparent until the patient develops circinate retinopathy, macular star, or serous retinal detachment (Figs. 10-9 and 10-11). The vascular supply of the exophytic tumors may be derived from the blood vessels of the optic nerve, the choroid, and the retina (Figs. 10-8 to 10-13). Lesions arising within the optic nerve head may be mistaken for papilledema (Fig. 10-13). The endophytic lesions may be associated with vitreous strands and neovascular ingrowth from the tumor surface into the vitreous (Figs. 10-3, 10-6, 10-8, and 10-12). Vitreoretinal traction near the tumor may cause a retinal hole and retinal detachment (Fig. 10-3). Loss of central vision secondary to contraction of a preretinal vitreous membrane may be the presenting complaint of patients with angiomatosis retinae as well as other peripheral vascular abnormalities (Fig. 10-6).

Fluorescein angiography may assist in the detection of minute angiomas that might be overlooked ophthalmoscopically (Fig. 10-6, *E* and *F*). There may be minimal extravascular leakage of dye from these minute tumors. As the tumor enlarges and is associated with dilatation and tortuosity of the major retinal vessels, angiographic evidence of arteriovenous shunting of blood through portions of the tumor becomes manifest (Figs. 10-2 to 10-4). Leakage of fluorescein occurs from the capillaries within the tumor as well as from the surrounding retinal capillaries. Large depositions of yellowish exudate in the macular area remote from the site of the angioma are usually unassociated with angiographic evidence of retinal vascular permeability changes in the macular area. Angiographic evidence of arteriovenous shunting is difficult or impossible to demonstrate in those lesions arising in or near the optic nerve head.

266

Histopathologically, these angiomas are composed of an aggregation of large histologically normal capillaries that are separated from each other by variable numbers of vacuolated stromal cells of uncertain origin (Figs. 10-12 and 10-13). These angiomas may occur as well-defined elevated tumors (Fig. 10-12, *A* and *B*) or as small placoid lesions arising either superficially (Fig. 10-12, *E*) or deep (Fig. 10-12, *F*) in the retina. Later, large foamy cells containing lipid accumulate between the capillaries (Fig. 10-13). These probably are secondary to chronic leakage of lipid-rich exudate from the capillaries comprising the tumor. Glial proliferation, exudation, hemorrhage, and retinal detachment are late secondary changes.

Untreated retinal angiomatosis usually leads to total retinal detachment, absolute glaucoma, and loss of the eye. Obliteration of the small isolated peripheral angiomas with light coagulation, cryopexy, or diathermy is possible. If not judiciously applied, however, this therapy may be followed by extensive retinal detachment, vitreous hemorrhage, retinitis proliferans, and retinal hole formation. A variety of modes of therapy have been proposed to avoid these complications. Most authors agree that it is preferable to use frequent applications of low-intensity therapy rather than a single application of high-intensity treatment. Xenon and argon photocoagulation are probably the most effective means of treatment of relatively small lesions. The ruby laser should not be used for this treatment. Successful obliteration of relatively small peripheral angiomas is usually possible with either photocoagulation or cryotherapy and will result in reattachment of the retina and resolution of intraretinal exudation. The degree of improvement of visual acuity is variable and probably depends primarily on the duration of the macular exudation. Photocoagulation of angiomas located on or surrounding the temporal margin of the optic nerve head is difficult to perform without destroying useful central vision (Figs. 10-8, 10-9, and 10-11). Photocoagulation of selected portions of the tumor may be successful in temporarily reducing the degree of intraretinal and subretinal exudation (Fig. 10-11). The long-term prognosis for central vision in these papillary and peripapillary tumors, however, is poor. Photocoagulation of lesions involving the optic nerve head should not be done in patients with normal visual acuity.

Fig. 10-2. Macular exudation and retinal detachment secondary to a retinal capillary angioma. A 24-year-old white man developed a field defect in his left eye. His past medical history and family history were normal. His visual acuity in the right eye was 20/15 and in the left eye was 20/800.

A, There was yellowish exudative material in the retina in the left macular area. A shallow serous detachment in the retina extended into the temporal periphery of the left eye.

B, Inferotemporally there was a one-and-one-half-disc-diameter-size nodular red tumor of the retina. The tumor was supplied by a single dilated retinal artery and was drained by two dilated tortuous retinal veins. Note the fine network of capillaries that connect these large vessels on the surface of the tumor. Note, also, the serous detachment and circinate retinopathy surrounding the tumor.

C, The arterial phase angiogram revealed rapid arteriovenous shunting of the dye through the tumor mass. Note dye in the vein *(arrow)* draining the tumor before complete perfusion of the retinal artery superior to the tumor.

D and **E,** Later angiography revealed evidence of leakage of dye from the vessels within the tumor as well as from the retinal capillary bed immediately surrounding the tumor.

F, The retinal angioma was treated with photocoagulation. Six months later the macular exudation had improved. The retinal detachment had disappeared. The patient developed retinitis proliferans in the region of the angioma and subsequently developed a tear and rhegmatogenous detachment, which was later repaired with a scleral buckling procedure.

(**A** to **E** from Gass.[1])

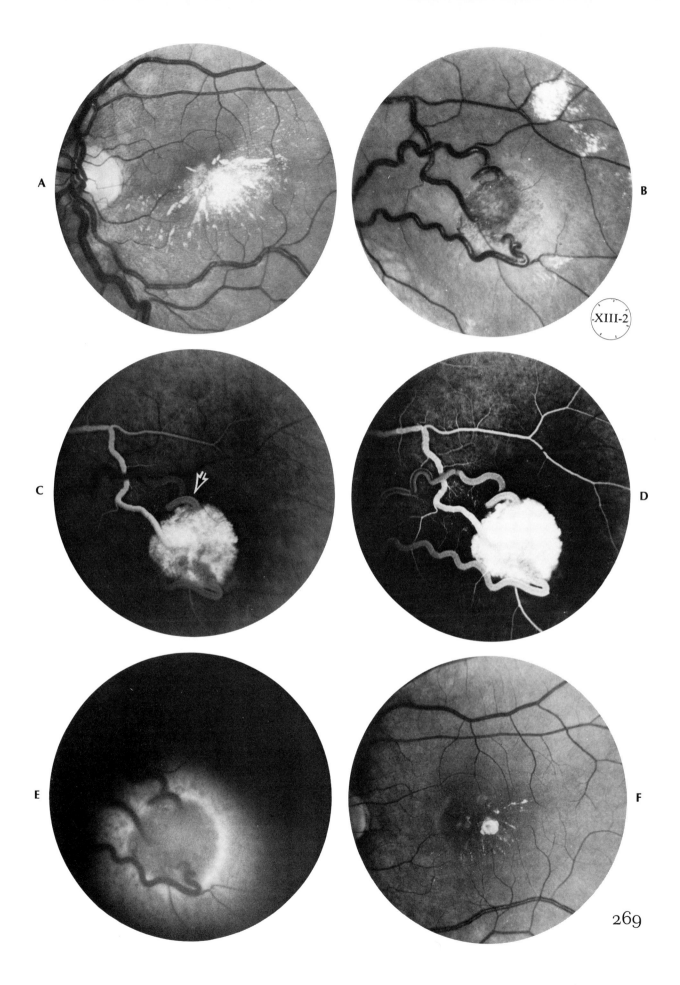

Fig. 10-3. Rhegmatogenous retinal detachment, the presenting manifestation of retinal angiomatosis. A 21-year-old white girl gave a 5-week history of floaters and a 2-day history of loss of the lower field of vision in her left eye. Her past history and family history were unremarkable. Funduscopic examination of the right eye was normal.

A, There was a bullous detachment of the retina superiorly in the left eye. At 12 o'clock at the equator there was a small red endophytic retinal angioma supplied by a dilated retinal artery and drained by a dilated tortuous retinal vein. An area of retinitis proliferans extended from the surface of the tumor into the vitreous. Just posterior to the angioma there was an irregular, well-circumscribed retinal tear (*arrows*).

B to **D,** Fluorescein angiography revealed rapid perfusion of the retinal angioma as well as new vessels extending from the angioma into the vitreous (*arrows*). Note the avascularity on the angiogram in the region of the retinal tear. The retinal angioma was treated with transscleral cryotherapy and a localized Silastic sponge buckle. On the first day postoperatively the retina was flat. There was no secondary exudative or hemorrhagic detachment during the early postoperative course.

E, One year after surgery the retina was flat and the angioma and retinitis proliferans were no longer evident within the white scar on the apex of the radial buckle (*arrows*).

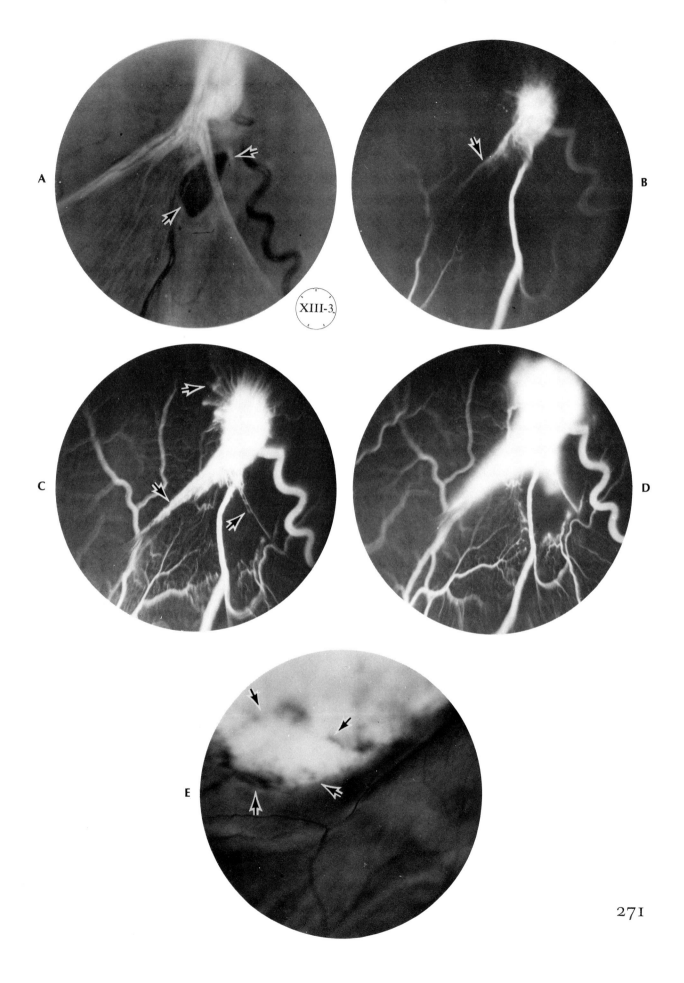

Fig. 10-4. Bullous detachment of the retina secondary to retinal angiomatosis. A 16-year-old white boy was seen in July 1965, because of loss of vision in his left eye. When he was 10 years of age, a school examination disclosed poor vision in his right eye. The diagnosis was "scar tissue in the back of the eye." He was 20/20 in the left eye at that time and had no trouble until August 1964, when he noted an inferior field defect. His local physician noted retinal detachment associated with three large retinal tumors at 11, 12, and 1 o'clock. The right eye was blind at that time and its fundus was not visible because of a cataract and pupillary membrane. The diagnosis at that time was retinal angiomatosis with secondary retinal detachment. Photocoagulation and cryotherapy were used to treat the lesions with no apparent effect on them. He developed a massive exudative detachment and was referred to the Bascom Palmer Eye Institute.

A and **B,** Superior to the left optic disc there was a large exophytic, orange-red retinal angioma *(black and white arrows)* with surrounding serous and yellowish exudative detachment of the retina. In the far periphery between 12 and 1 o'clock there were two other smaller angiomas with pigmentary changes secondary to previous photocoagulation and cryotherapy. Prominent dilated tortuous retinal vessels led to each of these three angiomas. On the surface of the 11 o'clock angioma there was a nest of fine capillaries lying between two large dilated retinal vessels *(black arrow)*.

C, An early angiogram revealed evidence of an arteriovenous shunt from the large dilated retinal artery *(black arrow)* through the small capillary cluster on the inner surface of the 11 o'clock angioma into a smaller retinal vein *(black and white arrow)*.

D and **E,** Later angiography revealed massive leakage of fluorescein into the substance of the retinal angioma. Transscleral cryotherapy to this mass was unsuccessful in reattaching the retina.

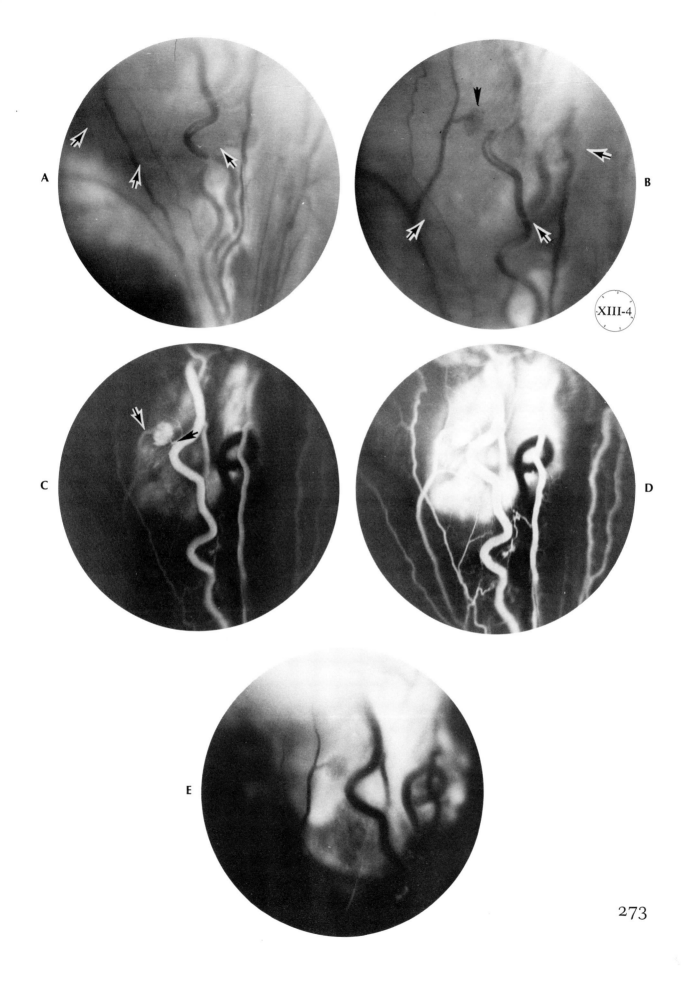

273

Fig. 10-5. Cystoid macular edema and macular distortion secondary to a preretinal vitreous membrane as the presenting manifestation of retinal angiomatosis. A healthy 28-year-old white man was seen at the Bascom Palmer Eye Institute in January 1973, with a 1-year history of distorted vision in his left eye. His local physician had diagnosed central serous retinopathy. His past medical history and family history were unremarkable. Visual acuity in the right eye was 20/20 and in the left eye was 20/80.

A, There were fine retinal folds extending into the macular area from a localized area of contraction of a preretinal vitreous membrane along the superotemporal vessels of the left eye *(arrows)*. There was cystoid macular edema. A few intraretinal and subretinal yellowish exudates were present inferior to the macula.

B, Inferiorly and temporally there was a large yellowish, exudative, balloonlike detachment of the retina. Two orange-red exophytic retinal angiomas were present in the 5 o'clock meridian. They were partly obscured by the opacification of the retina. A broad pigmented demarcation line surrounded the margins of the detachment. There was slight dilatation of the inferotemporal retinal vessels leading toward the area of detachment. There was pronounced dilatation of the retinal vesssels in the region of the angiomas.

C and **D,** Fluorescein angiography revealed prompt perfusion of the retinal angiomas and demonstrated dilatation and tortuosity of the retinal vessels in the area of the detachment. There was leakage of dye from the angiomas as well as from the retinal vessels in the area of the detachment. *Arrows* indicate the site of the small retinal angioma. The posterior margin of the larger angioma is just visible in the lower right hand corner of the angiogram.

E, Late angiogram showing cystoid macular edema *(arrow)* and staining of the retina in the region of the preretinal membrane. The patient was treated initially with argon laser with no effect whatsoever. In April 1973, heavy applications of xenon photocoagulation were placed over the two retinal angiomas.

F, By September 1973, the retina had reattached. There was partial destruction of the two retinal angiomas. The cystoid macular edema persisted and the visual acuity had not improved. The preretinal membrane had largely separated from the surface of the retina and had contracted into a ball along the superotemporal vessels *(arrow)*. Retreatment of the angiomas will be considered if improvement of the cystoid macular edema does not occur over the next 6 months.

274

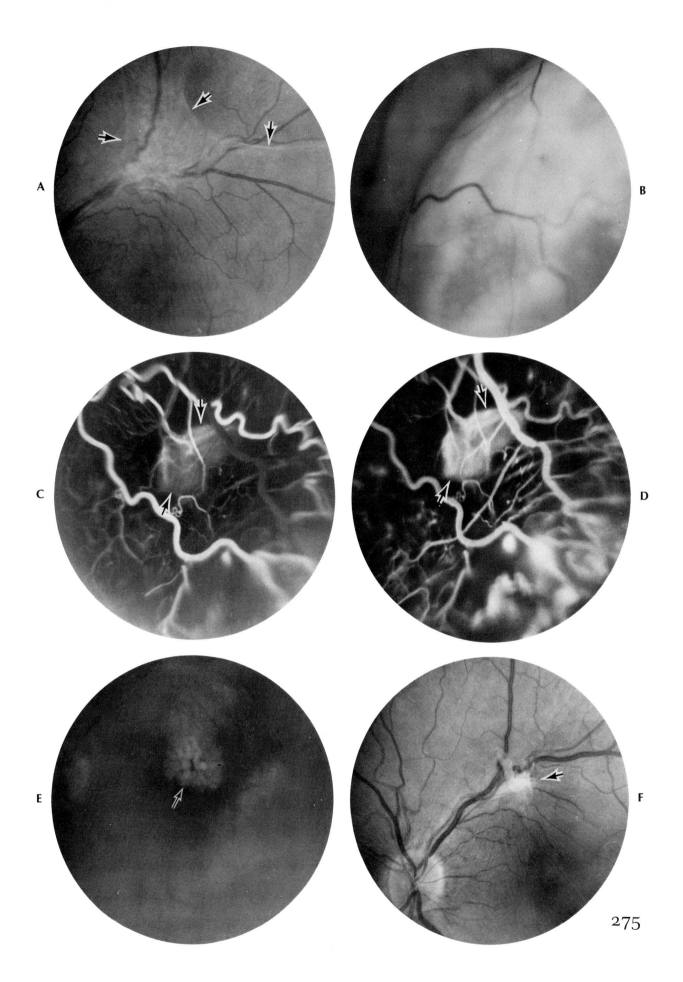

Fig. 10-6. Macular pucker secondary to retinal angiomatosis. A 23-year-old white woman was examined in February 1966, because of recent loss of central vision in the right eye. Her past medical history and family history were unremarkable. Visual acuity in the right eye was 20/70; in the left eye it was 20/15.

A, Ophthalmoscopic examination of the right eye revealed dilated tortuous retinal vessels on the temporal side of the fundus. The paramacular vessels were pulled centrally by a semitransparent preretinal vitreous membrane (*black and white arrows*). The optic nerve head was swollen. There were many new vessels present on the optic nerve head and surrounding retina (*black arrows*). There was a small retinal angioma in the left eye (see **E** and **F**).

B, At the equator, superotemporally, there was an oval-shaped, round, orange-reddish retinal angioma that was supplied by a dilated retinal artery and drained by a dilated tortuous retinal vein. Subretinal exudation surrounded the tumor. There was blood on the surface of the tumor.

C, Fluorescein angiography revealed extensive leakage of dye from the tumor. The tumor in the right eye was treated with cryopexy and photocoagulation. By June 1966, the preretinal membrane had detached from the macular surface and the visual acuity had improved. The peripheral angioma was destroyed.

D, When she was last seen in January 1972, the patient's visual acuity in the right eye was 20/25+3. The preretinal membrane had peeled from the surface of the retina and remained attached to the optic nerve head (*arrow*).

E, The small retinal angioma (*arrow*) noted in 1966 was approximately the same size.

F, Fluorescein angiography in the left eye confirmed the vascular nature of this small reddish retinal tumor. Over a period of years, this small tumor may exhibit growth and may eventually develop arteriovenous fistulization.

(From Gass.[2])

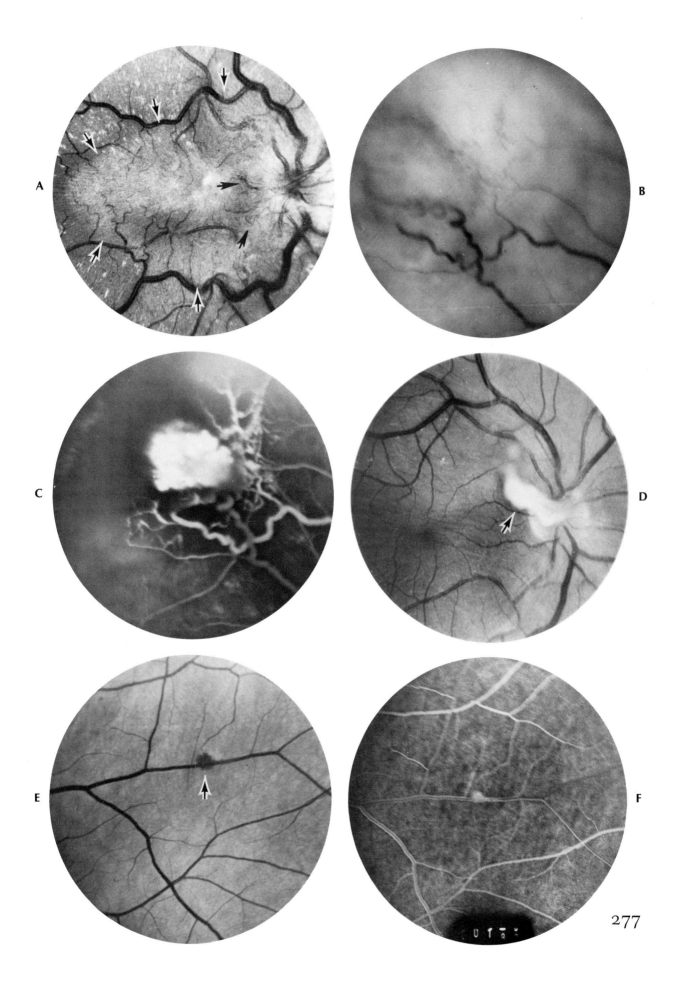

Fig. 10-7. Vermiform enlargement of the retinal vessels secondary to a large retinal angioma. A 21-year-old white boy was examined initially in 1968 and gave a 2-year history of decreased vision in the left eye. Visual acuity in the right eye was 20/20 and in the left eye it was light perception. A neurologic examination was normal.

A and **B,** Ophthalmoscopic examination of the left eye revealed an exudative detachment of the retina superiorly. There was considerable dilatation and tortuosity of the major retinal vessels.

C, In the far periphery, superiorly, there was a large orange-red exophytic retinal tumor (*arrows*).

D to **F,** Fluorescein angiography revealed a slight delay in filling of the retinal vein that drained the peripheral tumor and dilatation and permeability alterations in the capillaries of the optic nerve head and retina in the area of the vermiform enlargement of the major retinal vessels. One year later the retina was totally detached and was against the back surface of the lens. The patient developed angle-closure glaucoma and the eye was enucleated.

G, Histopathologic examination revealed a total retinal detachment and a capillary angioma of the retina in the far periphery (*arrows*).

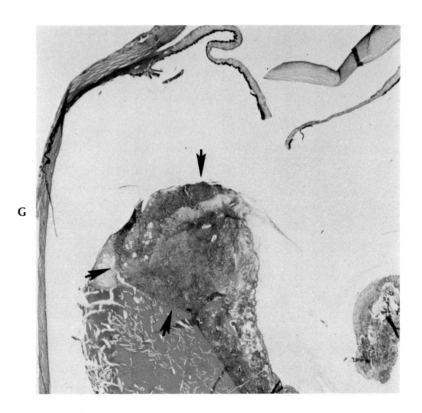

G

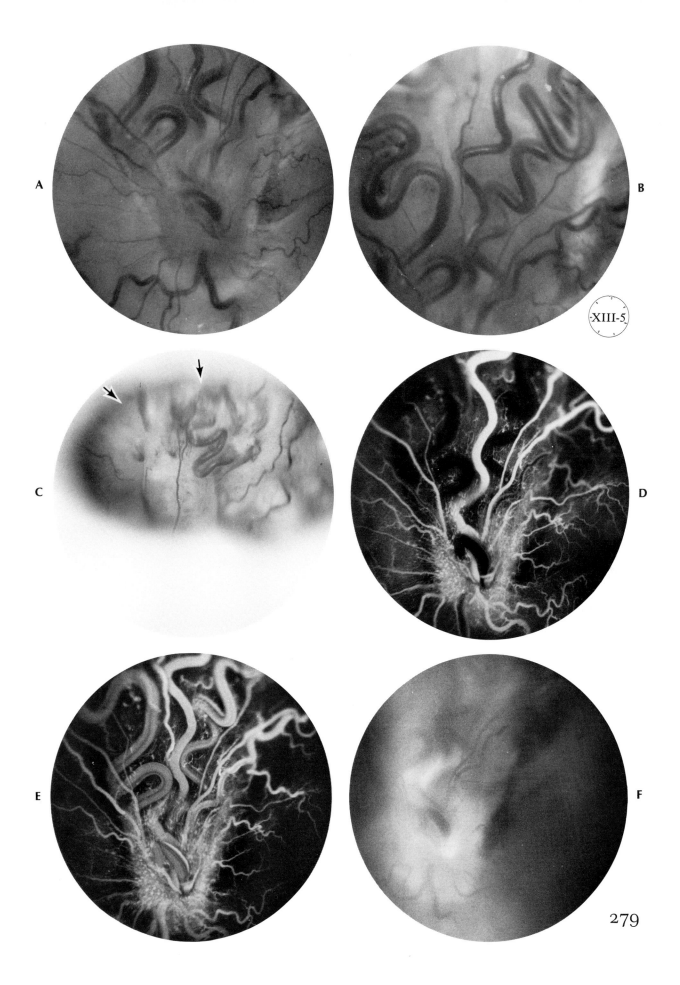

Fig. 10-8. Endophytic angiomatosis of the retina and optic nerve head. A 44-year-old white man had a routine eye examination in 1963. His local physician noted a hemangioma of the left optic nerve head at that time. Visual acuity was 20/20 in both eyes. He was followed until 1966 when xenon photocoagulation was used to treat the surface of the tumor. Immediately after the photocoagulation, he developed a dense central scotoma. His past history was unremarkable. His father died of epilepsy and progressive weakness and ataxia. He was examined initially at the Bascom Palmer Eye Institute in August 1968. His visual acuity in the right eye was 20/20 and in the left eye was 20/200.

A, In the left fundus he had a yellowish-orange tumor arising from the temporal half of the optic nerve head and adjacent retina. There was a small amount of surrounding sub-retinal serous and circinate exudate. A wisp of tissue extended from the inferior surface of the tumor into the vitreous (*arrow*).

B and **C,** Angiography revealed prompt perfusion of the retinal tumor and staining during the later phases.

D, By July 1970, the tumor had enlarged slightly, the subretinal exudate had increased, and the visual acuity had dropped to 20/400.

E, By July 1972, there was further enlargement of the temporal aspect of the tumor (*arrow*) and there were cystic macular changes as well as a large area of serous detachment and circinate retinopathy. Argon-laser photocoagulation was done but had no effect on the degree of the retinal detachment. No further treatment was recommended since the detachment did not extend beyond the posterior pole.

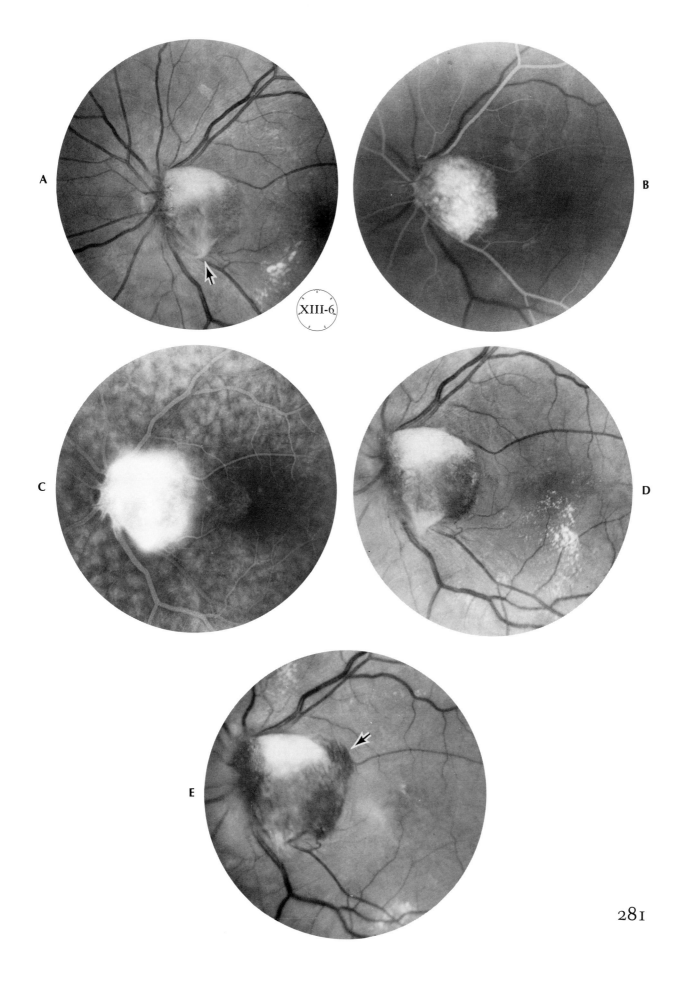

XIII-6

281

Fig. 10-9. Retinal detachment secondary to a juxtapapillary exophytic retinal angioma. A 30-year-old physician gave a 6-year history of a paracentral scotoma in his right eye. The scotoma had recently enlarged and he had noted decrease in his central vision associated with micropsia and metamorphopsia. His past medical history and family history revealed no phakomatoses. Maternal cousins had retinitis pigmentosa. Visual acuity in the right eye was 20/30 and in the left eye was 20/15.

A and **B,** Funduscopic examination in the right eye revealed a round, orange tumor involving the outer retinal layers and the inferotemporal edge of the optic disc *(arrows)*. A cystic retinal detachment extended inferiorly from the optic disc. There was yellowish subretinal and intraretinal exudate at the margins of this detachment. A shallow serous detachment of the retina extended into the macular region. There were dilated retinal capillaries overlying and extending down into the tumor.

C to **E,** Fluorescein angiography revealed evidence of dilation of the retinal capillaries overlying the tumor as well as dilation and permeability alterations extending into the area of long-standing retinal detachment. Some of the dilated tortuous capillaries overlying the tumor extended through the full-thickness of the retina into the tumor.

F, Between October 1969 and March 1970, he had three applications of photocoagulation to the area of the exophytic tumor as well as to the dilated capillaries extending from the inferior margin of the optic disc. There was reabsorption of the subretinal exudate, and when he was last seen on May 14, 1970, his visual acuity in the right eye was 20/50. There was still some circinate exudation superior to the macula *(arrow)*. The chances are great that this patient will develop further exudative changes from this exophytic vascular tumor and will lose additional central vision.

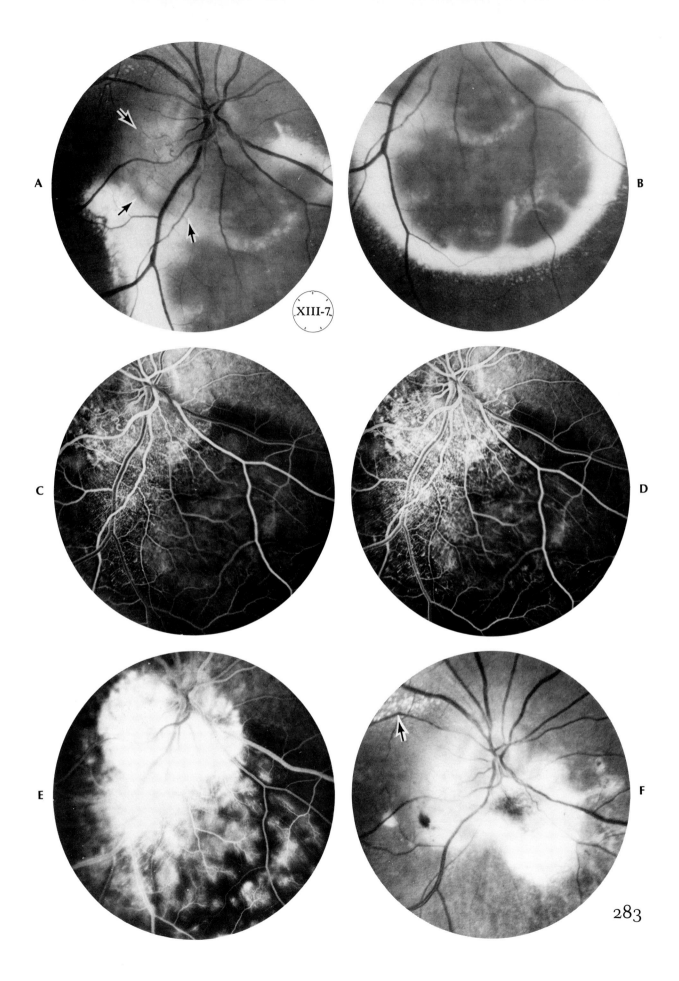

Fig. 10-10. Large juxtapapillary exophytic retinal angioma misdiagnosed as choroidal hemangioma and malignant melanoma of the choroid. A 46-year-old woman was seen at the Bascom Palmer Eye Institute in December 1969. She gave a 10-year history of blurred vision in the right eye.

A, A fundus painting made in 1959 revealed a large nonpigmented tumor arising from the temporal aspect of the right optic disc. At that time the two diagnoses entertained were choroidal melanoma and choroidal hemangioma. Her past medical history revealed hypertension. There was no family history of neurophakomatoses.

B, In December 1969, a large red globular tumor arose from the outer layers of the retina at the temporal margin of the optic disc in the right eye. Note that many of the large retinal vessels disappear into the surface of the tumor. Portions of the tumor appeared yellow rather than reddish orange. Subretinal exudates surrounded the tumor. A broad rim of pigment epithelial changes indicative of previous exudative retinal detachment surrounded the temporal margin of the tumor.

C, The arteriovenous phase angiogram revealed rapid perfusion of this exophytic retinal vascular tumor. Note the many dilated retinal capillaries on the surface of the tumor.

D, Late angiogram revealed massive leakage of dye into the tumor as well as into the subretinal exudate surrounding it. There were no retinal tumors in the left eye.

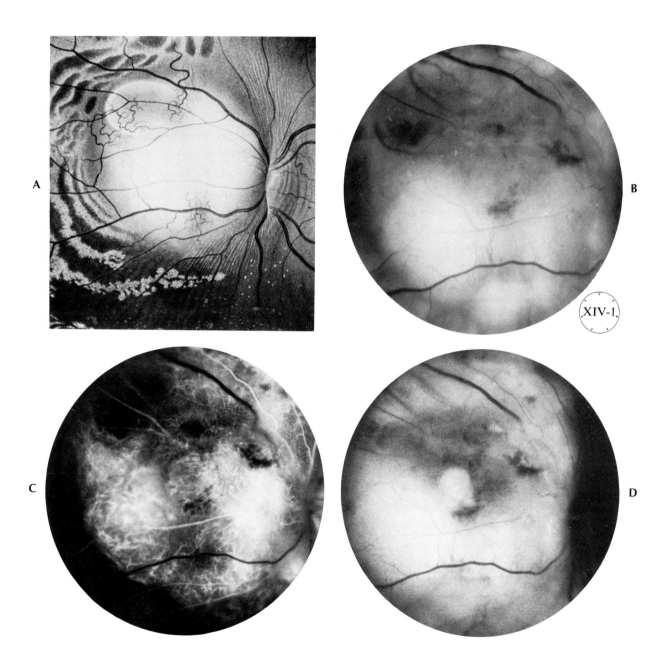

Fig. 10-11. Juxtapapillary exophytic retinal angiomatosis misdiagnosed as being papilledema. A 31-year-old white woman was referred to the Bascom Palmer Eye Institute in November 1970, because of a 5-month history of intermittent headaches and papilledema. Earlier in 1970 she had been hospitalized for thorough evaluation. Her neurologic examination was normal. Skull x-ray examination and carotid arteriograms were normal. Her past medical history and family history were normal. Visual acuity in both eyes was 20/20.

A, The retina surrounding the optic nerve head between 7 and 1 o'clock appeared thickened *(arrows)*. Many fine capillaries were visible within this portion of the retina as well as within the temporal half of the optic nerve head. A serous detachment extended into the macula. There was circinate retinopathy and a partial star figure. The left fundus was normal.

B, The early arteriovenous angiogram revealed a well-circumscribed, fine, vascular network confined to the area of swelling of the retina along the temporal margin of the optic nerve head *(arrows)*. Note that most of the capillaries lie deep within the retina. There was no evidence of pigment epithelial or retinal abnormality outside the immediate area of the slightly elevated optic nerve head tumor.

C and **D,** Angiography revealed evidence of leakage of dye from the capillaries within this tumor. Note the multiloculated pattern of cystoid edema along the tumor margins.

E, She subsequently developed chronic serous detachment of the macula and her visual acuity decreased to 20/50 in the right eye. On August 24, 1972, argon laser treatment was placed over a portion of the surface of the tumor to reduce the macular exudation.

F, By December 1972, visual acuity had improved to 20/20. Much of the subretinal exudate had disappeared. A repeat angiogram at this time revealed little change in the vascular pattern noted previously. The patient subsequently developed further loss of central vision caused by macular exudation and a second course of photocoagulation treatment was given. The prognosis for central vision in this patient with a retinal hamartoma involving the papillomacular bundle is quite poor.

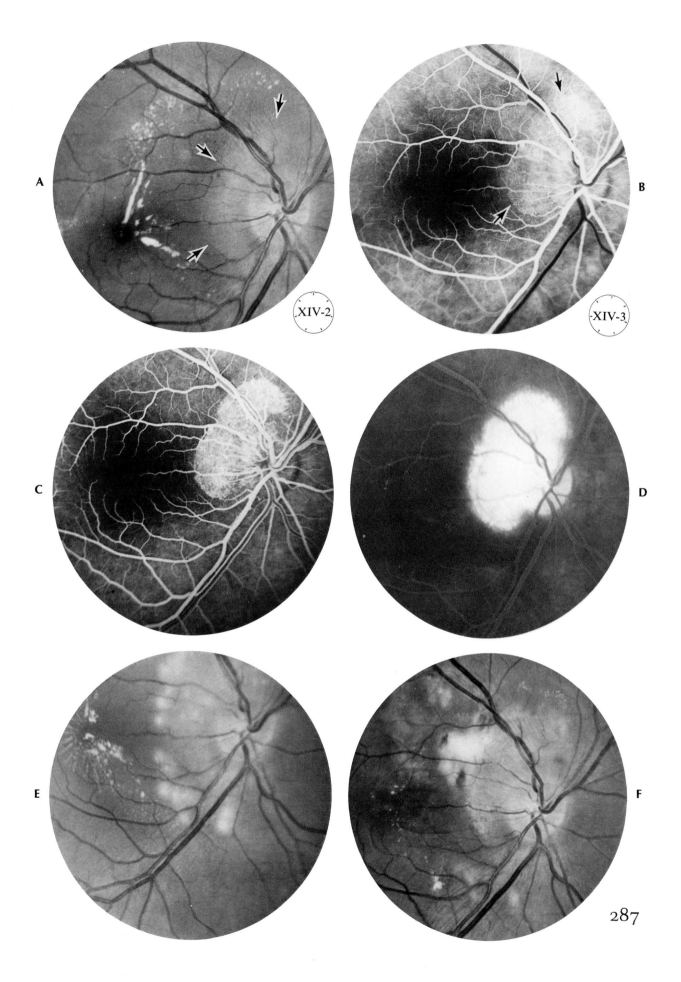

Fig. 10-12. Histopathologic condition of preexudative phase of retinal angiomas in von Hippel–Lindau disease. A 48-year-old white man complained of paresthesia of the arms and legs. His mother had died of a brain tumor at 40 years of age. His father died of unknown cause at 60 years of age. The patient's neurologic examination was normal. His cerebrospinal fluid protein level was 300 milligrams percent A myelogram revealed a block at the level of the first cervical vertebra, and a right brachial arteriogram revealed a large vascular tumor at the level of the brainstem. Cerebellar hemangioblastoma was found at craniotomy. The patient died soon thereafter. An autopsy revealed multiple cysts of the right kidney and pancreas.

A, Gross examination of the right eye revealed two nodular retinal angiomas. The larger one *(arrow)* measured 1.5 millimeters in diameter. The retinal vessels leading to both angiomas were dilated. There were no retinal exudates or retinal detachment. Two similar angiomas were present at the equatorial region of the left eye.

B, Histopathologic condition of the tumor depicted in **A**. Note the dilated feeder vessels *(arrow)* supplying the capillary tumor, which has replaced the normal retinal architecture and is protruding into the vitreous cavity.

C, High-power view of the tumor depicted in **B**. The tumor was composed of capillary-sized blood vessels lined by flattened endothelial cells. Most of the interstitial cells separating the capillaries were clear polygonal cells. There were occasional large glial and small multinucleated giant cells.

D, Strands of fibroglial tissue and capillaries were present on the surface of the tumor and extended into the vitreous *(arrow)*.

E, A small capillary angioma was present on the surface of the optic nerve head *(arrows)*.

F, At the nasal margin of the optic disc there was a small capillary angioma in the depth of the retina adjacent to the retinal pigment epithelium *(arrows)*. There was communication between this vascular lesion and the capillaries in the optic nerve head and the choriocapillaris at the margins of the optic disc.

(From Nicholson.[3])

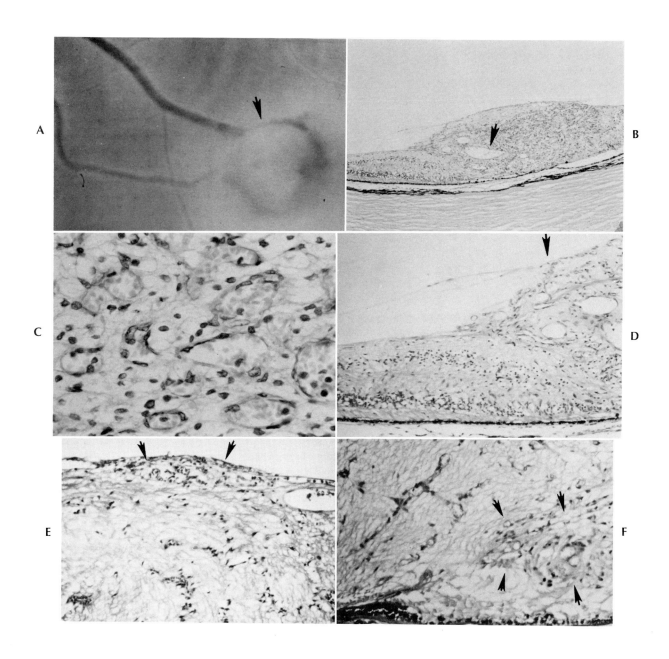

289

Fig. 10-13. Bilateral exophytic capillary angiomas of the optic nerve head and peripapillary retina simulating chronic papilledema. A 29-year-old white Army enlisted man first noted blurred vision in his right eye in early 1959.

A and **B,** Ophthalmoscopic examination revealed bilateral papilledema and peripapillary retinal exudates. A carotid arteriogram and pneumoencephalogram showed evidence of a small intracranial mass in the region of the infundibulum. In December 1959, a craniotomy was done and a biopsy was taken in the region of the infundibulum. The tissue was composed of mature, well-developed, cerebral gray matter that initially was interpreted as a hamartoma. At the time Dabezies and co-workers reported that the patient had a hypothalamic hamartoma. In June 1961, the patient was rehospitalized for treatment of a retinal detachment in the right eye. Visual acuity in the left eye was 20/20. The optic disc changes persisted. The patient was again hospitalized in August 1963, because of failing vision in his left eye. By this time, the right eye was blind. The patient's past medical history was unremarkable. The patient's mother died of an angioblastic meningioma. A niece and nephew had surgical removal of pheochromocytomas. A nephew had bilateral optic nerve head lesions said to be identical to those of this patient. On this admission, the patient's visual acuity in the left eye was 20/200. There was a total retinal detachment in the right eye. The optic nerve head was swollen

C, In the left eye there was evidence of a vascular tumor *(arrows)* involving the optic nerve head and the outer portions of the peripapillary retina. Yellowish exudates surrounded the optic nerve head. It was at this time that the diagnosis of retinal angiomatosis was first considered as the basis of the bilaterally swollen nerve heads. In January 1964, the right eye was enucleated.

D, Histopathologic examination of the right eye revealed a capillary angioma *(arrows)* involving the outer layers of the circumpapillary retina and the optic nerve head. There was extensive cystic degeneration of the surrounding retina. The retinal pigment epithelium in the peripapillary area was degenerated and in some areas was hyperplastic. The rod and cone layer was completely degenerated.

E, High-power view of the tumor showing considerable compression of the capillaries by large balloon cells filled with foamy cytoplasm.

F, There were bizarre astrocytic cells *(arrows)* scattered within the capillary angioma.

(**A** from Dabezies[4]; **C** from Gass[5]; **D** from Gass[5] and Darr.[6])

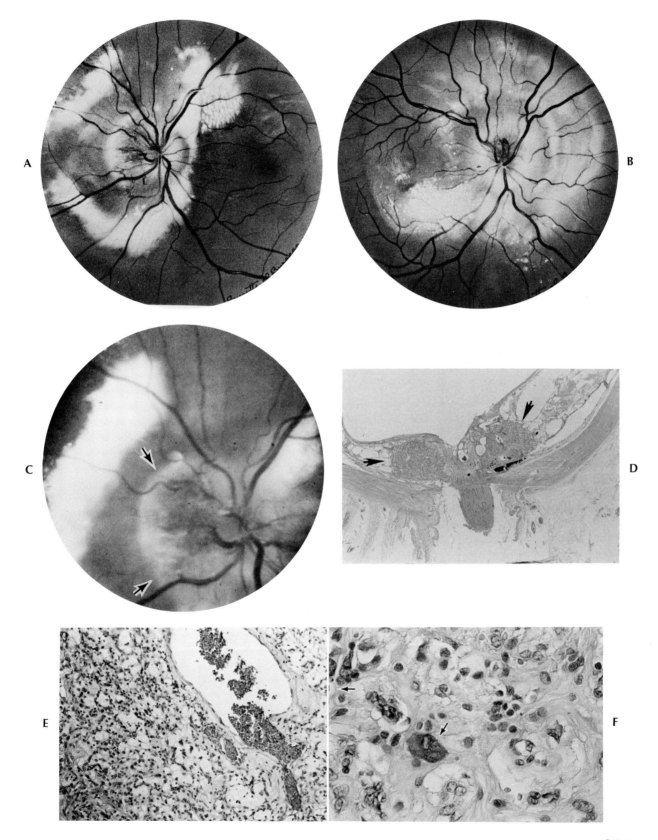

REFERENCES

1. Gass, J. D. M.: Ruby laser and xenon photocoagulation of macular lesions. Proc. XXI Int. Congr. Ophthalmol., Mexico, 1970, Amsterdam, Excerpta Medica Foundation, p. 504.
2. Gass, J. D. M.: Photocoagulation of macular lesions, Trans. Am. Acad. Ophthalmol. Otolaryngol. **75:**580-608, 1971.
3. Nicholson, D. H., Green, W. R., and Kenyon, K. R.: Angiomatosis retinae. Light and electron microscopic study, Am. J. Ophthalmol. (To be published.)
4. Dabezies, O., Walsh, F., and Hayes, G.: Papilledema with hamartoma of hypothalamus, Arch. Ophthalmol. **65:**174-180, 1961.
5. Gass, J. D. M.: The phakomatoses. In Smith, J. L. (editor): Neuro-Ophthalmology. Vol. II. Symposium of the University of Miami and the Bascom Palmer Eye Institute, St. Louis, 1965, The C. V. Mosby Co., p. 262.
6. Darr, J. L., Hughes, R. P., and McNair, J. N.: Bilateral peripapillary retinal hemangiomas. A case report, Arch. Ophthalmol. **75:**77-81, 1966.

SUGGESTED READINGS

Duke-Elder, S.: System of ophthalmology, St. Louis, 1967, The C. V. Mosby Co., vol. 10, pp. 738-754.

Hoeve, J. Van der: Eye symptoms in phakomatoses, Trans. Ophthalmol. Soc. U. K., **52:**380-401, 1932.

Jesberg, D. O., Spencer, W. H., and Hoyt, W. F.: Incipient lesions of von Hippel–Lindau disease, Arch. Ophthalmol. **80:**632-640, 1968.

Oosterhuis, J. A., and Rubinstein, K.: Haemangioma at the optic disc, Ophthalmologica **164:**362-374, 1972.

Reese, A. B.: Tumors of the eye, New York, 1951, Paul B. Hoeber, Inc., Harper & Row, Publishers, pp. 368-377.

Welch, R. B.: Von Hippel–Lindau disease: The recognition and treatment of early angiomatosis retinae and the use of cryosurgery as an adjunct to therapy, Trans. Am. Ophthalmol. Soc. **68:**367-424, 1970.

CHAPTER ELEVEN

Cavernous hemangioma
of the retina

Cavernous hemangioma of the retina and optic nerve head is a specific vascular hamartoma that should be differentiated from other retinal vascular malformations, including retinal telangiectasis, angiomatosis retinae, and racemose angioma. It is familial and may occur in association with one or more intracranial cavernous hemangiomas as well as with angiomatous hamartomas of the skin and perhaps other organs. The tumor may arise from either the retina or optic nerve head as a sessile tumor composed of clusters of thin-walled saccular aneurysms filled with dark venous blood. These aneurysms present the appearance of grapes projecting from the inner surface of the retina (Figs. 11-1 and 11-2) and optic nerve head (Fig. 11-3). Small clumps of isolated capillary aneurysms are often around the main tumor mass. Plasmaerythrocytic separation within the aneurysms is common. The caliber of the major retinal vessels is unaffected by the tumor. Exudation from the tumor vessels is rare. Although minor changes in the size and shape of the aneurysms occur (Fig. 11-2, A and F), the tumor has no significant growth potential. Hemorrhage into the vitreous or subretinal space may occur rarely.

Fluorescein angiography demonstrates that the vascular tumor is relatively isolated from the retinal circulation (Figs. 11-1 to 11-3). Perfusion of the hamartoma occurs but is delayed and appears incomplete. Plasmaerythrocytic layering within the saccular aneurysms is conspicuous in the later phases of angiography. Extravascular leakage of the dye from the tumor vessels does not occur.

Three types of vascular hamartomas of the skin have been associated with this entity (Fig. 11-4). A slightly raised cutaneous lesion composed of multiple small saccular aneurysms, very similar to that seen in the retinal lesion, occurred in one patient with retinal and central nervous system involvement (Fig. 11-4, B). Multiple small, nodular, smooth, round, red lesions were noted in another patient (Fig. 11-4, C). These lesions are believed to represent cherry angiomas. A poorly circumscribed, slightly elevated tumor consisting of a tangle of various sized blood vessels was present on the chin of one patient (Fig. 11-4, D). Similar but smaller lesions were noted on the arms and hands of another patient and her identical twin sister (Fig. 11-1). The latter two types of cutaneous angiomas occur commonly in the normal population and their presence in these patients with cavernous hemangioma of the retina may prove to be no more than coincidental findings.

Histopathologically the retinal and optic nerve head tumors are composed of multiple, thin-walled, dilated blood vessels that replace the normal architecture of the inner half of the retina (Fig. 11-5, A) and optic nerve head (Fig. 11-5, C). The vascular spaces vary in size and their walls are composed of endothelium and in some places a thin layer of stroma. Many of the vessels abut each other and their lumens are interconnected, often by small orifices. The internal limiting membrane of the retina overlying these tumors is thinned and in places may be missing. Some of the dilated vessel walls are in continuity with the vitreous.

Cavernous hemangiomas involving the central nervous system, or cavernomas, present as purple-red mulberry or honeycomb lesions in either the pre-Rolandic area of the cerebral cortex or along the surface of the midbrain, brainstem, and cerebellum (Fig. 11-5, F). Although they occur uncommonly compared to other vascular hamartomas, they have attracted considerable clinical interest—first, because they may be the underlying cause of convulsions or severe intracranial hemorrhage and second, because they are often amenable to surgical excision.

Other vascular malformations that must be considered in the differential diagnosis include retinal telangiectasis, retinal angiomatosis (von Hippel's disease), and racemose angioma of the retina. Retinal telangiectasis, sometimes referred to as Leber's miliary aneurysms, is perhaps the most difficult to clearly differentiate from cavernous hemangioma, particularly when the latter is composed of relatively small clusters of aneurysms as illustrated in Fig. 11-2. Retinal telangiectasis is a congenital anomaly affecting the structure and integrity of the intrinsic retinal vasculature, whereas cavernous hemangioma of the retina is a localized vascular tumefaction (hamartoma) that is partly isolated from the normal retinal vascular tree (Fig. 11-6).

The relative isolation of cavernous hemangioma from the retinal circulation may be an important factor in the rarity of exudation and hemorrhage from this tumor. Telangiectasis typically occurs unilaterally in healthy males, whereas cavernous hemangioma appears to be more common in females. The familial occurrence of telangiectasis has been reported only rarely (see Chapter 9). Although the natural course of retinal telangiectasis is variable, progressive vascular dilatation and intraretinal and subretinal exudation occur as a rule. Focal aneurysmal dilatation of the arterioles and venules, as well as the capillaries may be pominent. Leber referred to these changes as "miliary aneurysms." Retinal telangiectasis is the primary underlying cause of massive yellowish exudative detachment of the retina, or Coats' disease. Contrary to the findings in cavernous hemangioma, fluorescein angiography in telangiectasis demonstrates that the affected retinal vessels are in the mainstream of retinal blood flow. During the preexudative stage of telangiectasis, angiography demonstrates prompt perfusion of the capillary bed, which usually shows a normal pattern except for irregular dilatation. Partial disappearance of the capillary bed and dilatation and tortuosity of the adjacent segments of the capillary bed are probably late secondary changes occurring after prolonged exudation. Angiography demonstrates that leakage of dye from the capillaries in telangiectasis is the rule even during the early stages of the disease; it is the exception in cavernous hemangioma.

The vascular tumor, angiomatosis retinae (von Hippel's disease), is sufficiently characteristic that it is easily distinguished from cavernous hemangioma (see Chapter 10). Racemose angioma of the retina is characterized by the presence of dilated tortuous retinal vessels often with direct anastomosis between one or more major retinal veins and arteries. It may be associated with similar arteriovenous anomalies of the central nervous system, particularly in the midbrain (Wyburn-Mason syndrome). It is another retinal vascular anomaly that appears to be distinctly different from cavernous hemangioma (see Chapter 12).

The treatment of choice in patients with cavernous hemangioma of the retina and optic nerve head is uncertain. Treatment is probably unnecessary in patients showing no evidence of significant vitreous or subretinal hemorrhage. If hemorrhage occurs, photocoagulation, cryopexy, or diathermy should prove successful in destroying the lesion.

Cavernous hemangioma of the retina can be considered as one of the neurophakomatoses whose mode of inheritance is probably autosomal dominant.

Fig. 11-1. Cavernous hemangioma of the retina. A 30-month-old white girl developed right esotropia at 6 months of age. Her general health and physical examination were normal except for the presence of a few spider angiomas on her hands and wrists. She had a variable exotropia of 40 prism diopters. Fixation with the right eye was unsteady. The eyes were of equal size. An identical twin sister was normal except for similar spider angiomas on the hands.

A and **B,** In the upper temporal quadrant of the right eye there was an irregularly elevated vascular mass. This was composed of dilated, oval or rounded, thin-walled, saccular blood vessels that gave the appearance of a mass of grapes lying on the inner retinal surface and protruding into the vitreous. The tumor extended from the ora serrata almost to the macular area.

C, Early arteriovenous phase. The camera was focused on the surface of the large aneurysms. A large retinal artery was displaced superonasally by the tumor *(right arrow).* A small arteriole coursed over the surface of the aneurysm *(left arrow).*

D, Several minutes after dye injection there was further perfusion of the tumor and absence of dye in the center of the retinal vein draining the tumor *(arrow).*

E, Approximately 30 minutes after dye injection there was still incomplete perfusion of the tumor. Note the level of dye in the large tumor cyst *(arrow).* The patient was lying on her left side in the operating room during the angiographic study.

F, One hour after dye injection this photograph was made without the blue and yellow filter used in angiography and with the patient in the recumbent position. The blood in the dependent portion of the large aneurysms is completely obscured by fluorescein dye present in the overlying plasma *(arrow).* A single row of photocoagulation applications surround the tumor nasally.

(From Gass.[1])

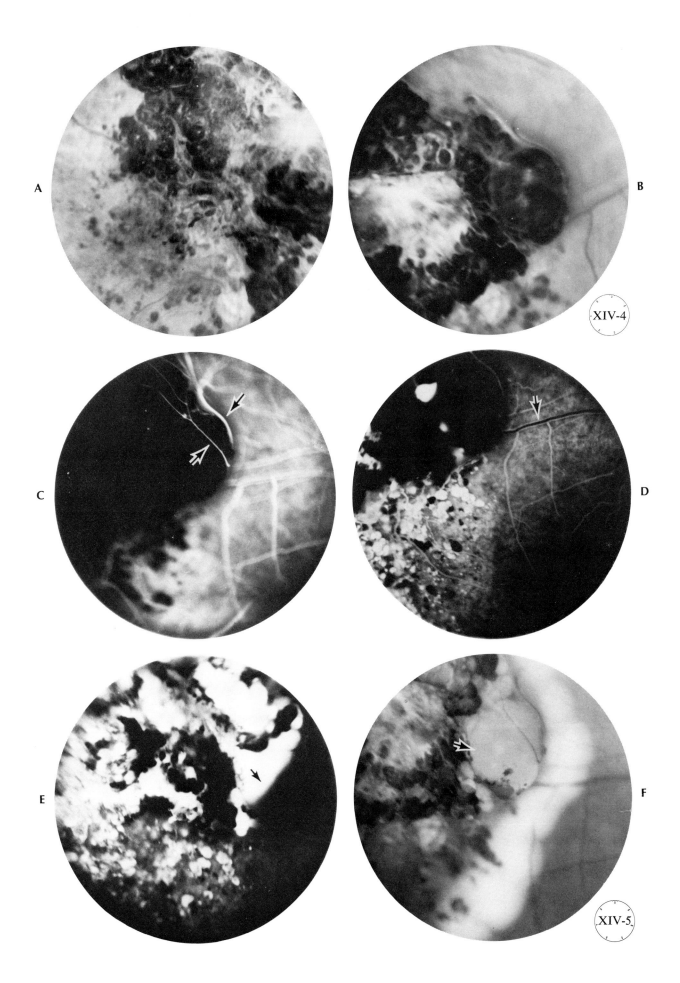

Fig. 11-2. Cavernous hemangioma of the retina discovered in a patient hospitalized because of a generalized seizure. A 27-year-old woman was well until she experienced a grand mal seizure while sleeping. After hospitalization her general physical examination was normal except for the presence of a retinal vascular lesion in her right eye. Skull x-ray films and carotid arteriogram were normal. An electroencephalogram revealed low voltage in the left cerebral hemisphere. No cause for the seizure was found and she remained asymptomatic thereafter. During her adulthood she noted several small slightly raised vascular tumors of the face and legs. They increased in size slowly and several were removed with cautery. Her father had idiopathic epilepsy since 27 years of age and required hospitalization on numerous occasions for control. His last hospitalization for seizure control occurred at the age of 49 years. Blood was found in his spinal fluid. He gradually deteriorated over a period of months and died. The autopsy, which did not include the eyes, revealed focal cavernous hemangiomas in the midbrain, pons, and cerebellum (Fig. 11-5, *F*). The woman was examined initially at the Bascom Palmer Eye Institute at 33 years of age. She had a stellate, angiomatous hamartoma of the right chin (Fig. 11-4, *C*) and several prominent cherry angiomas of the thigh (Fig. 11-4, *D*). Her eye examination showed normal results except for the fundus of the right eye.

A and **B,** She had a slightly elevated sessile retinal vascular tumor composed of clusters of saccular aneurysms of various sizes arising from tortuous venous channels. The tumor was drained by the inferior nasal retinal vein, which was of normal caliber. A small subretinal or deep retinal hemorrhage was present *(arrows)*. The color stereophotograph was made 4 years after **A** and **B.** Note that the hemorrhage is gone and that minor changes have occurred in the size of the dilated vascular spaces.

C, Arteriovenous phase. Note the relative lack of perfusion of the tumor despite early perfusion of the venous branches passing through the tumor *(arrows)*.

D, Early recirculation phase. The failure of many of the aneurysms to contain dye is indicative of the sluggish blood flow within this tumor.

E, One hour angiogram. There was incomplete perfusion of the tumor, including many of the small aneurysms. Note evidence of plasma layering *(arrows)* and absence of evidence of extravascular escape of dye.

F, The same tumor 5 years after that in **A** and **B.** The small subretinal hemorrhage present in **A** is no longer present. Note the minor changes in location and size of the dilated vascular channels that have occurred during the 5 years.

(From Gass.[1])

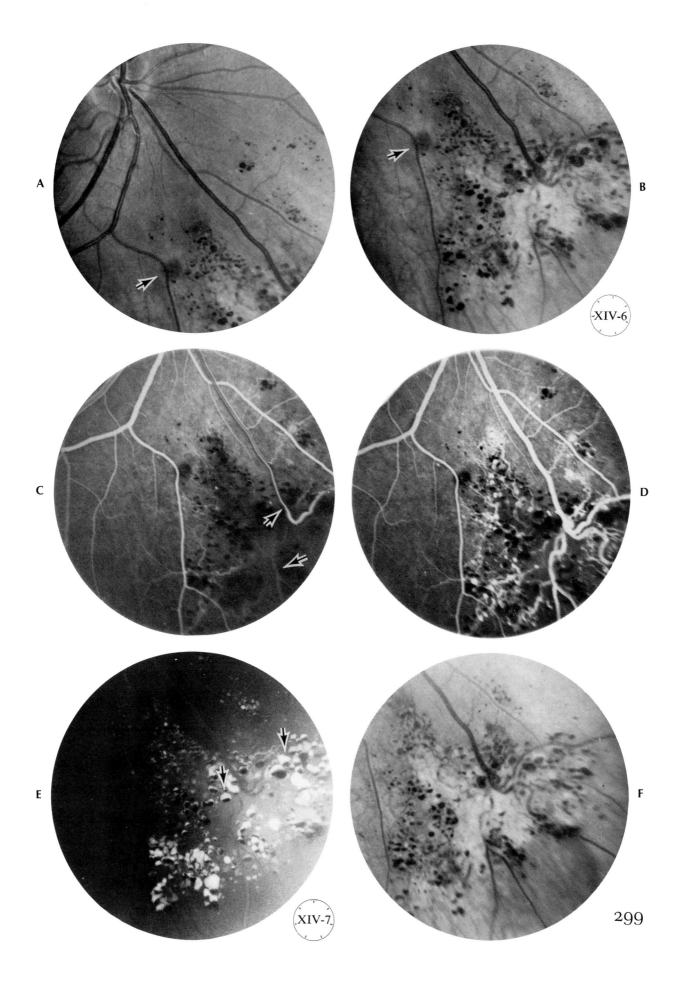

A

B

-XIV-6

C

D

E

XIV-7

F

299

Fig. 11-3. Cavernous hemangioma of the optic nerve head. A 51-year-old white woman was examined initially at the Wilmer Eye Institute at the age of 45 years for evaluation of a lesion of the right optic nerve head. This was discovered by an optometrist during a routine eye examination. Her local ophthalmologist believed it was probably a malignant tumor and recommended enucleation of the eye. Another made a diagnosis of a "blood clot." The patient was asymptomatic. Her past history showed emphysema and hemoptysis. Her family history was normal. Her uncorrected visual acuity in each eye was 20/15. On central field examination there was a slight enlargement of the blind spot in the right eye.

A, On October 30, 1964, ophthalmoscopic examination revealed a cavernous hemangioma of the optic nerve head. Note the plasma-erythrocytic separation in the large saccular aneurysm *(arrow)*.

B, In October 1973, the large aneurysm *(large arrow)* is now smaller and again plasma-erythrocytic separation is present. Note the small aneurysms in the superficial layers of the retina and optic nerve head *(small arrow)*.

C to **F,** Angiography revealed delay in perfusion of the tumor mass, incomplete perfusion of some of the saccular aneurysms, plasma layering, and absence of evidence of extravascular escape of dye. Note that angiography shows in some aneurysms evidence of plasma-erythrocytic separation, which is not evident in the color photography.

(From Gass.[1])

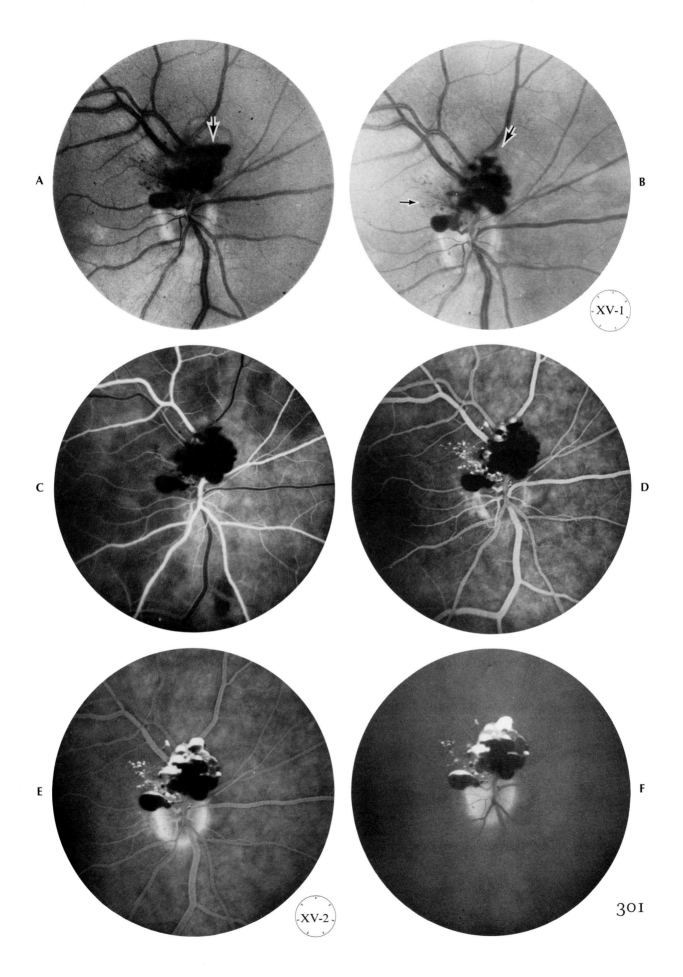

A

B

C

D

E

F

Fig. 11-4. Cutaneous angiomatous hamartomas associated with cavernous hemangioma of the retina.

A, This small cavernous hemangioma of the retina was discovered in a young man in his twenties during a routine eye examination.

B, At the same time a slightly raised cutaneous angioma was noted on one arm. This tumor was composed of multiple small saccular aneurysms of varying size lying beneath the epithelium. Its appearance was very similar to the retinal tumor. Several years later the patient began to experience generalized convulsive seizures that were well controlled with medications. He was followed by the same ophthalmologist until 54 years of age. No change occurred in either the retinal or cutaneous angioma. One of the patient's five children developed headaches, projectile vomiting, and generalized seizures at 5 years of age. He had cutaneous angiomas of the face, leg, and foot. He died soon after surgical excision of a vermiform, purplish, cavernous hemangioma in the region of the third and lateral ventricles.

C, This raised red cherry angioma of the thigh was excised from the patient in Fig. 11-2. Note the prominent feeder vessel (*arrow*).

D, This slightly raised stellate hemangioma of the chin was present in the patient in Fig. 11-2. There were prominent feeder vessels (*arrows*) surrounding the tumor.

E, Histopathologic condition of the lesion shown in **D** revealed a raised, well-circumscribed, subepithelial cavernous hemangioma that was supplied by several large underlying blood vessels (*arrows*).

(**A** and **B** courtesy Dr. L. L. Calkins, Prairie Village, Kansas.)

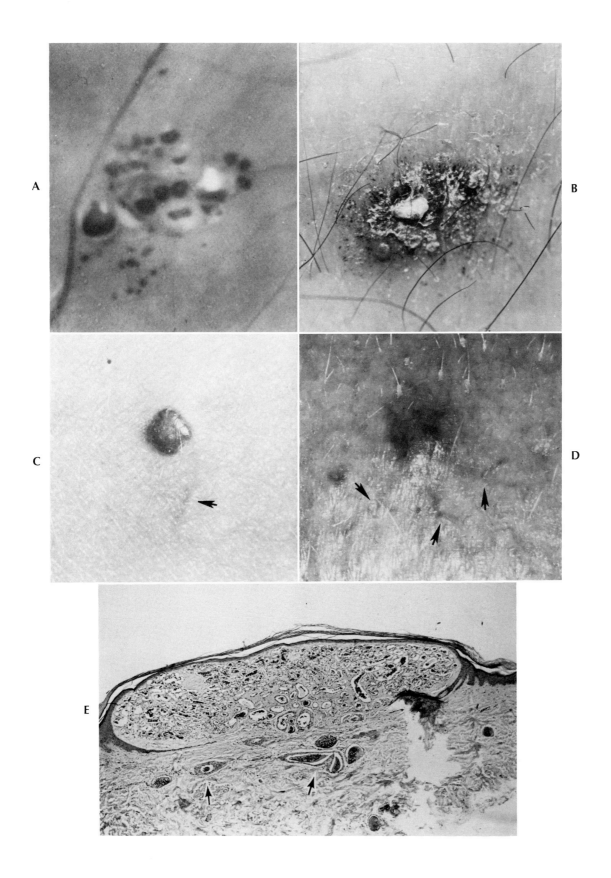

303

Fig. 11-5. Histopathologic findings in cavernous hemangioma of the retina and optic nerve.

A, Histopathologic condition of cavernous hemangioma of the retina in a 2-year-old girl whose eye was enucleated with the mistaken diagnosis of retinoblastoma. The sessile retinal tumor was composed of multiple, thin-walled, dilated blood vessels that replace the inner half of the retina. *Arrow* indicates pigment-laden macrophages in the subretinal space. The retinal detachment was artifactitious.

B, High-power view of lesion in **A**. Note the dilated endothelium-lined aneurysms interconnected by narrow channels *(arrows)*. These relatively isolated vascular saccules account for the sluggish circulation and plasma-erythrocytic separation demonstrated angiographically in these lesions.

C, Histopathologic condition of cavernous hemangioma of the optic nerve head and adjacent retina.

D and **E,** Histopathologic condition of a retrobulbar cavernous hemangioma of the optic nerve head. This was an incidental finding in the optic nerve of a 3-month old white girl who was born prematurely with a birth weight of 2 pounds, 14 ounces. She was in an incubator for 2 weeks. At 2½ months of age she had a cleft palate, severe mental retardation, bilateral buphthalmos and a retrolental membrane bilaterally. The eyes were enucleated because of the possibility of retinoblastoma. Histopathologic examination revealed bilateral funnel-shaped retinal detachments with vitreous organization in addition to the cavernous hemangioma of the optic nerve. After enucleation, right and left carotid arteriograms revealed multiple abnormal superficial venous structures that were most conspicuous in the region of the superior longitudinal sinus during the venous phase.

F, Cavernous hemangioma of the midbrain in the father of the patient in Fig. 11-2.

(**A** from Hogan and Zimmerman[2] and Gass[1]; **B** from Gass[1]; **C** from Davies and Thumin[3]; **D** and **E** from Spencer[4]; **F** from Gass[1] from AFIP Neg. No. 70-6110, hematoxylin and eosin, × 7.)

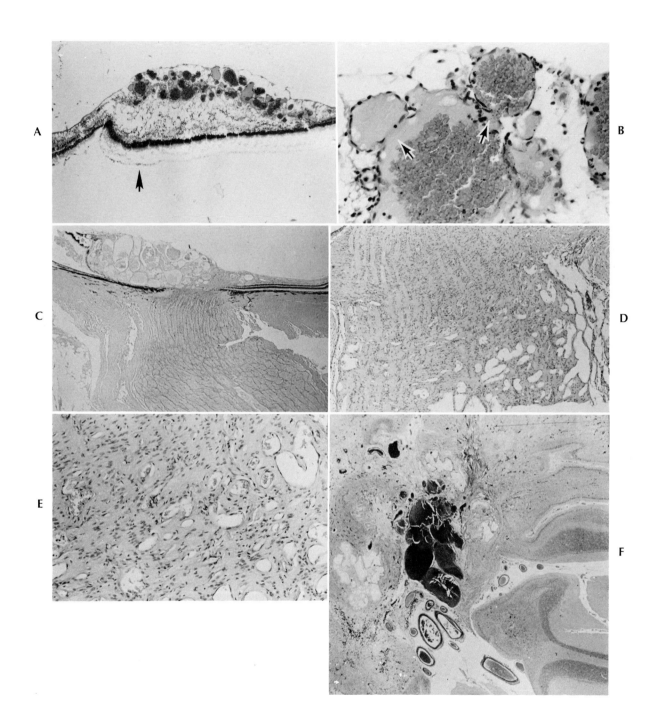

305

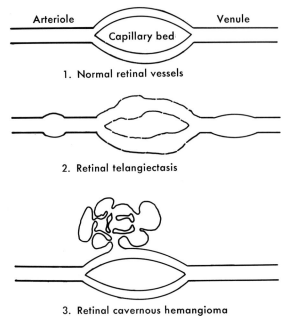

Arteriole   Venule

Capillary bed

1. Normal retinal vessels

2. Retinal telangiectasis

3. Retinal cavernous hemangioma

Fig. 11-6. Diagram showing (1) normal retinal vessels, (2) diffuse and focal vascular dilatation and permeability alteration in retinal telangiectasis, and (3) localized vascular malformation (hamartoma) arising from the capillary bed in cavernous hemangioma. (From Gass.[1])

REFERENCES

1. Gass, J. D. M.: Cavernous hemangioma of the retina, Am. J. Ophthalmol. **71:**799-814, 1971.
2. Hogan, J. M., and Zimmerman, L. E. (editors): Ophthalmic pathology, ed. 2, Philadelphia, 1962, W. B. Saunders Co., p. 533.
3. Davies, W. S., and Thumin, M.: Cavernous hemangioma of the optic disc and retina, Trans. Am. Acad. Ophthalmol. Otolaryngol. **60:**217-218, 1956.
4. Spencer, W. H.: Primary neoplasms of the optic nerve and its sheaths: Clinical features and current concepts of pathogenetic mechanism, Trans. Ophthalmol. Soc. U. K. **70:**490-528, 1972.

SUGGESTED READINGS

Amalric, P., and Biau, C.: L'Angiographie fluorescéinique chez l'enfant, Arch. Ophthalmol. (Paris) **28:**55-60, 1968.
Gautier-Smith, P. C., Sanders, M. D., and Sanderson, K. V.: Ocular and nervous system involvement in angioma serpiginosum, Brit. J. Ophthalmol. **55:** 433-443, 1971.
Wessing, A.: Fluorescein angiography of the retina: Textbook and atlas (von Noorden, G. K., translator), St. Louis, 1969, The C. V. Mosby Co., p. 132.

CHAPTER TWELVE

Congenital retinal arteriovenous malformations (racemose aneurysm, cirsoid aneurysm, and arteriovenous aneurysm)

A wide variety of congenital malformations of the major retinal vessels (Fig. 12-1) may occur, and in some patients they may be associated with similar vascular malformations of the extracranial and intracranial tissues (Fig. 12-1, *F*). These vascular anomalies may be familial. The retinal anomaly is often unilateral and may be confined to one portion of the retina and optic nerve head or it may involve the entire retina. The affected retinal vessels are typically enlarged, tortuous, and often more numerous than is normal (Fig. 12-1, *A* to *D*). Direct arteriovenous anastomosis is often present and the participating artery and vein are similar in color (Fig. 12-1, *A* to *C*). White sheathing of the vessels may occur (Fig. 12-1, *A*). There is no pulsation of the affected vessels. Retinal hemorrhage and exudation are infrequent. Visual function may or may not be affected. Visual loss generally parallels the extent of the vascular anomaly. Visual function is usually stable. Dilatation and tortuosity of the major retinal vessels may simulate closely those seen in retinal angiomatosis (see Fig. 10-7). In retinal angiomatosis however, arteriovenous fistulization always occurs through a capillary angioma in the peripheral fundus. Retinal arteriovenous anomalies may be associated with similar ipsilateral arteriovenous malformations of the face, orbit, optic nerve, maxilla (Fig. 12-1, A to C), pterygoid fossa, mandible, basifrontal area, the Sylvian fissue (Fig. 12-1, E and F), posterior fossa, and rostral midbrain. Wyburn-Mason stressed the association of retinal and midbrain lesions. The incidence of associated ocular and central nervous system lesions is unknown. Relatively mild alterations of the retinal vessels may occur in association with large central nervous system lesions (Fig. 12-1, E and F); the reverse is probably true also.

Fig. 12-1. Congenital retinal arteriovenous malformations associated with similar extracranial and intracranial vascular malformations. A 13-year-old white girl developed mobility and pulsations of her right upper first permanent molar at 9 years of age. This was associated with a bruit over the right maxillary area. Except for some evidence of left facial weakness and a positive Babinski test on the right, her neurologic examination was normal. Her right pupil reacted poorly to light. Visual acuity in the right eye was finger counting only. Ophthalmoscopic examination of the right eye revealed a vascular malformation of the retina and optic disc. The left eye was normal. Roentgenographic studies demonstrated widespread erosion of the walls of the right maxillary antrum and evidence of a soft tissue mass in the right antrum. Arteriography of the right carotid artery revealed a vascular mass involving the right maxillary area and multiple aneurysms of the right ophthalmic artery. The right external carotid artery was ligated and the maxillary tumor was excised. Postoperatively the right internal carotid artery was ligated and the patient developed a transient left hemiparesis. This patient was reported by Ladow et al.[1] in 1964. The retinal changes were misinterpreted as von Hippel's disease. At age 13 years the right eye was blind and the vision was 20/20 in the left eye.

A to **C,** Ophthalmoscopic examination of the right eye revealed gross dilatation and tortuosity of the superonasal retinal artery *(arrows)* and vein, which were in direct communication. A smaller arteriovenous aneurysm whose walls were opacified extended into the macular area. There were no retinal hemorrhages or exudates.

D, Fluorescein angiography confirmed the arteriovenous nature of this malformation.

E and **F,** A 27-year-old white woman was well until she developed a generalized seizure. She had a bruit over the right eye and right cartotid area. Her neurologic examination was normal except for the presence of a right homonymous sector field defect.

E, Ophthalmoscopic examination revealed considerable tortuosity of the major retinal vessels in both eyes. The veins were primarily affected. No arteriovenous anastomoses were identified.

F, Right carotid arteriography revealed a large arteriovenous malformation in the Sylvanian area.

(**A** to **D** courtesy Mr. Johnny Justice, Jr., Houston, Texas, and Dr. R. D. Mulberger, Philadelphia.)

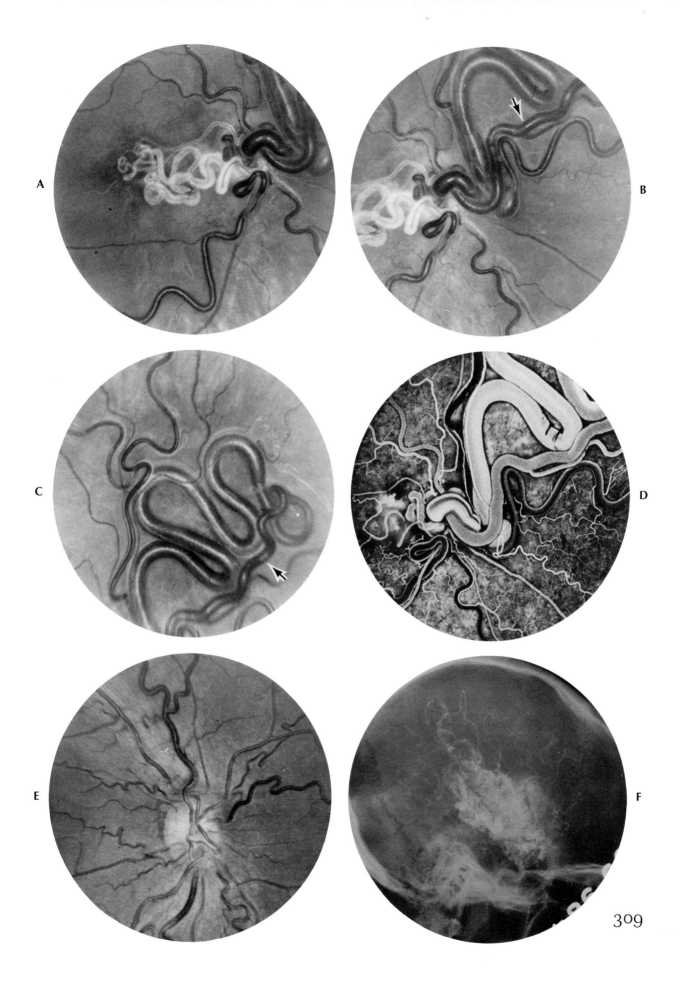

309

REFERENCE

1. Ladow, C. S., Henefer, E., and McFall, T. A.: Central hemangioma of the maxilla with von Hippel's disease: A report of a case, J. Oral Surg. **22:**252-259, 1964.

SUGGESTED READINGS

Archer, D. B., Deutman, A., Ernest, J. T., and Krill, A. E.: Arteriovenous communications of the retina, Am. J. Ophthalmol. **75:**224-241, 1973.

Brock, S., and Dyke, C. G.: Venous and arteriovenous angiomas of the brain, clinical and roentgenographic study of 8 cases, Bull. Neurol. Instit. **2:** 247-293, 1932.

Bonnet, P., Dechaume, J., and Blanc, E.: L'Anévrysme cirsoïde de la rétine. (Anévrysme racémeux). Ses relations avec l'anévryme cirsoïde de la face et avec l'anévrysme cirsoïde du cerveau, J. Med. Lyon **18:**165-178, 1937.

Hoyt, W. F., and Cameron, R. B.: Racemose angioma of the mandible, face, retina and brain, J. Oral Surg. **26:**596-600, 1968.

Wyburn-Mason, R.: Arteriovenous aneurysm of midbrain and retina, facial naevi and mental changes, Brain **66:**163-203, 1943.

Walsh, F. B., and Hoyt, W. F.: Clinical neuro-ophthalmology, Baltimore, 1969, The Williams & Wilkins Co., pp. 1690-1694.

CHAPTER THIRTEEN

Retinal astrocytic hamartomas

Retinal astrocytic hamartomas are rare developmental tumors that are usually discovered in the second and third decades of life. They may or may not be associated with other manifestations of tuberous sclerosis (Figs. 13-1 to 13-8).

RETINAL ASTROCYTIC HAMARTOMAS ASSOCIATED WITH TUBEROUS SCLEROSIS

Bourneville's syndrome, or tuberous sclerosis, is one of the heritable phakomatoses that is transmitted in an irregular dominant fashion. Most of these patients are mentally deficient and suffer from epilepsy. They typically have multiple astrocytic hamartomas of the cerebrum and retina, nodular fibroangiomatous hamartomas of the face (adenoma sebaceum), subungual fibromas, and hamartomas of other organs including the kidneys, heart, lungs, liver, thyroid gland, epididymis, and uterus (Figs. 13-1 to 13-4). The retinal tumors are typically globular, white, well-circumscribed, elevated lesions arising from the inner surface of the retina and optic nerve head. Multiple lesions are common. Early in life the tumors may be semitranslucent and they may be mistaken for retinoblastoma (Fig. 13-2). Later in life they assume a more densely white color and multiple nodular areas of calcification occur and give the lesion a mulberry appearance (Figs. 13-1, E and F, and 13-2, F). Clear cystic spaces may be present within the tumors (Fig. 13-3). The tumors show varying degrees of fine vascularization that is more evident angiographically than ophthalmoscopically. The tumor blood vessels are permeable to fluorescein (Figs. 13-2 to 13-4). In addition to nodular retinal tumors flat or slightly elevated white circular or oval astrocytic hamartomas of the inner retinal layers are common. These show less tendency to undergo calcific degeneration. Retinal astrocytic hamartomas generally show minimal evidence of growth and no treatment is indicated. Rarely, however, secondary exudative detachment or growth, or both, may be sufficient to cause visual loss (Fig. 13-5, E and F).

The fossilized mulberry tumors of the optic nerve head should be distinguished from hyaline bodies of the optic nerve head. The latter are calcified masses of extracellular material unrelated to astrocytic hamartomas.

Histopathologically these tumors are composed of astrocytes, some of which are elongated fibrocytes containing small oval nuclei (Fig. 13-5, A and D). Other tumors are composed of large bizarre pleomorphic astrocytic cells (Fig. 13-5, E and F). Cystic areas containing serous exudate and blood as well as areas of calcific degeneration may be present (Fig. 13-5, B and C).

A careful search should be made for the various manifestations of tuberous sclerosis in any patient presenting with a white retinal tumor. This is of particular importance in children because of the similarity in clinical appearance of astrocytic hamartomas and retinoblastoma. As is true with the other phakomatoses many patients have only a few of the manifestations of the disease. The multinodular tan or pink lesions of adenoma sebaceum are usually most prominent over the malar area. They may be mistaken for acne vulgaris. Larger more discrete soft, yellow-brown tumefactions simulating pigmented cutaneous nevi are common, particularly in the brow area (Figs. 13-1, A, 13-2, A, and 13-3, A). Multiple hamartomas of the kidneys are often present in these patients, and they may be of sufficient size to produce albuminuria, elevation of the serum urea nitrogen, and abnormal radiographic findings. Skull x-rays in adult patients may reveal localized radiodensities secondary to calcified cerebral hamartomas and sclerotic plaques in the calvaria.

These radiodensities are referred to as "brain stones" (Fig. 13-1, C). Cystic changes in other bones, particularly the phalanges, and irregular cortical thickening often in the metatarsal and metacarpal bones are other roentgenographic changes that are frequently found in patients with tuberous sclerosis.

RETINAL ASTROCYTIC HAMARTOMAS UNASSOCIATED WITH TUBEROUS SCLEROSIS

Globular white tumors identical to those occurring in tuberous sclerosis may occur in the absence of any other manifestations of that disease (Figs. 13-6 to 13-8). They may occasionally be exophytic (Figs. 13-5, E, and 13-8) rather than endophytic in nature. I have seen one patient in whom a presumed retinal astrocytic hamartoma spontaneously disappeared (Fig. 13-7).

Fig. 13-1. Tuberous sclerosis (Bourneville's syndrome).

A, A 18-year-old man with adenoma sebaceum had Jacksonian seizures since early childhood. A single, mulberry, partially calcified, astrocytic hamartoma was present at the superior margin of the right optic disc (see **E**). A large nodular opacity was located eccentrically in the midcortex of the lens bilaterally. Visual acuity was normal. He had albuminuria and distinct enlargement of both kidneys. Skull x-ray examination revealed multiple calcified astrocytic hamartomas ("brain stones") (see **C**).

B, This 35-year-old white woman was admitted to the urology service for evaluation of hypertension and questionable polycystic kidneys. Renal enlargement was found on arteriography to be caused by the multiple renal vascular hamartomas. Adenoma sebaceum, subungual fibromas (see **D**), intracranial calcification, cystic lesions of the long bones, and a mulberry lesion of the peripheral retina (see **F**) were also found. Note the relatively few but typical fibroangiomas of the skin in the nasolabial area.

C, Skull x-ray film of patient shown in **A** showing multiple calcified astrocytic hamartomas (*arrows*) characteristic of tuberous sclerosis. These opacities are caused by calcific plaques in the calvaria and by calcification of intracerebral astrocytic hamartomas.

D, Subungual fibroma (*arrow*) in a patient with tuberous sclerosis (see **B**).

E, Partly calcified mulberry astrocytic hamartoma involving the optic nerve head margin and retina in a patient with tuberous sclerosis (see **A**).

F, Peripheral calcified mulberry astrocytic hamartoma of the retina in a patient with tuberous sclerosis (see **B**).

(From Gass: **A,** 1a; **B,** 1b; **C** and **D,** 1c; **E** and **F,** 1d.)

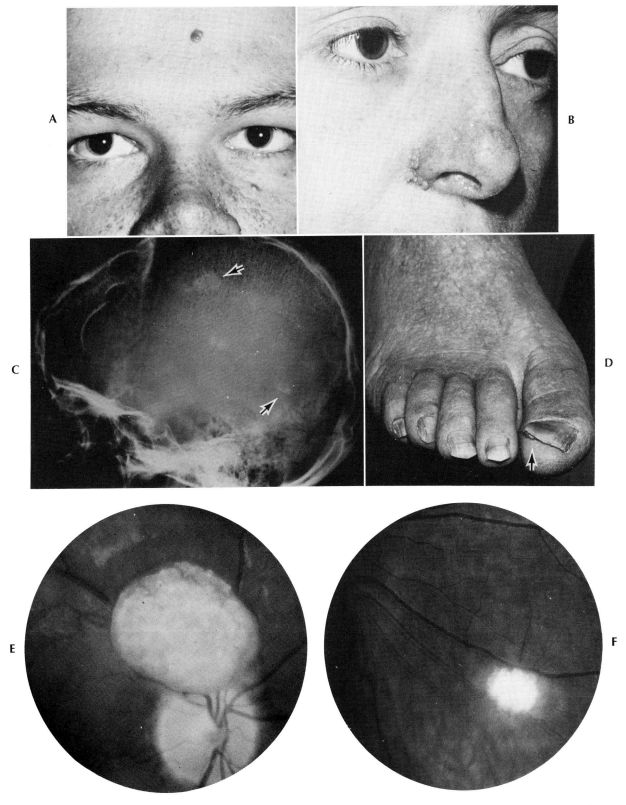

315

Fig. 13-2. Noncalcified retinal astrocytic hamartoma in a boy with tuberous sclerosis. A 3-year-old black male was first examined at 9 months of age because of seizures. The diagnosis at that time was idiopathic epilepsy. By 3 years of age he had evidence of mental retardation. Retinal tumors were noted bilaterally. Skull x-ray findings were normal.

A, There were scattered raised slightly pigmented lesions *(arrows)* on the face. A biopsy of one of these lesions revealed a fibroangioma compatible with tuberous sclerosis.

B, Ophthalmoscopic examination of the right eye revealed a highly elevated round semitranslucent lesion protruding from the anterior surface of the retina. Fine folds radiated from the tumor. A large retinal artery was barely discernible through the translucent tumor. Three other similar tumors were present in the right and left eye.

C to **E,** Angiography revealed evidence of a fine blood vascular network within and surrounding the base of the tumor. There was leakage of dye from the blood vessels within the tumor.

F, When the boy was 13 years of age, examination revealed that the tumor was slightly smaller and that its central portion was calcified and mulberry in appearance *(arrows)*.

(From Gass: **A,** le; **B,** 1f.)

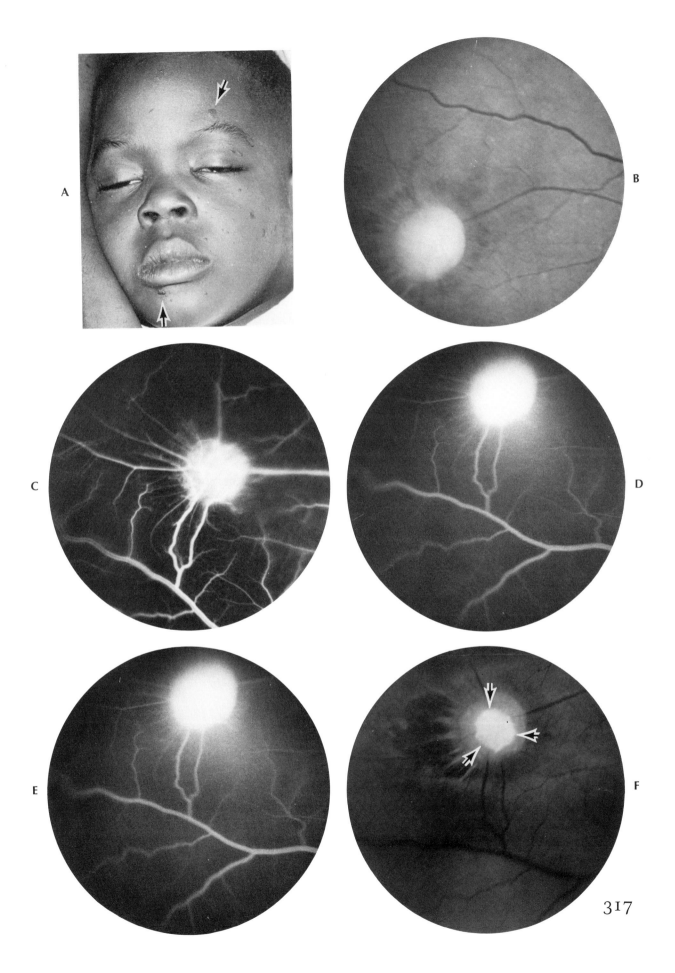

317

Fig. 13-3. Partly calcified cystic astrocytic hemartoma in tuberous sclerosis. A 9-year-old white girl was the product of full-term normal pregnancy and delivery. Her family history was normal. She developed generalized seizures between 2 and 3 years of age but had had no seizures since that time. She was not mentally retarded.

A, External examination revealed adenoma sebaceum and in addition a number of fairly large elevated slightly pigmented lesions on the forehead and upper lip *(arrows)*.

B, Multiple subungual fibromas *(arrow)* were present.

C, Ophthalmoscopic examination of the right eye revealed a multiloculated cystic, partly calcified hamartoma of the retina at the inferior margin of the right optic disc. Two mulberry-like areas of calcification were present within the larger cystic lesion. Another smaller hamartoma was present inferior to the macula. Note the small hamartomas within the nerve head substance superiorly *(arrow)*.

D, Fluorescein angiography demonstrated dilatation of the capillary network in the optic nerve head as well as evidence of an extensive capillary network within the large astrocytic hamartoma inferiorly.

E, Angiography revealed leakage of dye from the capillaries within the astrocytic hamartomas. Note the leakage of dye from the translucent hamartomas extending from the superior pole of the optic disc.

F, The late angiogram showed extensive staining of the astrocytic hamartomas.

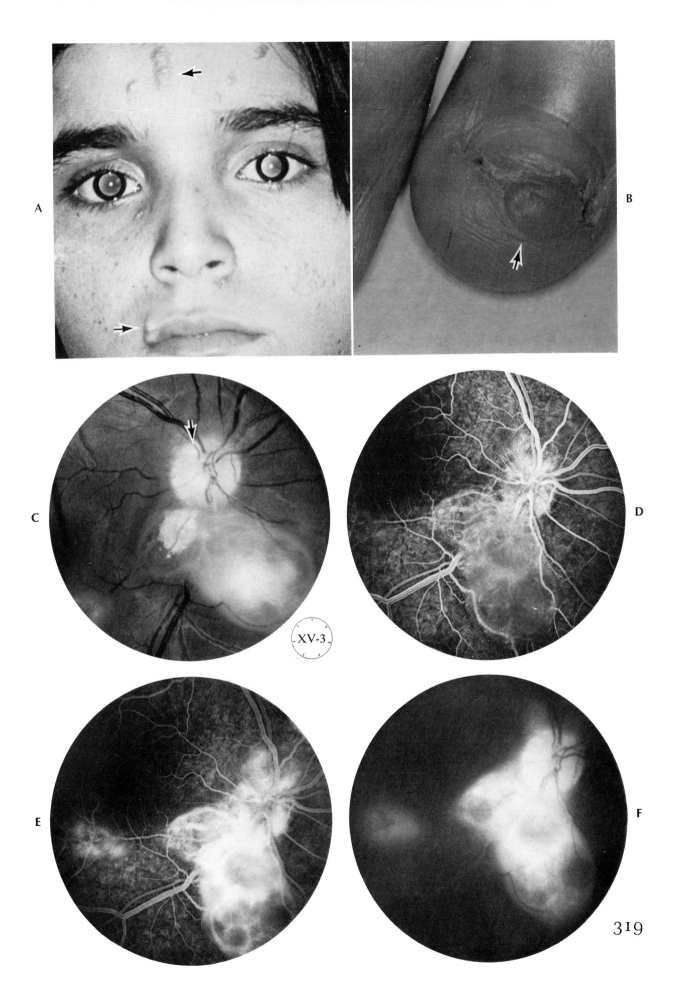

Fig. 13-4. Multiple astrocytic hamartomas of the optic nerve head and retina in tuberous sclerosis. A 35-year-old white female gave a life-long history of generalized seizures well controlled with medication. She had five mentally retarded children. Her family history was otherwise normal.

A, She had prominent adenoma sebaceum and subungual fibromas of the fingers and toes. Vision in the right eye was 20/25 and in the left eye was 20/30.

B, Funduscopic examination of the left eye revealed multiple endophytic astrocytic hamartomas of the retina. The lesions were elevated, globular, and semitranslucent. Retinal vessels could be seen through some of these tumors. Several of the tumefactions showed evidence of early calcification *(arrow)*.

C and **D,** Angiography revealed the presence of a capillary network within the hamartomas. These capillaries were permeable to fluorescein dye and there was evidence of fluorescein diffusion into the vitreous in the late phases of angiography.

E, A semitranslucent tumor showing early calcification *(arrow)* was present in the periphery of the fundus. Note the similarity of this lesion to a small retinoblastoma (see Fig. 14-3).

F, Angiography showed evidence of staining of this lesion.

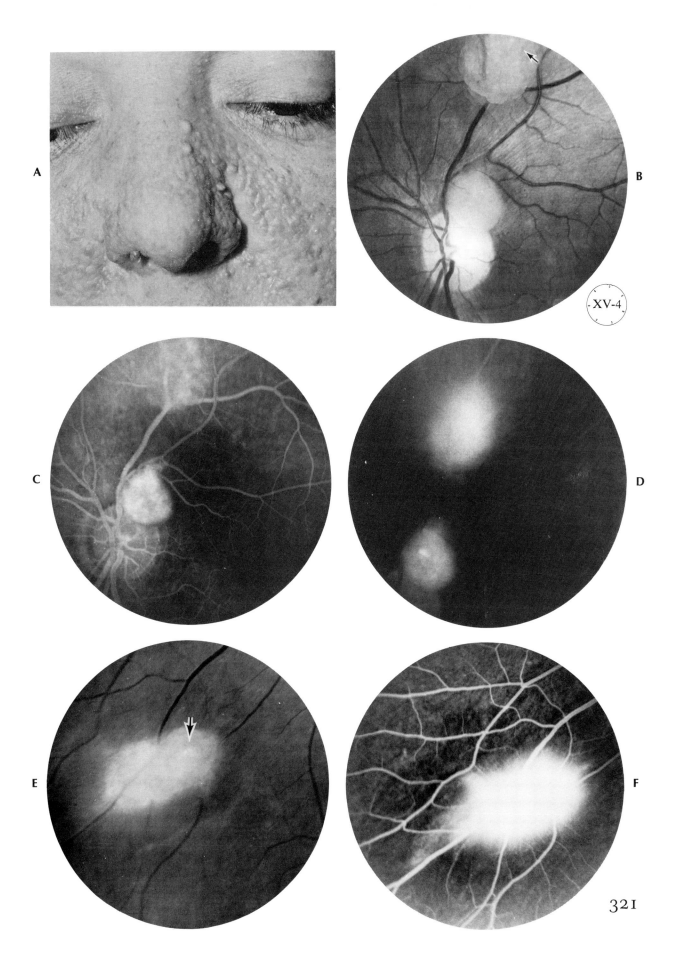

321

Fig. 13-5. Histopathologic condition of retinal astrocytic hamartomas.

A, Endophytic noncalcified retinal astrocytic hamartoma in an infant whose eye was enucleated because of suspected retinoblastoma. She subsequently developed evidence of tuberous sclerosis.

B, Calcified astrocytic hamartoma of the optic disc and adjacent retina in a 17-year-old white boy with adenoma sebaceum. The calcified central portion of the tumor was lost in sectioning.

C, High-power view of the tumor in **B** showing the large astroglial cells at the outer margin of the calcified tumor.

D, Endophytic noncalcified astrocytic hamartoma of the peripheral retina from the same patient in **B.**

E, A 12-year-old white girl with adenoma sebaceum, seizures, and mental retardation was noted to have an elevated white retinal tumor about six disc diameters in size in the macula of one eye. She had a strong family history of tuberous sclerosis. Eighteen months later the eye was blind and painful and was enucleated. Histopathologic examination revealed a funnel-shaped retinal detachment and a large exophytic astrocytic hamartoma of the retina (*arrows*).

F, High-power view of the lesion depicted in **D** showing large bizarre pleomorphic astrocytic cells.

(**A** from McLean,[2] AFIP Accession No. 219942; **B** to **D** from Zimmerman and Walsh,[3] AFIP Accession No. 511046; **E** and **F** courtesy Dr. R. P. Shaver, Oklahoma City, Okla.)

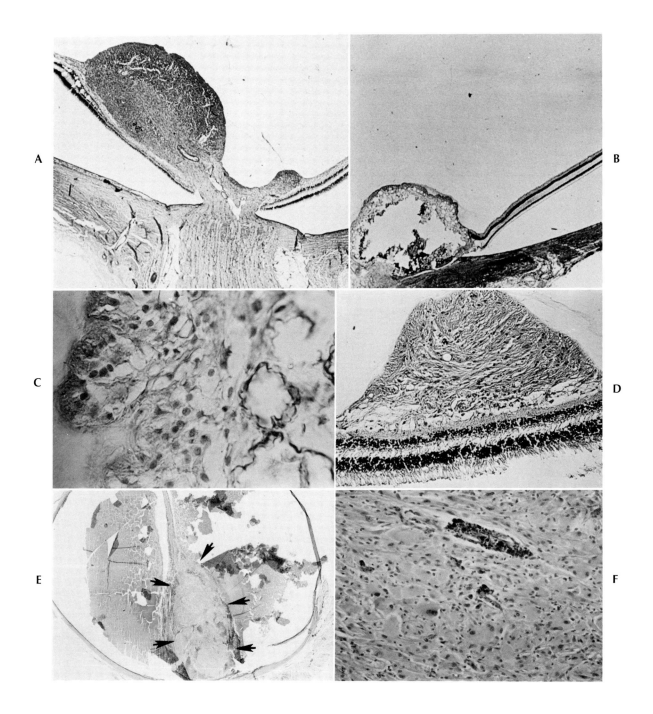

Fig. 13-6. Cystic astrocytic hamartoma of the retina in a patient without other evidence of tuberous sclerosis. On routine eye examination a 10-year-old white girl had a tumor in the left fundus. A maternal aunt had an eye enucleated for causes unknown at 30 years of age. The patient gave no history and had no physical findings of tuberous sclerosis. Skull x-ray findings were normal. Her vision in the right eye was 20/20 and in the left eye was 20/15. Funduscopic examination of the right eye was normal.

A, There was a white finely polycystic tumor arising from the inner retinal layers just superior to the left macular area. It was unassociated with exudative changes. Note that most of the retinal vessels are hidden within this cottony tumor.

B to **D,** Fluorescein angiography revealed a network of retinal vessels within the depth of this tumor. There was some evidence of leakage of dye from these vessels during the later phases of angiography.

E, A poor-quality fundus photograph taken 9 years later showed evidence of slight growth of this tumor.

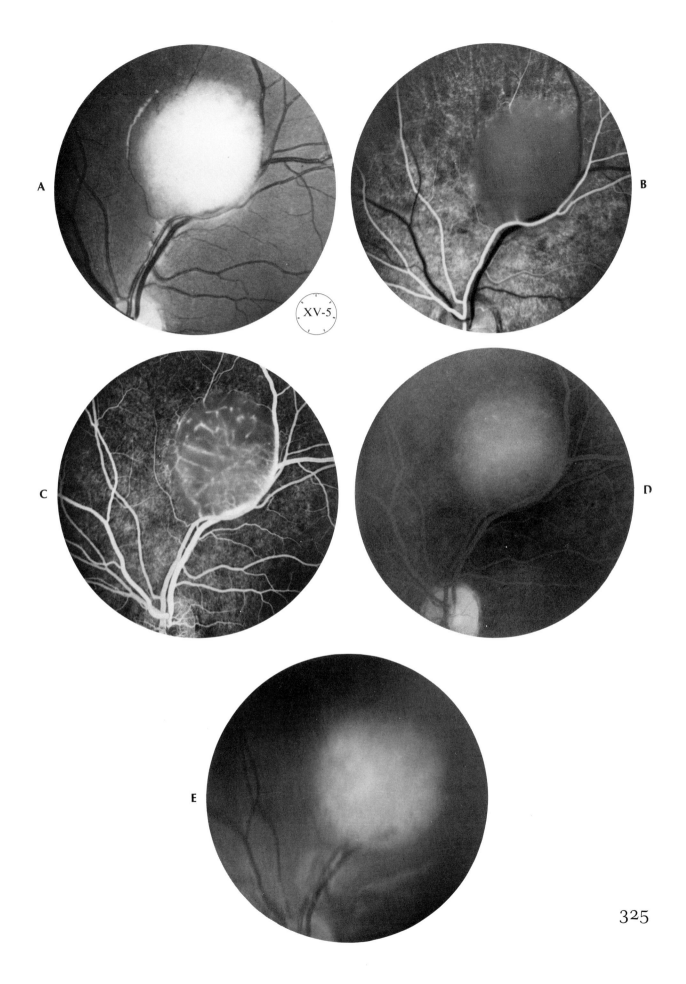

XV-5

325

Fig. 13-7. Endophytic retinal tumor simulating an astrocytic hamartoma of the retina. A 38-year-old white woman was examined on December 28, 1970, because of a 3-month history of blurred vision in her left eye. Her past history showed convulsions unassociated with fever at 1 year of age. Her past medical history was otherwise unremarkable. On her legs the patient had flat, brown "suntan spots" that were not typical of café-au-lait spots. Her vision in the right eye was 20/20−1. Amsler grid revealed slight metamorphopsia superior to fixation in the left eye. Funduscopic examination of the right eye was normal.

A, In the left eye there was an elevated white tumor located in the retina inferior to the macula. There were many blood vessels present within this tumor, which partly obscured most of the major retinal vessels.

B to **D,** Fluorescein angiography outlined an extensive vascular network within this tumor. There was some leakage of dye from the vessels of this tumor. The clinical impression was an unusually vascularized astrocytic hamartoma of the retina. Skull and chest x-ray findings were normal. The patient was examined again on October 11, 1971, and there was no change in the appearance of the lesion. She returned on September 15, 1973, and the lesion had disappeared, leaving only a minor disturbance in the retina in the area of the tumor. Because of the spontaneous disappearance of the lesion, it is doubtful as to whether this indeed did represent an astrocytic hamartoma.

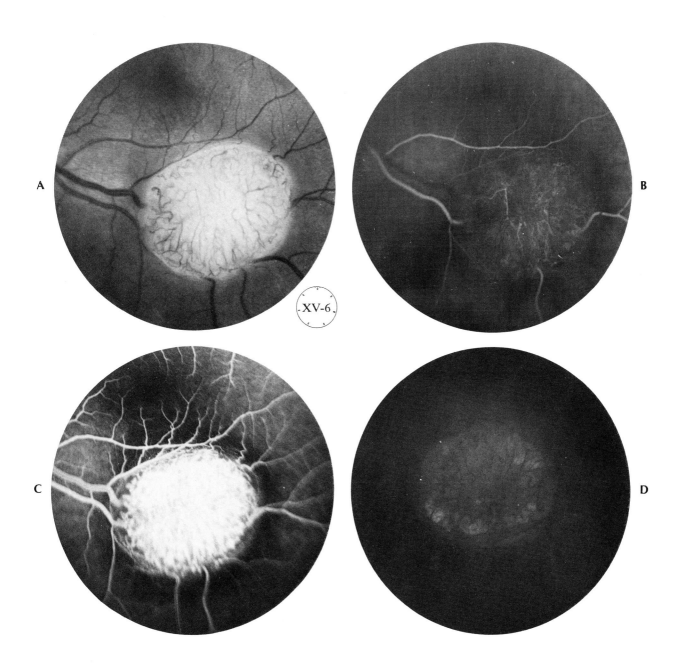

Fig. 13-8. Large calcified exophytic astrocytic hamartoma of the retina in a patient without other evidence of tuberous sclerosis. A 15-year-old white boy gave an 8-year history of defective vision in the right eye. This was first noted while he was firing a gun. The central scotoma in the right eye had remained unchanged since that time. His family history and past history were unremarkable for any other diseases. Visual acuity in the right eye was 20/300 and in the left eye was 20/15.

A, Funduscopic examination in the right eye revealed a large elevated white tumor composed of many semitranslucent globules, some of which were white and appeared calcified. The tumor appeared to arise primarily in the outer retinal layers and to extend into the subretinal space. There was one clear cystic area present within the tumor (*arrow*). The tumor encroached on the temporal aspect of the optic nerve head. The pattern of retinal vessels overlying the tumor was relatively normal. Some of the larger blood vessels dipped down into the depth of the tumor.

B to **D,** Angiography revealed an extensive capillary network that extended down into the tumor. There was leakage of dye from this network and staining of the tumor. Note the dye pooled within the cystic area (*arrow*).

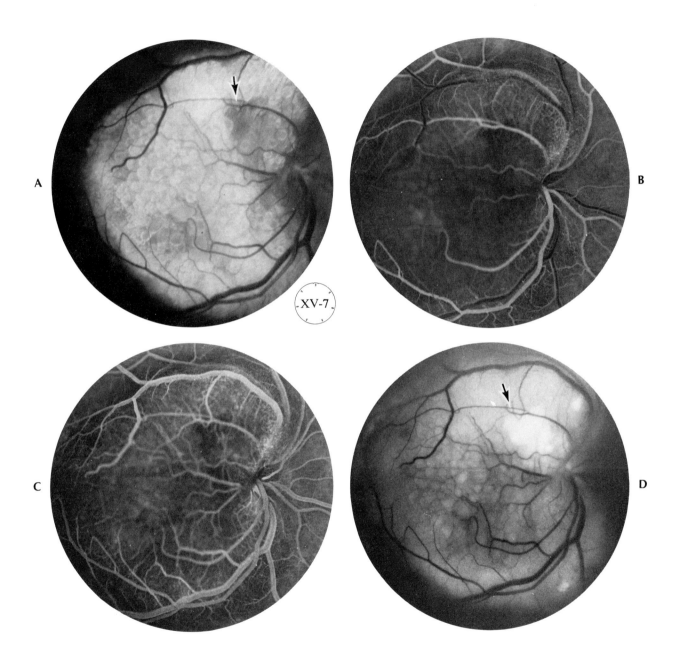

XV-7

REFERENCES

1. Gass, J. D. M.: The phakomatoses. In Smith, J. L. (editor): Neuro-ophthalmology Vol. II. Symposium of the University of Miami and the Bascom Palmer Eye Institute, St. Louis, 1965, The C. V. Mosby Co., 1a-244, 1b-227, 1c-235, 1d-231, 1e-225, and 1f-230.
2. McLean, J. M.: Glial tumors of retina in relation to tuberous sclerosis, Am. J. Ophthalmol. 41:428-432, 1956.
3. Zimmerman, L. E., and Walsh, F. D.: Clinicopathological conference, Am. J. Ophthalmol. 42:737-747, 1956.

SUGGESTED READINGS

Boniuk, M., and Hawkins, W. R.: Transscleral migration of pigment following cryotherapy of intraocular glioma, Trans. Am. Acad. Ophthalmol. Otolaryngol. 75:60-69, 1971.

Parkhill, E. M., and Benedict, W. L.: Gliomas of the retina, A histopathologic study, Am. J. Ophthalmol. 24:1354-1373, 1941.

Reese, A. B.: Tumors of the eye, New York, 1963, Paul B. Hoeber, Inc., Harper & Row, Publishers, pp. 173-177.

CHAPTER FOURTEEN

Retinoblastoma

The congenital multicentric retinal neoplasm call retinoblastoma is the most common intraocular tumor of childhood. It is detected most frequently in the patient about the age of 2 years. It rarely is diagnosed after the age of 7 years. There is no significant sex or race predilection. It occurs bilaterally in approximately 25 to 35 percent of patients. Two-thirds of the children present because of leukokoria. Most of the others present because of strabismus. The typical funduscopic picture is that of one or more white or pearly pink, either endophytic or exophytic retinal masses (Figs. 14-1 to 14-3). The endophytic tumors are often cauliflower in configuration and multiple tumor nodules may be scattered along the inner retinal surface or within the vitreous (Fig. 14-2). Blood vessels are usually visible within the tumor mass. In the exophytic tumors the secondary irregular dilatation of the retinal blood vessels may occasionally be mistaken for that seen in retinal telangiectasis (see Chapter 9). The large blood vessels in retinoblastoma characteristically dip into the depth of the tumor (Fig. 14-1), whereas they do not in retinal telangiectasis. Scattered chalky white areas of calcification occur frequently within retinoblastomas (Fig. 14-3). Rubeosis iridis, hypopyon, keratic precipitates, hyphema, cataract, glaucoma, buphthalmos, and proptosis are other manifestations of the disease in its more advanced form. Bone-free radiographic techniques will detect the presence of intraocular calcification in over 50 percent of eyes harboring retinoblastoma.

Fluorescein angiography has been of no value in differentiating small retinoblastomas (Fig. 14-3) from astrocytic hamartomas. They both contain a capillary network that is permeable to fluorescein. Angiography may be of some benefit in differentiating large retinoblastomas from highly elevated exudative detachments secondary to retinal telangiectasis (Figs. 9-4 and 9-5). Angiography often demonstrates evidence of blood vessels within the depth of retinoblastoma, whereas in retinal telangiectasis the abnormal retinal vascular network is confined to the inner surface of the large exudative mass.

In approximately 75 percent of patients, retinoblastoma is the result of a somatic mutation. In the others it is the result of a germinal mutation and it is transmitted as an irregularly dominant trait with incomplete penetrance. Bilateral retinoblastoma is always the result of a germinal mutation or inherited retinoblastoma. A retinoblastoma survivor who himself has proved hereditary retinoblastoma has a 50 percent chance that some of his children will be affected. A sporadically-affected person has a 25 percent chance that some of his children will be affected. Healthy parents with one affected child run a low (approximately 6 percent) risk of producing more affected children. A detailed family history and ophthalmoscopic examination of the parents and siblings for evidence of regressed retinoblastoma should be part of the evaluation of all patients with retinoblastoma (Fig. 14-4).

Retinoblastomas can be destroyed with x-ray irradiation, chemotherapy, diathermy, light coagulation, and cryotherapy. Only the first two methods, however, provide widespread treatment to the retina that may contain tumor nodules too small for ophthalmoscopic visualization. Until recent years, x-ray irradiation of the entire retina, combined in advanced cases with supplemental chemotherapy, has been the conservative treatment of choice in treating retinoblastoma. Photocoagulation and cryotherapy have been reserved primarily for treating those small lesions that fail to respond to x-ray irradiation therapy. More recently, however, local therapy with photocoagulation, cryotherapy, and cobalt applicators has been used as primary mode of therapy by some physicians in the treatment of selected patients with small tumors. After therapy all patients must be examined with the indirect ophthalmoscope and scleral depression under general anesthesia at frequent intervals for evidence of recurrence. Recurrence of tumor is relatively rare after the age of 3 years.

The reported 5-year survival rate after therapy of retinoblastoma is as high as 95 percent in those patients with relatively small tumors (four disc diameters or smaller) located at or behind the equator. In those with massive tumors involving over half of the retina and with vitreous seeding, the reported survival rate is approximately 30 percent.

Microscopically these tumors are composed primarily of undifferentiated neuroblastic cells with hyperchromatic nuclei and scanty cytoplasm (Fig. 14-1, *E* and *F*). Cellular differentiation may be seen in the form of Flexner-Wintersteiner rosettes (Fig. 14-1, *F*). Tumors containing large numbers of true rosettes are believed to have a better prognosis. Seeding of the tumor along the inner retinal surface and vitreous as well as in the subretinal space is common (Fig. 14-2, *C*). The tumor may invade the choroid. It shows a distinct tendency to invade the optic nerve head and optic nerve. In a study done at the Armed Forces Institute of Pathology by Dr. MacKenzie and Dr. Zimmerman[1] the mortality in those patients where the retinoblastoma did not extend into the optic nerve head was 8 percent compared to a mortality of 64 percent in those patients with extension of the tumor into the optic nerve beyond the plane of transection. Approximately 50 percent of patients who died as the result of retinoblastoma show evidence of spread of the tumor from the eye to the brain via the subarachnoid space. For this reason enucleation of any eye suspected of harboring a retinoblastoma should always include a large segment of the optic nerve. Hematogenous spread of tumor cells in retinoblastoma may occur by invasion of the choroidal as well as the retinal vessels. Choroidal invasion occurs in over 50 percent of serial-sectioned eyes with retinoblastoma, and this finding does not necessarily carry with it a grave prognosis since there is evidence that over 50 percent of such patients will survive. There is, however, a strong relationship between eyes showing extensive areas of choroidal invasion and death from the tumor.

Spontaneous regression of retinoblastoma may occur. Calcified remnants of the tumor may be visible ophthalmoscopically (Fig. 14-4). Spontaneous resolution of large retinoblastomas may lead to phthisis bulbi.

Fig. 14-1. Exophytic retinoblastoma. A 1-year-old white boy was seen because of a white pupillary reflex.

A and **B,** Funduscopic examination of the right eye revealed a large white globular exophytic retinal tumor involving much of the temporal half of the fundus. Note the dilatation and tortuosity of the retinal vessels leading toward the tumor. Many of the retinal vessels dip into the surface of the tumor.

C and **D,** Fluorescein angiography revealed evidence of extensive leakage of dye from the blood vessels within the tumor. The clinical diagnosis was retinoblastoma and the eye was enucleated.

E, Histopathologic examination revealed an exophytic retinoblastoma. There were large blood vessels near the surface as well as in the depth of the tumor.

F, In a few areas the tumor was well differentiated and showed typical Flexner-Wintersteiner rosettes *(arrow)*.

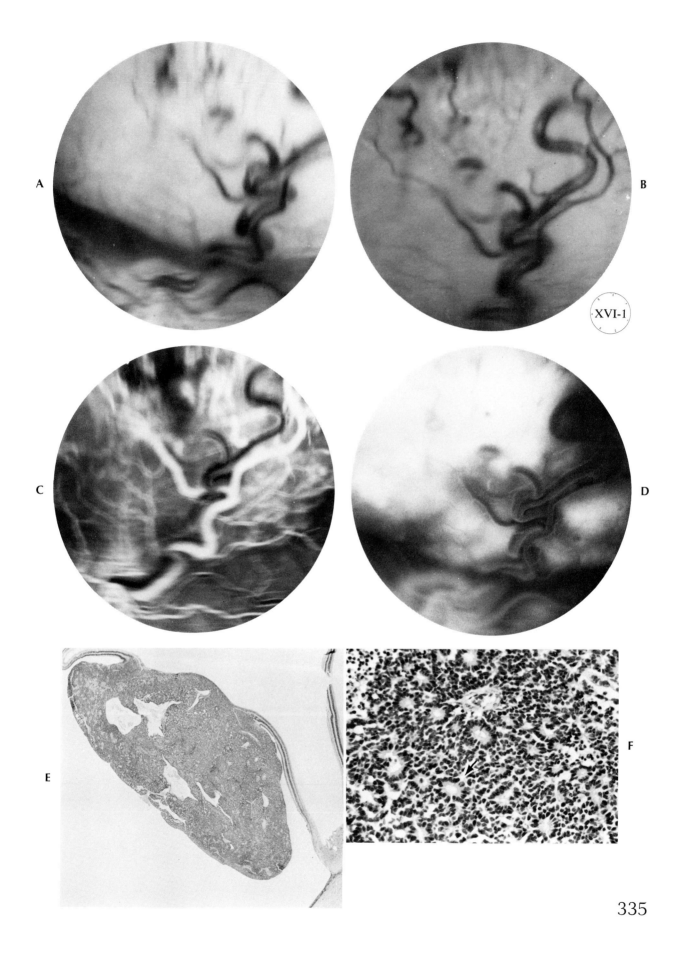

Fig. 14-2. Vitreous seeding in retinoblastoma. A 5-year-old white boy was examined because of 1-month glaucoma in the left eye. The past history and family history were normal. Funduscopic examination of the right eye was normal. In the left eye he had a large endophytic retinoblastoma in the periphery of the fundus.

A, Posteriorly there were scattered nodules of retinoblastoma along the inner surface of the retina.

B, The hypofluorescent areas *(arrows)* on the angiogram indicate the sites of the preretinal nodules of retinoblastoma. The clinical diagnosis was retinoblastoma and the eye was enucleated.

C, Histopathologic examination revealed an endophytic undifferentiated retinoblastoma with many tumor nodules scattered along the inner retinal surface. The centers of some of the nodules were necrotic *(arrow)*.

D and **E,** A 2-year-old white boy was seen because of leukokoria.

D, Ophthalmoscopic examination revealed a highly elevated multilobular white tumor with gross distortion of the normal retinal vascular pattern. Large vessels dipped in and out of the tumor. There were free-floating tumor nodules within the vitreous cavity *(arrows)*. These latter two findings should clearly differentiate this tumor from Coat's disease secondary to retinal telangiectasis.

E, Late angiogram shows extensive staining of the tumor. The intravitreal tumor nodules are outlined as hypofluorescent areas *(arrows)*.

F, The eye in **D** and **E** was enucleated, and histopathologic examination revealed a massive endophytic retinoblastoma with free-floating tumor nodules *(arrows)*. There was extensive necrosis of the inner portions of this highly vascular tumor.

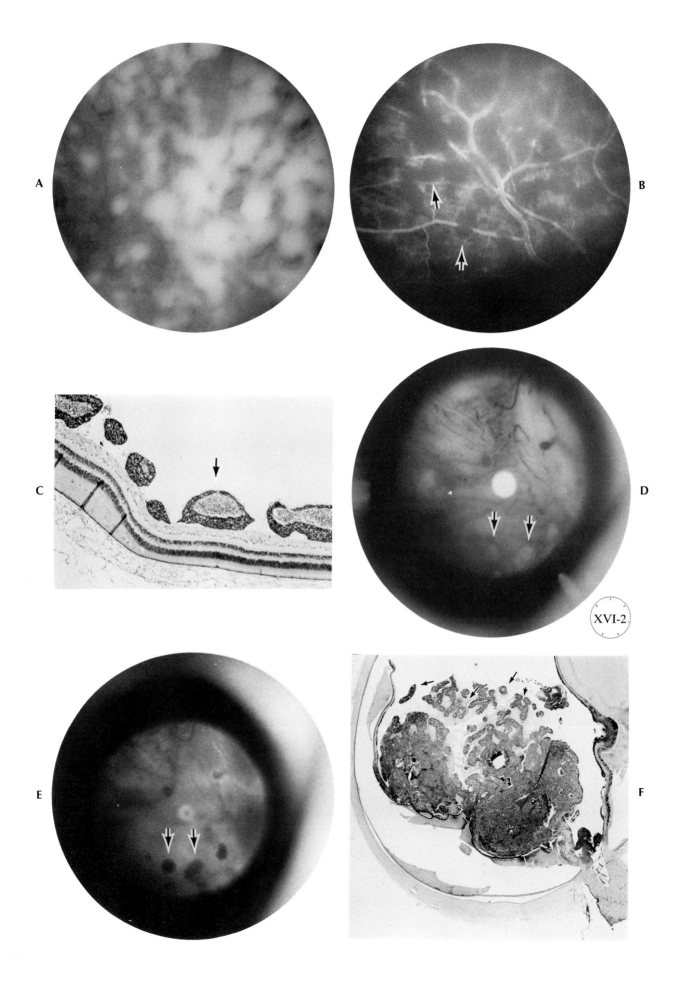

A

B

C

D

XVI-2

E

F

Fig. 14-3. Small retinoblastoma showing calcification. A 4-year-old Indian child had enucleation of his left eye 1 month prior to examination at the Bascom Palmer Eye Institute. Histopathologic examination of that eye revealed retinoblastoma with invasion of the optic nerve. He was referred for treatment of a solitary lesion noted in the right eye. The family history showed a retinoblastoma in a 6-year-old brother who had an enucleation of one eye at 8 months of age. Two other siblings were living and well. His father, 28 years of age, had generalized seizures as a child. The mother's history was normal (see Fig. 14-4). A maternal aunt had a facial rash and generalized seizures and died at 30 years of age.

A, Ophthalmoscopic examination revealed an elevated white tumor with areas of calcification *(arrow)* located superonasal to the optic disc. The remainder of the fundus was normal.

B to **D,** Fluorescein angiography revealed a fine capillary network within and immediately surrounding the tumor. There was widespread leakage of dye from these vessels. This patient died of widespread metatasis several months later. The clinical and angiographic appearance of this solitary nodule is quite similar to that of astrocytic hamartomas in the retina (see Fig. 13-4, *B* and *E*). It is of interest that this child with hereditary retinoblastoma also had a family history suggesting tuberous sclerosis.

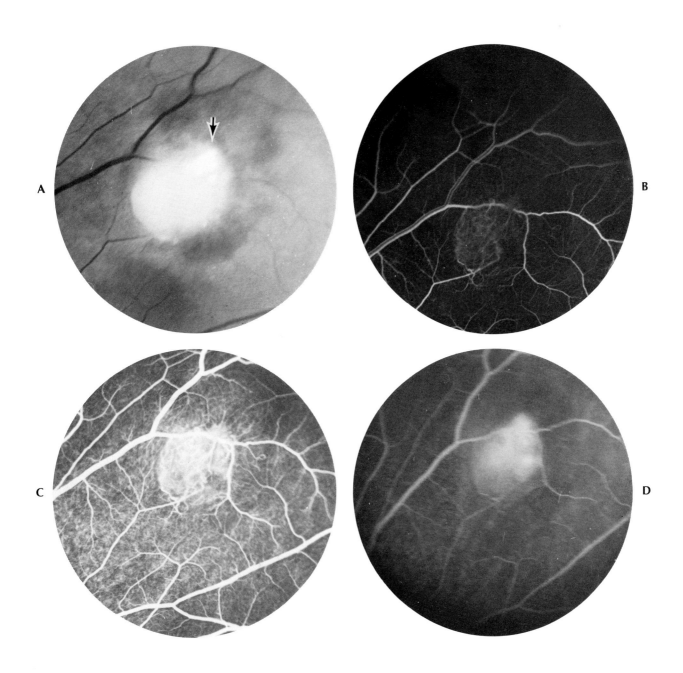

339

Fig. 14-4. Regressed retinoblastoma in the mother of two children with retinoblastoma. This 23-year-old Indian woman, the mother of the patient illustrated in Fig. 14-3, was asymptomatic.

A, On the temporal edge of the right macula there was a chorioretinal scar secondary to regressed retinoblastoma. Note the clublike calcified opacity (*arrow*) lying in the atrophic retina, which lies in the depth of the lesion. There is sheathing of the retinal vein draining this area.

B, Arteriovenous phase showing early filling of the retinal arteries and choroidal circulation.

C, Later stage showing network of retinal and underlying choroidal vessels.

D, Dye leakage from both the retinal and choroidal vessels is evident in the area of the atrophic lesion.

E and **F,** Two other areas of regressed retinoblastoma in the same patient.

(**A** to **D** from Gass.[2])

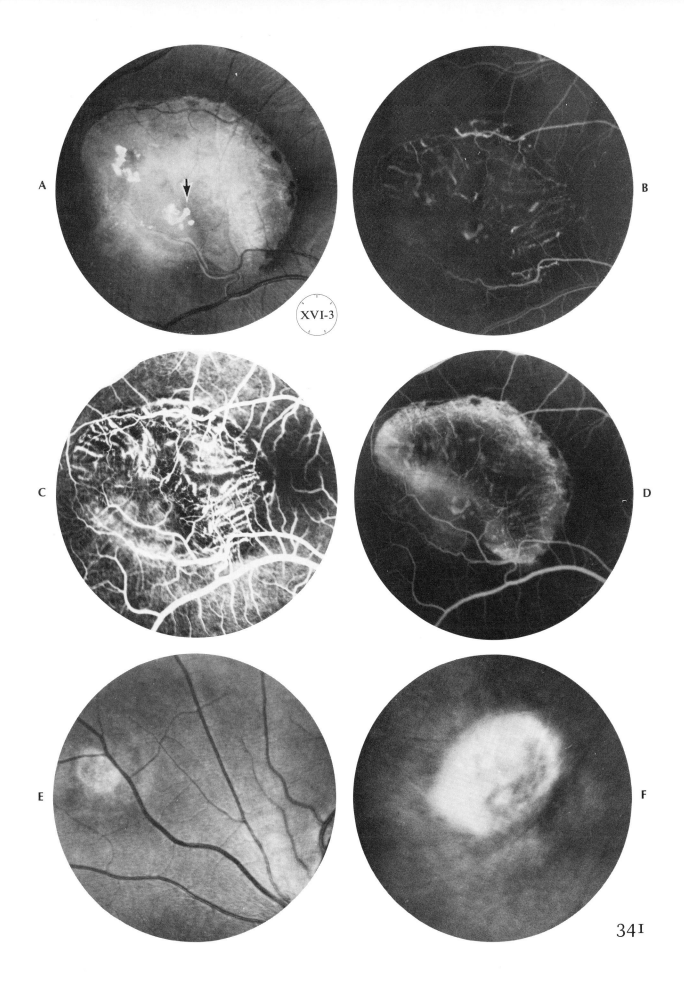

REFERENCES

1. Zimmerman, L. E.: Registry of ophthalmic pathology. Trans. Am. Acad. Otolaryngol. **65:**51-113, 1961.
2. Gass, J. D. M.: Stereoscopic atlas of macular diseases, St. Louis, 1970, The C. V. Mosby Co., p. 191.

SUGGESTED READINGS

Bedford, M. A., Bedotto, C., and MacFaul, P. A.: Retinoblastoma: A study of 139 cases, Brit. J. Ophthalmol. **55:**19-27, 1971.

Boniuk, M., and Girard, L. J.: Spontaneous regression of bilateral retinoblastoma, Trans. Am. Acad. Ophthalmol. Otolaryngol. **73:**194-198, 1069.

Ellsworth, R. M.: Treatment of retinoblastoma, Am. J. Ophthalmol. **66:**49-51, 1968.

Francois, J., and Matton-Van Leuven, M. T.: Recent data on the heredity of retinoblastoma. In Boniuk, M. (editor): International symposium on ocular tumors, Houston, Texas, 1962: Ocular and adnexal tumors, St. Louis, 1964, The C. V. Mosby Co., pp. 123-141.

Hopping, W., and Meyer-Schwickerath, G.: Light coagulation treatment in retinoblastoma. In Boniuk, M. (editor): International symposium on ocular tumors, Houston, Texas, 1962: Ocular and adnexal tumors, St. Louis, 1964, The C. V. Mosby Co., pp. 192-196.

Meyer-Schwickerath, G.: The preservation of vision by treatment of intraocular tumors with light coagulation, Arch. Ophthalmol. **66:**458-466, 1961.

Redler, L. D., and Ellsworth, R. M.: Prognostic importance of choroidal invasion in retinoblastoma, Arch. Ophthalmol. **90:**294-296, 1973.

Reese, A. B.: Tumors of the eye, New York, 1963, Paul B. Hoeber, Inc., Harper & Row, Publishers, pp. 84-161.

Reese, A. B.: Persistent hyperplastic primary vitreous, Am. J. Ophthalmol. **40:**317-331, 1955.

Reese, A. B., and Blodi, F. C.: Retinal dysplasia, Am. J. Ophthalmol. **33:**23-32, 1950.

Reese, A. B., Hyman, G. A., Tapley, N., and Forrest, A. W.: The treatment of retinoblastoma by x-ray and triethylene melamine, Arch. Ophthalmol. **60:**897-906, 1958.

Reese, A. B., and Straatsma, B. R.: Retinal dysplasia, Am. J. Ophthalmol. **45:**199-211, 1958.

Rubin, M. L., and Kaufman, H. E.: Spontaneously regressed probable retinoblastoma. Report of a case, Arch. Ophthalmol. **81:**442-445, 1969.

Stallard, H. B.: The conservative treatment of retinoblastoma. In Boniuk, M. (editor): International symposium on ocular tumors, Houston, Texas, 1962: Ocular and adnexal tumors, St. Louis, 1964, The C. V. Mosby Co., pp. 171-191.

Ts'o, M. O., Fine, B. S., and Zimmerman, L. E.: The nature of retinoblastoma. II. Photoreceptor differentiation: An electron microscopic study, Am. J. Ophthalmol. **69:**350-359, 1970.

Ts'o, M. O., Zimmerman, L. E., and Fine, B. S.: The nature of retinoblastoma. I. Photoreceptor differentiation: A clinical and histopathologic study, Am. J. Ophthalmol. **69:**339-349, 1970.

Zimmerman, L. E.: Retinoblastoma, Med. Ann. D. C. **38:**366-374, 1969.

**CHAPTER
FIFTEEN**

Iris tumors

A small number of hamartomatous, neoplastic, and inflammatory iris tumors have been studied with fluorescein angiography at the Bascom Palmer Eye Institute. To date, fluorescein angiography has been of limited value as an aid to the diagnosis of these tumors.

Several techniques have been used in fluorescein angiography of lesions in the anterior segment. The fundus camera may be used, but it is not ideally suited for anterior segment photography because of low magnification, severe peripheral aberration, inadequate depth of field, and obscured picture frame margins. Matsui et al.[1,2] have reviewed the various techniques employed for angiography of the anterior segment and they have described an improved technique of their own.

IRIS NEVI AND MELANOMAS

Nevi and melanomas are the most common iris tumors. The clinical and histopathologic distinction between the two is not always easy. Nevi, in general, are small slightly raised tumors that arise in the anterior iris stroma (Fig. 15-1). They are congenital, but may not be visible until they acquire pigmentation in young adulthood. Their maximum period of growth occurs in childhood and young adulthood. They usually do not alter the shape and reaction of the pupil. They may, however, occasionally be large and more highly elevated and may affect the pupil. Iris nevi may be multiple and are more common in patients with multiple pigmented cutaneous nevi with or without other manifestations of neurofibromatosis. They are frequently present in patients with malignant melanoma of the choroid and ciliary body. They may involve the iris diffusely in melanosis oculi.

Iris nevi may remain stationary for years and then show evidence of growth. In addition to a change in the tumor size, shape, and color, other ipsilateral clinical features that suggest that an iris lesion may be a malignant melanoma are changes in pupillary size, shape, and reaction, iridocyclitis, glaucoma, heterochromia iridis, and hyphema (Figs. 15-2 to 15-5). Melanomas of the iris are typically nodular and highly vascularized (Figs. 15-2 and 15-5). Blood vessels within the tumor may be obscured by heavy pigmentation (Fig. 15-4). Occasionally the degree of vascularization in nonpigmented melanomas is so great that they may be misdiagnosed as hemangiomas (Fig. 15-5). Iris melanomas may invade the anterior chamber angle. An iris tumor may represent an anterior extension of a ciliary body melanoma (Fig. 15-4). One should always use gonioscopy, indirect ophthalmoscopy with scleral depression, and transillumination in patients with iris tumors to determine the extent of anterior chamber angle and ciliary body involvement. Some melanomas infiltrate the iris without producing a mass lesion. This type of melanoma should be suspected in patients presenting with unilateral heterochromia iridis, iridocyclitis, and glaucoma. Rarely an iris melanoma may undergo spontaneous necrosis and cause secondary glaucoma (Fig. 15-3).

Fluorescein angiography demonstrates minimal evidence of alteration of the normal iris vascular pattern and permeability in the presence of localized iris nevi (Fig. 15-1). Angiography in localized iris melanomas usually shows evidence of blood vessels within the tumor as well as evidence of abnormal leakage of dye from these vessels and those in the neighboring iris (Figs. 15-2 to 15-5).

Histopathologically there is no sharp division between an iris nevus and a malignant melanoma. Iris nevi are composed of small delicate spindle cells that on cut section often appear round. The commonest type of malignant melanoma of the iris is one composed of an admixture of these small nevoid spindle cells and spindle A cells. Some iris melanomas also contain spindle B cells. Epithelioid cells occur infrequently. Most melanomas invade the iris stroma and grow in a sheet along its surface as a cohesive cellular mass. Metastasis is extremely rare. It usually occurs in patients with rapidly growing iris tumors that histopathologically are composed of less cohesive epithelioid as well as spindle cells. The rarity of metastasis dictates conservative management of patients suspected of iris melanomas. No treatment is indicated in the absence of clear-cut history of growth. A review of old portrait photographs of the patient may prove helpful in detecting growth. Stereophotographs are valuable in following iris tumors. If evidence of growth occurs and if the lesion does not extend into the ciliary body, excisional biopsy is indicated. If the tumor extends into the anterior chamber angle and ciliary body, the treatment depends on many factors, including the extent of the angle and ciliary body involvement, the age of the patient, and the rate of growth. If the angle is involved for 90 degrees or less, and if growth has been documented, excisional iridocyclectomy might be considered. This procedure, however, probably will prove to be useful only in treating the relatively slow-growing spindle cell tumors, which have virtually no potential for metastasis. If the anterior chamber angle is involved over a wide area and if this is associated with secondary glaucoma, enucleation is the treatment of choice.

OTHER IRIS TUMORS

Iris melanomas must be differentiated from other rare iris tumors, such as metastatic carcinoma (Fig. 15-6), juvenile xanthogranuloma (usually in infants or children with hyphema), pigment epithelial cysts, nonpigmented epithelial cysts, choristoma of the iris (aberrant lacrimal gland), dictyoma, leukemia, rhabdomyosarcoma, angiomas (Fig. 15-7), inflammatory tumors including sarcoidosis, syphilis, tuberculosis, iris abscess (Fig. 15-8), and foreign body granuloma.

Fig. 15-1. Pigmented lesion of the iris presumed to be a nevus. A 72-year-old white woman was seen for a routine eye examination in December 1970. Her visual acuity in both eyes was 20/40. The intraocular pressure was normal in both eyes.

A, There was a pigmented lesion of the iris *(arrow)* in the right eye. There was very slight distortion of the pupillary margin. Gonioscopy revealed the lesion did not extend into the angle. There was no abnormal pigmentation in the anterior chamber angle.

B to **D,** Fluorescein angiography revealed no evidence of abnormal vessels in the area of the tumor *(arrows),* which obscured the normal iris vessels from view. There was no evidence of staining in the vicinity of the tumor in late angiograms. The patient was last seen 2 years later. There was no change in the appearance of the lesion.

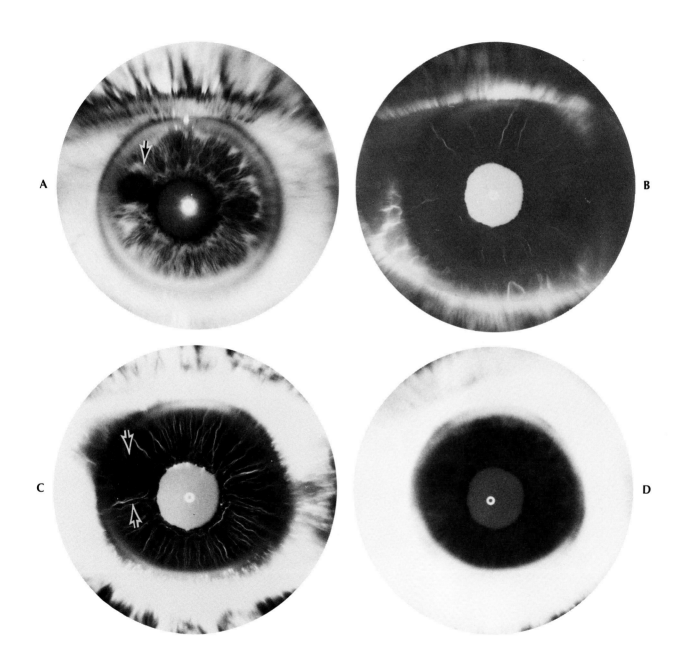

Fig. 15-2. Hyphema and secondary glaucoma: the presenting manifestation of a melanoma of the iris and ciliary body. A 30-year-old white man was well until he noted the sudden onset of decreased vision in his left eye. He gave a 6-year history of slight discoloration of the iris in the left eye. He was examined by his local physician who noted an anterior chamber hyphema and a steamy cornea in the left eye. The intraocular pressure was elevated.

A, When the patient was examined at the Bascom Palmer Eye Institute 2 months later, he had an elevated nonpigmented vascularized mass involving the iris of the left eye in the 7 o'clock meridian. On gonioscopy the mass appeared to barely extend into the angle. There was a small amount of blood on the anterior surface of the tumor. The intraocular pressure at that time was normal. The pupil was peaked toward the tumor.

B to **D,** Fluorescein angiography showed evidence of a vascularized tumor. There was staining of the tumor in the late photographs. Approximately 1 week later the patient had an iridocyclectomy with apparent complete excision of the tumor. Histopathologic examination revealed a very vascularized nonpigmented spindle B melanoma that involved the iris and the anterior portion of the ciliary body. His postoperative course was uneventful and he was asymptomatic when last seen 2 years later. The transient secondary glaucoma was presumably caused by the hyphema and was unrelated to widespread tumor invasion of the angle structures.

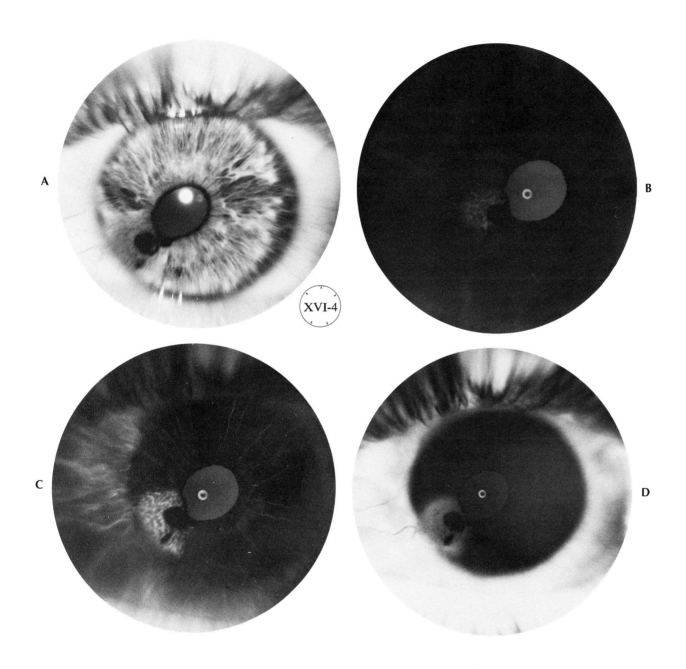

XVI-4

Fig. 15-3. Spontaneous hyphema and melanomalytic glaucoma secondary to spontaneous necrosis of a low-grade spindle cell melanoma of the iris and ciliary body. In October 1959, a 52-year-old white woman had a 5-day history of irritation in the left eye. Her local physician noted a spontaneous hyphema and abnormal pigmentation of the left iris. The patient had noted that the left eye had always been darker than the right eye and that there had been no recent change. She was seen initially at the Bascom Palmer Eye Institute 5 days after the onset of symptoms. Her visual acuity was 20/25 in both eyes. Gonioscopic examination revealed a small amount of blood in the angle of the left eye inferiorly. The intraocular pressure was 30 mm Hg in the left eye and was normal in the right eye.

A, An irregular brown hyperpigmented lesion associated with multiple focal areas of atrophy of the iris stroma and ectropion uvea was present on the left iris. The iris tumor extended from 4 to 10 o'clock. There was a slight elevated pigmented nodule at 6 o'clock in the periphery. There were some dilated tortuous vessels on the episclera from 3 to 6 o'clock. There was fine pigment dust scattered over the entire anterior surface of the iris. There was a noticeable ray in the anterior chamber. The tumor extended in a flat fashion into the angle inferiorly.

B, Early angiogram revealed disruption in the normal radial pattern of the iris blood vessels nasally.

C, There was irregular staining of the iris stroma and pooling of dye in the aqueous humor inferiorly. The small iris nodule appeared hypofluorescent in the late angiogram *(arrow)*. Follow-up examination 6 weeks later revealed minimal cells and ray. There was evidence of more atrophy of the flat portion of the pigmented tumor. The intraocular pressure was 14 mm Hg in each eye. The patient was followed elsewhere with chronic uncontrolled glaucoma and progressive atrophy of the iris in the area of the tumor. There was no evidence of further growth of the tumor until November 1972. At that time the eye was blind and there was evidence of pigmentation along some of the emissary channels at the limbus. The eye was enucleated.

D to **F,** Histopathologic examination revealed large areas of atrophy involving the full thickness of the iris nasally. There were scattered foci of small pigmented spindle cells *(arrows 1)* scattered within the iris stroma nasally. These focal areas of tumor were separated by large clumps of pigment-laden macrophages *(arrows 2)* that had replaced the normal iris stroma. The anterior surface of the iris temporally was covered with these macrophages. The trabecular meshwork and outflow channels were packed with these macrophages *(arrows 3)*. There was minimal invasion of the ciliary body. There was deep glaucomatous cupping of the optic disc, and the ganglion cell layer of the retina was completely atrophic. The histopathologic diagnosis was melanomalytic glaucoma secondary to spontaneous necrosis of a low-grade spindle cell melanoma of the iris and ciliary body.

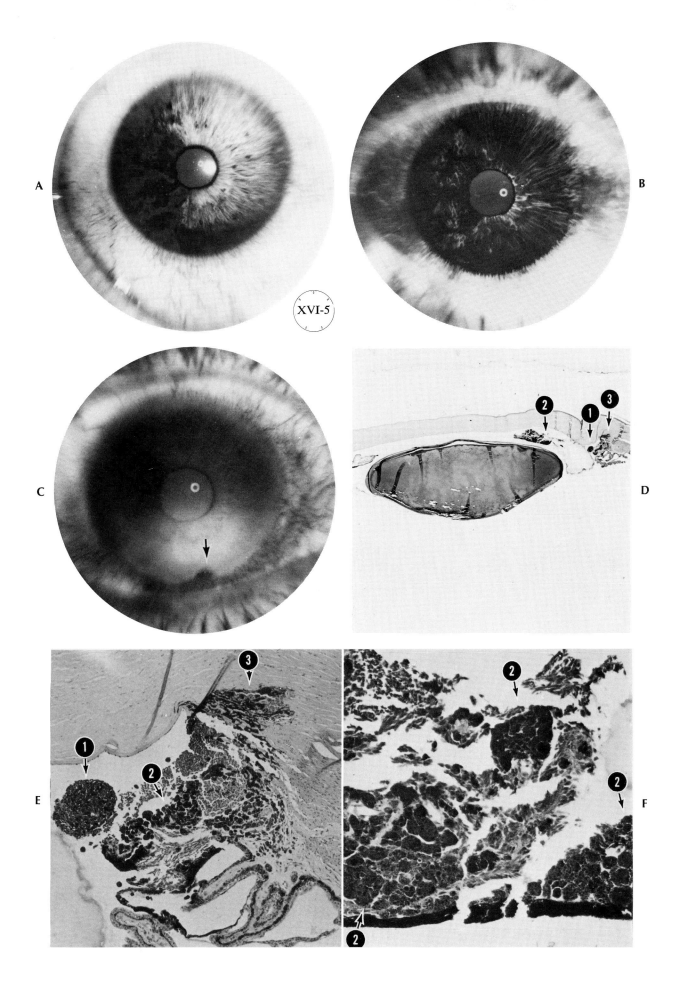

XVI-5

Fig. 15-4. Rapidly growing epitheloid cell melanoma of the iris and ciliary body. A 60-year-old white man had a 6-week history of an enlarging black mass in his left iris. His medical history was negative. His visual acuity in the right eye was 20/20 and in the left eye was 20/30. His applanation tension was 14 mm Hg in the right eye and 24 mm Hg in the left eye.

A, In the left eye he had a heavily pigmented lesion displacing the iris forward between 9 and 11 o'clock. The mass was in contact with the cornea peripherally. There were no visible blood vessels in the tumor. It indented the lens and extended back to the pars plana. Gonioscopy revealed some evidence of irregular hyperpigmentation of the trabecular meshwork.

B to **D,** Fluorescein angiography showed no evidence of blood vessels near the surface of the tumor, but there was diffusion of dye from its surface (*arrows*). Note the distortion and dilatation of the iris vessels extending from the flattened iris margin to the tumor.

E, The glaucoma worsened and the eye was enucleated. Histopathologic examination revealed an epithelioid cell melanoma involving the peripheral iris and the ciliary body. Tumor cells were present in the anterior chamber angle opposite the tumor.

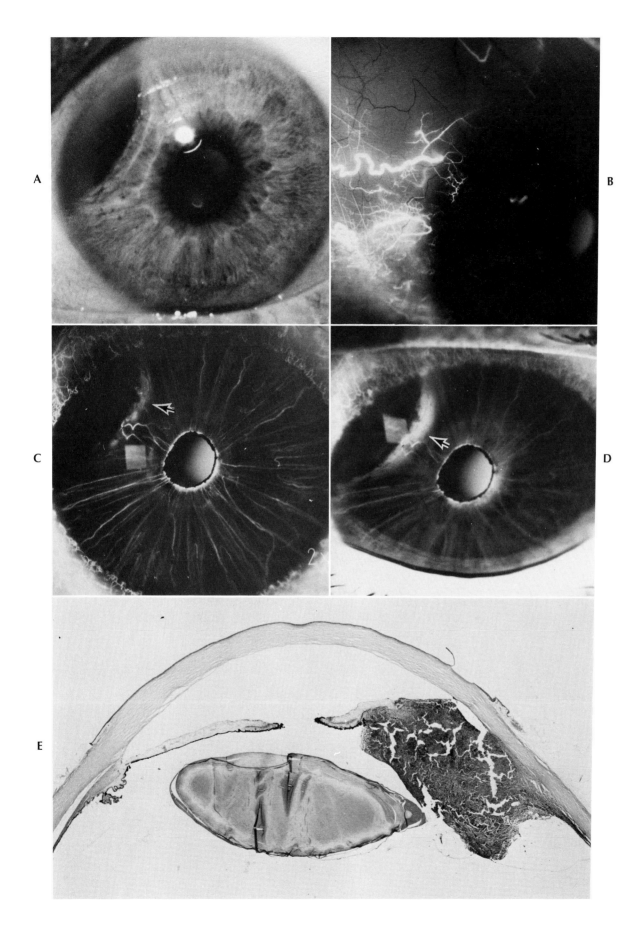

Fig. 15-5. Malignant melanoma of the ciliary body presenting as an amelanotic iris mass. A 73-year-old white man had uncomplicated cataract extraction in both eyes in May and June 1972. Postoperatively, indirect ophthalmoscopy revealed no evidence of choroidal detachments or abnormalities of the fundi.

A, On October 17, 1972, he developed a small pink lobulated iris mass projecting into the anterior chamber of the left eye between 7:30 and 9:30 o'clock. Note the prominent blood vessels.

B to **E,** Fluorescein angiography revealed a highly vascularized tumor that stained during the late phases of angiography. Note in **B** the blood vessels in the tumor filling prior to those in the iris. On dilated funduscopic examination there was a large brown, globular mass in the ciliary body in the lower nasal quadrant. On October 31, the anterior chamber mass was larger. Intraocular pressure was normal and the visual acuity was normal.

F, The eye was enucleated on December 19, 1972, and histopathologic examination revealed a fascicular malignant melanoma. Very vascular amelanotic melanomas of the iris may be misdiagnosed clinically as hemangiomas, which are extremely rare tumors of the iris.

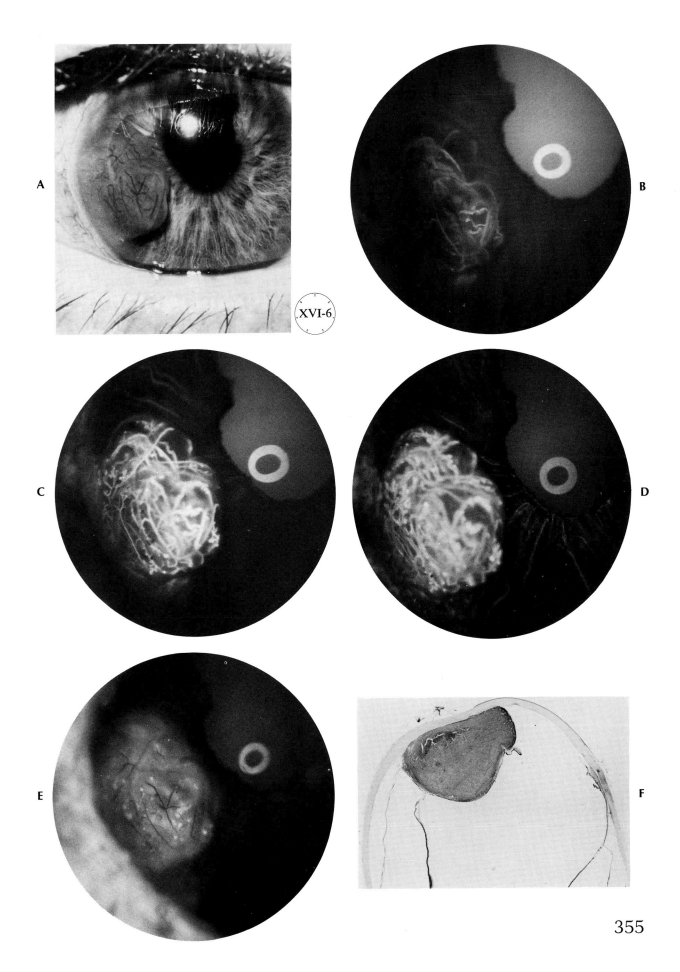

XVI-6

355

Fig. 15-6. Metastatic skin melanoma to the iris. A 51-year-old white man developed a malignant melanoma of the skin in the right axilla in February 1969. An axillary node dissection showed malignancy. In December 1969, a recurrent axillary mass showed malignant melanoma. In July 1969, the patient noted photophobia and redness of the right eye with secondary glaucoma and iritis. Over a period of months he gradually developed a small mass on the right iris. He was first seen at the Bascom Palmer Eye Institute on January 9, 1970. His visual acuity was 20/30 in both eyes.

A, In the right eye at 7 o'clock there was a 3 to 4 mm, pink yellowish, fleshy mass on the anterior surface of the iris extending into the angle. There were several mutton-fat keratic precipitates.

B and **C,** Angiography outlined a vascular network within the tumor *(arrows)*. The retroilluminated keratic precipitates are visible in the pupillary area.

D, Note the faint halo of fluorescein surrounding the tumor, which is stained with dye. There were several blotchy areas of staining of the iris stroma inferonasal to the tumor. The diagnosis was probable metastatic melanoma of the skin to the iris. On February 7, 1970, the patient died from diffuse melanomatosis.

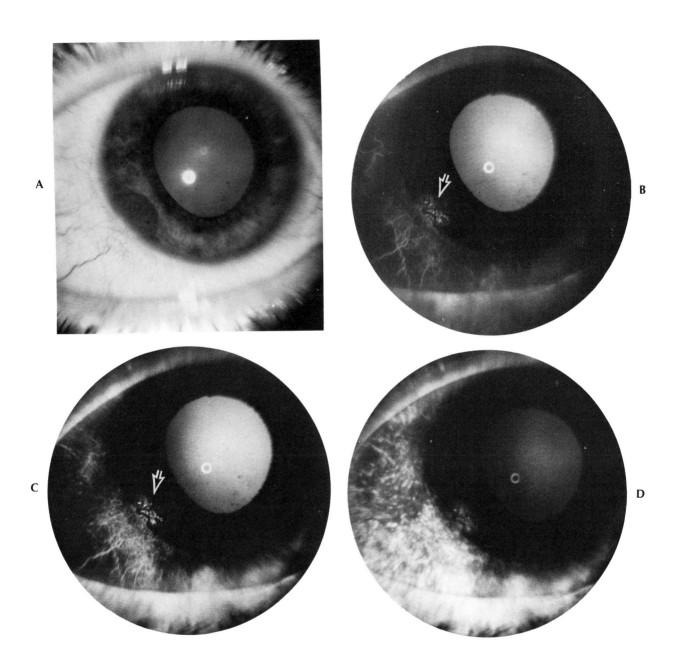

357

Fig. 15-7. Racemose angioma of the episclera and iris.

A and **B,** An incidental finding in the left eye of a middle-aged white man with no other ocular abnormality was the presence of an irregularly dilated tortuous episcleral artery that disappeared near the limbus and appeared to be in continuity with a similarly dilated mass of vessels within the depth of the iris stroma in the 9:30 o'clock meridian (*arrows*).

C to **E,** Fluorescein angiography demonstrated apparent continuity of the episcleral artery with a similarly dilated tortuous artery in the iris stroma (*arrows*). This artery appeared to be in direct continuity with a dilated tortuous vein in the 8 o'clock meridian. Other abnormalities in the iris vessels surrounded this lesion. This is believed to be a congenital vascular angiomatous tumor of the iris.

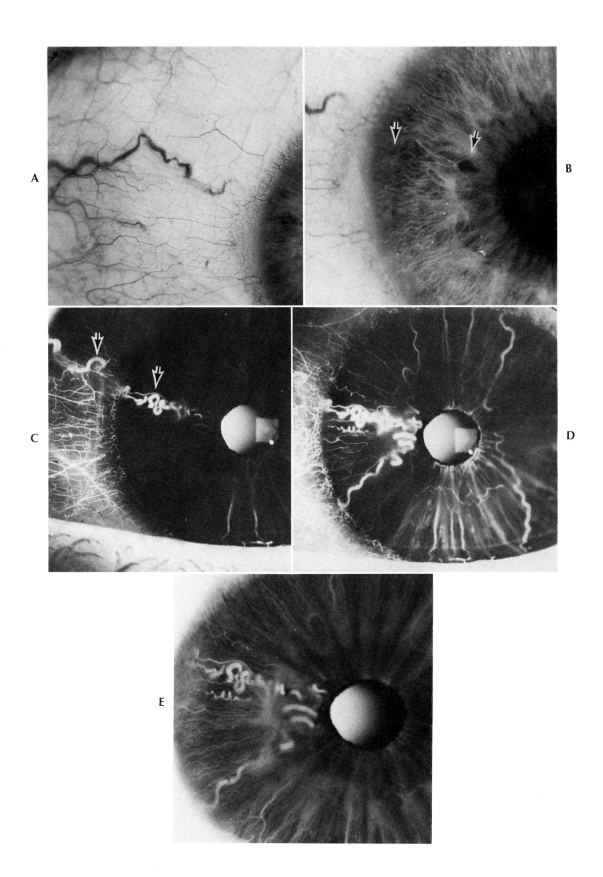

359

Fig. 15-8. Iris abscess simulating a malignant melanoma. A healthy 18-year-old boy with a past history of repeated episodes of dendritic keratitis in the left eye developed conjunctival injection, vesicular epithelial lesions of the cornea, a mild flare, and keratic precipitates in the anterior chamber of the left eye. The diagnosis was herpetic iridocyclitis. He was treated with topically applied cortisone, idoxuridine, and a mydriatic. Five weeks later he developed a rapidly growing lightly pigmented mass of the left iris and he was referred to the Bascom Palmer Eye Institute. His visual acuity in the right eye was 20/20 and in the left eye was 20/70. There was infection of the bulbar conjunctiva in the left eye, and slight irregular superficial stromal scarring of the cornea. The corneal epithelium was intact. The corneal sensation was decreased. There was a mild flare and a few keratic precipitates.

A, There was a tan-colored, well-circumscribed tumor arising from the iris surface between the positions of 1:00 and 2:00 o'clock (*arrows*). The anterior surface of the tumor was smooth and contained many dilated capillaries. The tumor extended to and flattened the pupillary margin. It did not extend into the anterior chamber angle. Posterior synechias were present near the pupillary margin of the tumor.

B to D, Fluorescein angiography of the anterior segment revealed a dense pattern of blood vessels within the iris tumor and leakage of dye from these vessels into the anterior chamber. There was extensive staining of the iris stroma surrounding the tumor during the late phases of the study. The primary clinical diagnosis entertained was malignant melanoma of the iris versus inflammatory pseudotumor of the iris secondary to herpes simplex. Despite intensive topical corticosteroid treatment, the tumor continued to enlarge. On March 9, 1971, an excisional biopsy of the iris tumor was performed.

E, Microscopic examination revealed a very cellular tumefaction that protruded from the anterior surface of the iris and eroded the pigment epithelium posteriorly. The tumor was composed of four concentric cellular layers. Centrally, there was a core of large necrotic polymorphonuclear leukocytes and scattered pigment granules (*zone 1*). A thin zone of melanin-laden macrophages surrounded the central area of necrosis (*zone 2*). Peripheral to this thin zone was a narrow zone of epithelioid cells and swollen, partly degenerated plasma cells (*zone 3*). Peripherally there was a thick zone of densely packed plasma cells and dilated capillaries that comprised the bulk of the tumor (*zone 4*).

F, High-power view of the four zones depicted in **E**. Special stains for fungi, bacteria, and acid-fast organisms in the specimen showed normal results. Electron microscopy failed to reveal evidence of virus particles. The histopathologic diagnosis was "localized iris abscess and granuloma."

(From Gass.[3])

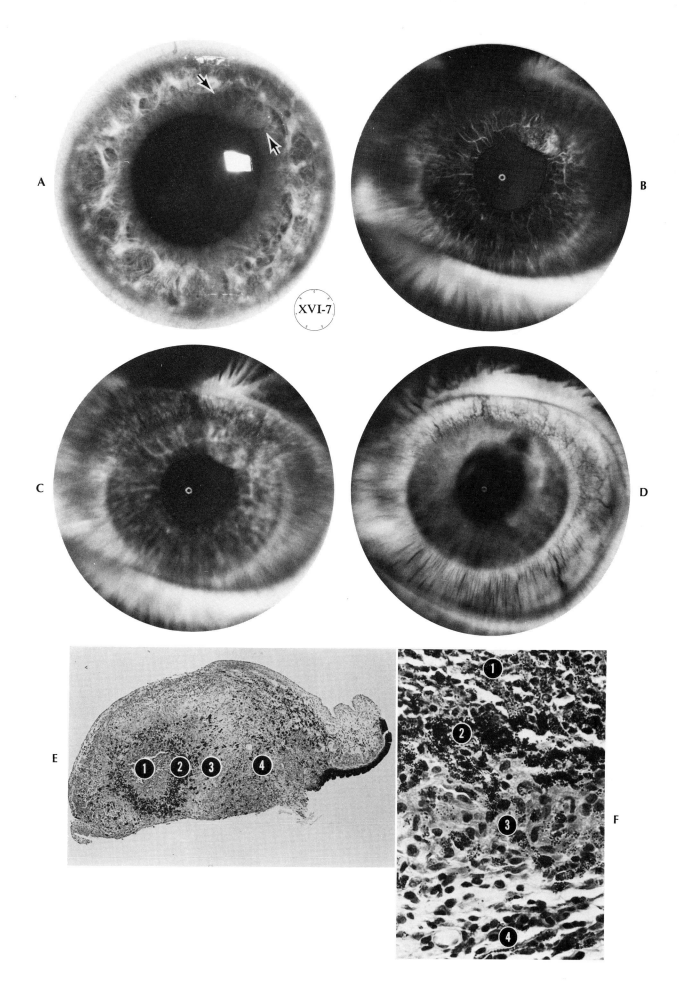

A

B

C

D

E

F

XVI-7

REFERENCES

1. Matsui, M., Parel, J.-M., Weder, H., and Justice, J., Jr.: Some improved methods of anterior segment fluorescein angiography. I. Basic system, Am. J. Ophthalmol. **74:**1075-1079, 1972.
2. Matsui, M., Weder, H., and Parel, J.-M.: Some improved methods of anterior segment fluorescein angiography. 2. Simultaneous stereoscopic photographic system, Am. J. Ophthalmol. **76:**54-59, 1973.
3. Gass, J. D. M.: Iris abscess simulating malignant melanoma, Arch. Ophthalmol. **90:**299-302, 1973.

SUGGESTED READINGS

Duke, J. R., and Dunn, S. N.: Primary tumors of the iris, Arch. Ophthalmol. **59:**204-214, 1958.

Greer, C. H.: Metastatic carcinoma of the iris, Brit. J. Ophthalmol. **38:**699-701, 1954.

Johnston, S. S., and Ware, C. F.: Iris involvement in leukemia, Brit. J. Ophthalmol. **57:**320-324, 1973.

Naumann, G., and Ruprecht, K. W.: Xanthom der Iris, Ophthalmologica **164:**293-305, 1972.

Reese, A. B., and Cleasby, G. W.: The treatment of iris melanoma, Am. J. Ophthalmol. **47:**118-125, 1959.

Rones, B., and Zimmerman, L. E.: The production of heterochromia and glaucoma by diffuse malignant melanoma of the iris, Trans. Am. Acad. Ophthalmol. Otolaryngol. **61:**447-463, 1957.

Rones, B., and Zimmerman, L. E.: The prognosis of primary tumors of the iris treated by iridectomy, Arch. Ophthalmol. **60:**193-205, 1958.

Woyke, S., and Chwirot, R.: Rhabdomyosarcoma of the iris. Report of the first recorded case, Brit. J. Ophthalmol. **56:**60-64, 1972.

Yanoff, M., and Scheie, H. G.: Melanomalytic glaucoma, Arch. Ophthalmol. **84:**471-473, 1970.

Zimmerman, L. E.: Clinical pathology of iris tumors, The Ward Burdick Award Contribution, Am. J. Clin. Path. **39:**214-228, 1963.

Zimmerman, L. E.: Ocular lesions of juvenile xanthogranuloma, Trans. Am. Acad. Ophthalmol. Otolaryngol. **69:**412-442, 1965.

INDEX

Harada's disease, simulated by
  idiopathic central serous choroidopathy, 178-179, 190-191
  leukemic infiltration of the choroid, 164-165
Hemangioma
  capillary, retina; *see* Angiomatosis, 9-10, 114-137
  choroid, cavernous
    cystoid retinal edema and degeneration, 114-116, 118-123
    diffuse, 116-117, 130-137
    fluorescein angiographic changes
      atypical, 126-127
      typical, 9, 115, 118-125
    histopathology, 115, 128-129
    localized, 114-116, 118-129
    macular detachment, 114-116, 118-123
    photocoagulation, 115-116, 118-119, 122-123
    pigment epithelial atrophy, surrounding, 114, 124-125
    pigment epithelial hyperplasia and metaplasia, 115-116, 128-129
    pseudoglioma, 116, 128-129
    pseudoretinitis pigmentosa, 114, 124-125
    radioactive phosphorus uptake study, 116
    retinal vascular permeability alterations, 115, 120-121
    simulated by
      angiomatosis retinae, 284-285
      posterior hypertrophic scleritis, 204-207
    Sturge-Weber syndrome, 116, 134-135
    transillumination, 115
    ultrasonography, 116, 126-127
    visual-field defects, 115
  iris, 345, 358-359
    amelanotic melanoma simulating, 344, 354-355
  optic nerve head, cavernous, 300-301, 304-305
  retina, capillary; *see* Angiomatosis retinae
  retina, cavernous, 293-306
    with cutanous lesions, 296-303
    with intracranial lesions, 298-299, 302-303
    photocoagulation, 295-297
    simulating retinal telangiectasis; *see* Retinal telangiectasis
    vitreous hemorrhage, 294, 304-305
Hematoma, intravitreal, simulated by a choroidal melanoma, 92-95
Hemorrhagic detachment, macula, retina, and retinal pigment epithelium; *see* Detachment
Herpes simplex iridocyclitis, associated with iris abscess, simulating a melanoma, 360-361
Heterochromia iridis, secondary to iris melanoma, 65, 344, 350-351
Hyaline bodies, optic nerve head, 312
Hyperfluorescence, types of, 5
Hyperplasia
  benign reactive lymphoid; *see* Lymphoid hyperplasia
  ciliary epithelium, 65
  pigment epithelium; *see* Pigment epithelium, tumors

Hypertrophy of the pigment epithelium; *see* Pigment epithelium, tumors
Hyphema
  secondary to iris melanoma, 344, 348-349
  secondary to retinoblastoma, 332
Hypofluorescence, causes of, 5-6
Hypopyon, retinoblastoma, 332

I

Inflammatory tumors simulating
  benign reactive lymphoid hyperplasia, 181, 208-211
  cysticercosis, 181-182, 212-213
  iris abscess, 360-361
  malignant melanoma of the uveal tract, 180-182, 200-215
  rheumatoid scleritis, 180-181, 200-207
Intracranial tumors related to intraocular tumors; *see* Angiomatosis retinae; Hemangioma, choroid, cavernous; Hemangioma, retina, cavernous; Retina, astrocytic hamartoma
Interpretation of fluorescein angiography, 4-10
Iridocyclitis, secondary to melanoma of iris and ciliary body, 65, 344-345, 356-357
Iris
  fluorescein angiography, techniques, 344
  tumors
    abscess, 360-361
    arteriovenous racemose angioma, 345, 358-359
    choristoma, 345
    dictyoma, 345
    hemangioma, 345
    juvenile xanthogranuloma, 345
    leukemia, 160
    melanoma; *see* Melanoma, iris
    metastatic skin melanoma, 356-357
    nevus, 344, 346-347
      diffuse, in melanosis oculi, 344
      fluorescein angiography, 344, 346-347
      gonioscopy, 344, 346-347
      histopathology, 344-345
      melanosis oculi, 344
      neurofibromatosis, 344
    rhabdomyosarcoma, 345
    sarcoidosis, 345
    syphilis, 345
    tuberculosis, 345

J

Juvenile xanthogranuloma, iris, 345
Juxtapapillary angiomatosis retinae, 265-266, 280-287
Juxtapapillary pigment epithelial and retinal hamartoma, 222-223, 234-239

L

Leber's miliary aneurysms; *see* Retinal telangiectasis
Leukemia
  choroid and ciliary body, 65, 160, 162-167
  histopathology, 166-169
  iris, 160, 345

366

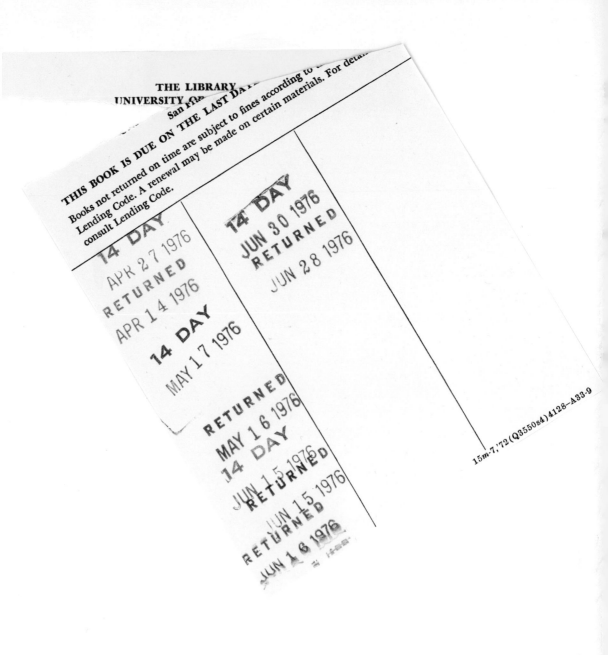

THE LIBRARY
UNIVERSITY OF
San Fr

THIS BOOK IS DUE ON THE LAST DAY
Books not returned on time are subject to fines according to
Lending Code. A renewal may be made on certain materials. For deta
consult Lending Code.

14 DAY
APR 27 1976
RETURNED
APR 14 1976

14 DAY
MAY 17 1976

14 DAY
JUN 30 1976
RETURNED
JUN 28 1976

RETURNED
MAY 16 1976
14 DAY
JUN 15 1976
RETURNED
JUN 15 1976
RETURNED
JUN 16 1976

15m-7;'72(Q3550s4)4128—A33-9